Head Injury Rehabilitation

Head Injury Rehabilitation: Children and Adolescents

edited by
Mark Ylvisaker, MA, CCC/Sp

**The Rehabilitation Institute
of Pittsburgh,
Pittsburgh, Pennsylvania**

 COLLEGE-HILL PRESS, San Diego, California

College-Hill Press
4284 41st Street
San Diego, California 92105

Library of Congress Cataloging in Publication Data
Main entry under title:

Head injury rehabilitation.

    Includes bibliographies and indexes.
    1. Head—Wounds and injuries—Complications and sequelae. 2. Brain-damaged children—Rehabilitation.
I. Ylvisaker, Mark, 1944-   [DNLM: 1. Brain
Injuries—in infancy and childhood. 2. Brain Injuries—rehabilitation. WS 340 H432]
RD521.H45   1985   617'.51044   84-29209

ISBN 0-88744-106-8 (soft)

Printed in the United States of America

THIS BOOK IS DEDICATED TO
HEAD INJURED CHILDREN AND THEIR FAMILIES

CONTENTS

CONTRIBUTORS

Kathleen M. Bachman, BS
Parent of a head injured child

Judy J. Barin, MSW
Social Services Department
The Rehabilitation Institute of
Pittsburgh, Pittsburgh,
Pennsylvania

Eleanore Barovitch, RN, BSN
Director of Rehabilitation Nursing
Services, The Rehabilitation
Institute of Pittsburgh, Pittsburgh,
Pennsylvania

Ronald Baxter, PhD
Director of Psychological Services,
The Rehabilitation Institute of
Pittsburgh, Pittsburgh,
Pennsylvania

Irvin Chamovitz, MD, FAAP
Consulting Neurologist, The
Rehabilitation Institute of
Pittsburgh, Pittsburgh,
Pennsylvania

Anna J. L. Chorazy, MD, FAAP
Medical Director, The
Rehabilitation Institute of
Pittsburgh, Pittsburgh,
Pennsylvania

Sally B. Cohen, MEd
Clinical Facilitator, The Cognitive
Rehabilitation Therapy Program
and Curriculum Coordinator,
Education Department, The
Rehabilitation Institute of
Pittsburgh, Pittsburgh,
Pennsylvania

Joseph A. Divack, MSW
Psychology Department, The
Rehabilitation Institute of
Pittsburgh, Pittsburgh,
Pennsylvania

Linda Ewing-Cobbs, MA
Department of Psychiatry and
Behavioral Sciences, The
University of Texas Medical
School, Houston, Texas

Jack M. Fletcher, PhD
Developmental Neuropsychology
Section, Texas Research Institute
of Mental Sciences, Houston,
Texas

Eva Marie R. Gobble, PhD, CRC
Director, Prevocational/Vocational
Program, The Rehabilitation
Institute of Pittsburgh, Pittsburgh,
Pennsylvania

Juliet Haarbauer-Krupa, MA, CCC/Sp
Cognitive Rehabilitation Therapist
Staff Speech-Language Pathologist,
The Rehabilitation Institute of
Pittsburgh, Pittsburgh,
Pennsylvania

Jeanne M. Hanchett, MD, FAAP
Pediatrician, The
Rehabilitation Institute of
Pittsburgh, Pittsburgh,
Pennsylvania

Kevin Henry, MEd
Cognitive Rehabilitation Therapist,
The Rehabilitation Institute of
Pittsburgh, Pittsburgh, Pennsylvania

James Herrle, BA
Rehabilitation Nursing Services, The
Rehabilitation Institute of Pittsburgh,
Pittsburgh, Pennsylvania

Audrey L. Holland, PhD
Departments of Communication and
Psychiatry, The University of
Pittsburgh, Pittsburgh, Pennsylvania

W. Lindsay Jacob, MD
Psychiatrist, The
Rehabilitation Institute of Pittsburgh,
Pittsburgh, Pennsylvania

Mata B. Jaffe, PhD, CCC/Sp
Assistant Director, Speech-Language
Therapy Department, The
Rehabilitation Institute of Pittsburgh,
Pittsburgh, Pennsylvania

Colleen M. Joyce, MEd
Education Department, The
Rehabilitation Institute of
Pittsburgh, Pittsburgh,
Pennsylvania

Jean L. Kozik, RN, BSN
Rehabilitation Nursing Services, The
Rehabilitation Institute of Pittsburgh,
Pittsburgh, Pennsylvania

Daniel Leger, RN Rehabilitation
Nursing Services, The Rehabilitation
Institute of Pittsburgh, Pittsburgh,
Pennsylvania

Harvey S. Levin, PhD
Division of Neurosurgery,
University of Texas Medical
Branch, Galveston, Texas

Jerilyn Logemann, PhD
Chairman, Department of
Communication Disorders,
Northwestern University,
Evanston, Illinois

Phyllis-Ann Mandella, RD
Director of Nutritional Services,
Rehabilitation Institute of Pittsburgh,
Pittsburgh, Pennsylvania

Joyce P. Mastrilli, OTR/L
Assistant Director, Occupational
Therapy Department, The
Rehabilitation Institute of Pittsburgh,
Pittsburgh, Pennsylvania

Cindy Black Molitor, LPT, MS
Physical Therapy Department, The
Rehabilitation Institute of Pittsburgh,
Pittsburgh, Pennsylvania

Lorelli Moser, MOT, OTR/L
Cognitive Rehabilitation Therapist
and Staff Occupational Therapist,
The Rehabilitation Institute of
Pittsburgh, Pittsburgh, Pennsylvania

Lynn O'Donnell, RN, BSN
Rehabilitation Nursing Services, The
Rehabilitation Institute of Pittsburgh,
Pittsburgh, Pennsylvania

**Dachling Pang, MD, FRCS(C),
FACS,** Assistant Professor of
Neurosurgery, University of
Pittsburgh School of Medicine,
Pittsburgh, Pennsylvania

James C. Pfahl, BS, CRC
Senior Rehabilitation Counselor

The Rehabilitation Institute of
Pittsburgh, Pittsburgh, Pennsylvania

Paul R. Polinko, MSW
Neurosurgical Social Worker
Children's Hospital of Pittsburgh,
Pittsburgh, Pennsylvania

Kathy Weider Rhoades, MEd
Education Department, The
Rehabilitation Institute of Pittsburgh,
Pittsburgh, Pennsylvania

Mason B. Scott, PhD
Psychology Department, The
Rehabilitation Institute of Pittsburgh,
Pittsburgh, Pennsylvania

Gloria J. Smith, OTR/L
Cognitive Rehabilitation Therapist
and Staff Occupational Therapist, The
Rehabilitation Institute of Pittsburgh,
Pittsburgh, Pennsylvania

Deborah M. Sullivan, MEd
Cognitive Rehabilitation Therapist,
Staff Occupational Therapist, The
Pittsburgh, Pittsburgh, Pennsylvania

Shirley F. Szekeres, MA, CCC/Sp
Cognitive Rehabilitation Therapist
and Assistant Director, Speech-
Language Therapy Department, The
Rehabilitation Institute of Pittsburgh,
Pittsburgh, Pennsylvania

Jan Titonis, MPH
Senior Program Coordinator for
Head Injury Programs, The
Rehabilitation Institute of Pittsburgh,
Pittsburgh, Pennsylvania

Anne S. Valko, MD, FAAP
Physiatrist/Pediatrician, The
Rehabilitation Institute of
Pittsburgh, Pittsburgh,

Dianna M. Welks, MEd
Education Department, The
Rehabilitation
Pennsylvania

Janette Yanko, RN, MN, CNRN
Neuroclinical Nurse Specialist,
Youngstown Hospital Association,
Youngstown, Ohio

Mark Ylvisaker, MA, CCC/Sp
Director, Speech-Language Therapy
Department, The Rehabilitation
Institute of Pittsburgh, Pittsburgh,
Pennsylvania

FOREWORD

I appreciate the opportunity to be among the first to congratulate the editor and contributors who have collaborated on this book.

It is timely, straightforward, and practical! The holistic approach and comprehensive material convey a sensitive and caring attitude focused on the young head injured survivor and the family, and all combine to make this a unique text.

As a parent of a severely head injured daughter, I would encourage families to own this book to have as a constant reference and source of needed information and support.

As Executive Director of the National Head Injury Foundation, I would recommend this book to all those who treat or serve young head injured individuals in rehabilitation-educational facilities or in their community environments.

The value of the integrated team approach is well documented within these pages and should serve as a model for those who might be encouraged to work with this population. Currently not enough attention is being given to the long-term varied effects of head injury on children and adolescents—effects that can be devastating to their development in our fast-moving and competitive world.

The authors are to be thanked for creating a valuable source of information and education that addresses assessment, treatment approaches, and management of head injury rehabilitation but focuses solely on children.

Marilyn Price Spivack
Executive Director
National Head Injury Foundation, Inc.

PREFACE

The tragedy of severe closed head injury begins with its sudden and fortuitous selection of victims, generally children or young adults who have an expectation of long life and unlimited possibilities. This tragedy then encompasses families, whose coping abilities are stretched to the limit, patients who only dimly understand why their lives must be changed in such dramatic ways, and a professional community inadequately equipped with appropriate programs and validated treatment techniques to meet this challenge.

Head injuries are more common than spinal cord injuries and all neurologic diseases with the exception of stroke. With the increasing sophistication of acute medical management, the rate of survival continues to grow. Survival rates are particularly high in children who, along with young adults, constitute the highest risk age group for head injury. Although the survival rates are high, recent research has questioned the traditional belief that the prognosis for full recovery is better in children than in adults with comparable injuries.

Despite the prevalence of head injury in children and adolescents and the growing awareness of the previously hidden cognitive and psychosocial deficits, the professional community has only recently begun to address their special rehabilitative needs. Until recently, children whose motor functioning returned quickly following an accident were prematurely returned to their community schools with no provision for special services and no comprehension of their hidden impairments. In many parts of the country, this practice continues. The common result is school failure, behavioral maladjustment, and family disruption.

Over the past decade, many excellent rehabilitation programs have been created for adult survivors of severe head injury. Creative treatment techniques have been fashioned, some of which have been shown to affect recovery in ways that were once thought to be impossible. A body of literature has also begun to emerge on adult head injury rehabilitation, based largely on conference proceedings or on the work being carried out in specific adult head injury programs.

Rehabilitation programs for head injured children are newer and fewer in number than adult programs. Furthermore, there are to date no comprehensive textbooks on the subject of pediatric head injury rehabilitation. Professional journals in key fields, such as special education and speech-language pathology, offer few publications in this area. Well-subscribed conferences and a large number of requests for unpublished therapy materials indicate a substantial need and desire for a book on pediatric head injury rehabilitation.

This book will be of interest to all rehabilitation and special education professionals who work with head injured children and adolescents and their families. Its comprehensiveness in scope carries with it the frustration of insufficient detail and depth in each of the specific areas covered. The contributors have struggled with this frustration and have compressed a large amount of useful information into a relatively small number of pages.

In addition to specific treatment principles and techniques, readers of this textbook will be exposed to an interdisciplinary approach to pediatric head injury rehabilitation that has evolved at The Rehabilitation Institute of Pittsburgh over years of working with this population. One of the threads that runs through the wide range of individual differences among head injured patients is depressed cognitive and psychosocial functioning, particularly in the areas of self-awareness, problem solving, judgment, attention, and general efficiency of information processing (including memory and thought organization). Rehabilitation programs must address these areas directly, and traditional treatments in noncognitive areas must also be modified in light of these characteristic impairments. Programs that are structured by rigidly defined professional boundaries cannot efficiently treat the cognitive and social fragmentation that commonly results from severe head injury. A collection of therapists focusing independently on diverse areas of dysfunction will not, when added together, constitute a total, coherent rehabilitation team capable of addressing in an integrated manner the fundamental needs of head injured patients.

These considerations argue for interdisciplinary rehabilitation programs and also explain the fact that most of the chapters in this text are multiply authored by professionals from diverse rehabilitation disciplines. For example, therapists treating perceptual disorders, language disorders, and memory and learning disorders must all address patients' lack of self-insight, impaired problem solving, inefficient attentional and processing mechanisms, and shallow social awareness, among other problems. Hence, themes that might otherwise be discussed in separate chapters by an occupational therapist, a speech-language pathologist, and a psychologist or special educator are here integrated under a general heading, cognitive rehabilitation therapy. Similarly, what distinguishes the physical restoration of head injured patients is the same collection of cognitive and psychosocial deficits that at the same time sets limits to treatment options and also requires therapists to broaden their traditional role definition. For this reason, the treatment of motor disorders is discussed in one integrated chapter by a physiatrist, a physical therapist, an occupational therapist, and a speech-language pathologist.

This book is intended to be a practical guide for professionals seeking concrete guidance in the difficult and frustrating search for effective treatment strategies for head injured patients. While maintaining a commitment to scholarship, the authors of the treatment chapters of this textbook have taken as their primary responsibility the clear presentation of a treatment philosophy as well as specific principles and techniques of remediation. It is a high recommendation for this book that most of these authors spend their long working days in the trenches, struggling to restore head injured patients and their families to a life of fulfillment and satisfaction.

There are more people responsible for this book than we can hope to acknowledge here. The contributors have devoted more early mornings, late evenings, and long weekends to this project than any of us care to remember. They are a dedicated and creative group of professionals committed to the highest standards of rehabilitative care and to learning from one another and their patients. The administrators of The Rehabilitation Institute of Pittsburgh have made this book possible through their ongoing support for excellence in rehabilitation and by providing the resources necessary for the completion of this large project. Sean Monagle and John Rosenbek offered invaluable editorial advice, as did Georgia Schneider, Larry Edelman, and Ken Seibert. Marsha Ihrig, Joy Spang, Mary Jane Teig, and Susan Arlen deserve rich thanks and praise for their tireless typing and retyping of the manuscript. I also thank Nancy Spears for her help in providing contributors with necessary reference materials. Finally, I express my deep gratitude to my wife Kathy, daughter Jessie, and son Ben for their support and willingness to live without a husband and father for many months.

Mark Ylvisaker

INTRODUCTION

Head Injury Rehabilitation: Children and Adolescents

Anna J. L. Chorazy

Children are not miniature adults. Although disorders similar in causality, diagnosis, and treatment affect both children and adults, it is the wide range of developmental phenomena that distinguishes the rehabilitation of head injured children and adolescents from that of adults. The development of objectives and effective techniques of rehabilitation is complicated not only by the biologic recovery processes taking place at different stages following the injury but also by the additional uncertainties of the process of biologic maturation of the brain, which is simultaneously influenced by multiple environmental factors. Pediatric rehabilitation professionals must never lose sight of the developmental process; it is a map providing a rough and sometimes primitive guide through the virgin wilderness of an undeveloped and now damaged brain. It is a template for establishing appropriate goals. Additionally, when working with children, it must be appreciated that they are integral members of a family, with parents, siblings, and grandparents who share a profound investment in the child's treatment program and outcome.

Trauma in the United States is the third leading cause of death, behind cardiovascular disease and cancer (Trunkey, 1983). It is the leading causes of death for those under 44 years of age. Accidents are the largest cause of morbidity and mortality during childhood (United States Center for Health Statistics, 1978). The causes of serious injury include possibly preventable environmental factors as well as uncontrollable chance. Age is a significant epidemiologic factor; the causes of injury, including head injury, differ according to the developmental stage of the child. Children are most appropriately grouped by developmental stage (Rivara, 1984): infants under 1 year, toddlers 1 to 2 years old, preschoolers 3 to 6 years old, school-aged children 6 to 12 years old, and teenagers 13 to 18 years old. If perinatal insults are excluded, the two main hazards for infants are accidental dropping and intentional abuse. As infants progress through active toddler and preschool stages, their risk of injuries from falls, especially in the home, increases significantly because judgment does not keep pace with developing motor skills. Most of these head injuries are relatively minor; serious falls, however, do occur, and abuse continues to be seen. Young children are involved in motor vehicle accidents both as pedestrians and, particularly when they are not properly restrained, as passengers. School-aged children show a marked increase in head injuries from recreational and sporting activities, such as bicycling, skating, and horseback riding. Falls continue to be an issue; more importantly, automobile-bicycle accidents are not uncommon. Among adolescents and young adults, assault, particularly among the lower socioeconomic groups, begins to emerge as an important cause of head injury. A dramatic increase in head injuries in this age group also occurs as a result of motor vehicle accidents with the adolescent as driver or passenger. Alcohol or drugs are often involved. Sporting and recreational injuries also increase, both in organized competitive activity and in unsupervised activity on the playing field. Many of the head injuries sustained in these activities are mild but not necessarily insignificant. Accidents involving motorcycles, motorbikes, and snowmobiles also add to the number of motor vehicle accidents (Cartlidge and Shaw, 1981; Rivara, 1984). Automobile and automobile-bicycle accidents have consistently been the primary cause of injury among head injured children and adolescents admitted to The Rehabilitation Institute of Pittsburgh. In addition, injuries among our patients have resulted from falls, from sport and recreational activities, and, most distressing of all, from gunshot wounds and child abuse.

It is difficult to obtain accurate statistical data for the incidence and prevalence of head injury. Many factors are responsible for this: (1) the lack of a universally accepted definition of head injury; (2) the lack of a universal system of terminology to code such injuries, reflecting current thinking regarding pathophysiology; (3) the lack of uniformity in characterizing the severity of head injury with respect to including the extremes of early fatalities and the very mildly head injured; and (4) the inclusion of diverse populations in reported studies (Jennett and Teasdale, 1981).

Because of these factors, epidemiologic data can only be estimated. Available sources indicate that 422,000 persons annually in the United States sustain a head injury and survive long enough to be admitted to a hospital, or 200 head injured persons per 100,000 population. Of all age groups, the 15 to 24 year old group has the highest frequency, but the rate is nearly as high in persons under 15 years of age. Males have a rate more than twice that of females. The major overall cause of head injury is motor vehicle accidents, which account for 49 per cent of the total number, followed by accidental falls (28 per cent). Most falls causing head injury occur in children under 15 years of age (Kalsbeek, McLaurin, Harris, and Miller,

1980). The National Head Injury Foundation (1983) estimates that nationwide there are 30,000 to 50,000 persons disabled each year by head injury; the Foundation terms head injury "the silent epidemic" because its frequency and disabling effects have largely been unrecognized by the professional community and the public.

In assessing the cost of head injury to society, Kalsbeek and co-workers (1980) reported both direct and indirect costs. (Direct cost is the expense of providing health care to the injured; indirect cost represents the patient's loss of productivity, and this was calculated on an annual basis only. Lifetime costs are not available.) The total cost of head injury in 1974 was reported as $2.43 billion. This study was published in 1980, at which time inflation had already increased the figure to $3.9 billion. The study did not include mild head trauma. Rimel, Giordani, Barth, Boll, and Jane (1981) reported that, of the mildly head injured patients who are described on discharge as being "completely normal," 59 per cent continue to have memory problems. Thirty-four per cent of those who had been employed prior to the injury had not returned to work three months post trauma. No comparable study has been reported for children. However, various authors have noted that children who sustain mild head injury do exhibit personality changes, irritability, school learning problems, headaches, and memory and attention deficits (Boll, 1983).

Length of stay in both acute care and rehabilitation settings is a critical factor in cost containment. At The Rehabilitation Institute of Pittsburgh, we have found that children transferred to our center from the nearby specialty children's hospital are usually transferred much sooner than those sent from general hospitals. The length of stay for these children is substantially shorter in the rehabilitation center, as well as in the acute care hospital. We speculate that earlier transfer for comprehensive rehabilitation may facilitate more rapid return of skills.

The dollar cost of head injury is truly staggering. The cost in terms of human suffering can be overwhelming, not only to the patient, but also to family members and friends. The coping skills of all involved, including the professional staff, are often taxed to the limit.

Rehabilitation of head injured children and adolescents requires a coordinated interdisciplinary approach. No single person has the skills to provide all that is required. An integrated program is needed to treat the physical, cognitive, and psychosocial fragmentation that typically results from severe head injury. Four threads knit the fabric of comprehensive rehabilitation for children:

- Concentrated, interdisciplinary attention to the reduction of discernible impairments

- Concern for all aspects of the total handicap, with a strong focus upon developing potential abilities and fostering adaptive compensation for lost or impaired function as well as psychosocial adjustment
- A climate that presents the child with acceptance, challenge, and encouragement toward independence
- Postdischarge follow-up, including the development of support within the child's own family and community

Long-term care extends beyond the four walls of our rehabilitation facilities and touches all aspects of the child's life (Bisdee, 1975). This textbook emerged from our staff's collective experience over the past 30 years in providing comprehensive rehabilitation for children with all types of congenital and acquired neurologic disabilities. It is hoped that the book will be a contribution to the improvement of treatment and the quality of life for head injured children.

REFERENCES

Bisdee, C. H. (1975). Rehabilitation: The way it is at the Home For Crippled Children. *Journal of the American Hospital Association, 49,* 83–86.
Boll, T. J. (1983). Minor head injury in children—out of sight but not out of mind. *Journal of Clinical Child Psychology, 12*(1), 74–80.
Cartlidge, N. E. F., and Shaw, D. A. (1981). *Head injury.* Philadelphia: W. B. Saunders.
Jennett, B., and Teasdale, G. (1981). *Management of head injuries.* Philadelphia: F. A. Davis.
Kalsbeek, W. D., McLaurin, R. L., Harris, B. S. H., III, and Miller, J. D. (1980). The national head and spinal cord injury survey: Major findings. *Journal of Neurosurgery* (Suppl.) *53,* 19–31.
National Head Injury Foundation (1983). *Head injury.* Framingham, MA: Author.
Rimel, R. W., Giordani, M. A., Barth, J. T., Boll, T. J., and Jane, J. A. (1981). Disability caused by head injury. *Neurosurgery, 9*(3), 221–228.
Rivara, F. P. (1984). Childhood injuries. III. Epidemiology of non-motor vehicle head trauma. *Developmental Medicine and Child Neurology, 26*(1), 81–87.
Trunkey, D. D. (1983). Trauma. *Scientific American, 249*(2), 28–35.
United States National Center for Health Statistics (1978). *Facts of life and death* (DHEW Publication PHS 79-1222). Hyattsville, MD: United States Public Health Service.

PART I
PATHOPHYSIOLOGY AND OUTCOME

Informed rehabilitation professionals must have an understanding of the disability that they attempt to treat. To be adequate, this understanding should encompass the nature of the brain injury, the natural history of the recovery process, and the likely constellations of deficits that characterize long-term outcome. A careful study of the first section of this text should provide clinicians with a firm basis of understanding on which to build solid treatment approaches.

In Chapter 1, Pang summarizes the current state of knowledge about the mechanisms of primary and secondary brain injury in standard accident-related closed head injuries and the pathophysiologic basis for several of the neurobehavioral syndromes commonly observed following head injury. Although research is far from complete in the case of these syndromes (e.g., the pathophysiology of memory and learning disorders), Pang provides an excellent condensation of relevant research findings.

There is a long-held belief that children recover more quickly and completely than adults from comparable injuries and that, short of very substantial damage to the brain, a child's prognosis for recovery is good. In Chapter 2, Ewing-Cobbs, Fletcher, and Levin summarize results of recent studies that call this belief sharply into question. Although research on the late effects of head injury in children is relatively sparse (much of it contributed by the authors of Chapter 2), there is a growing body of literature that describes more pervasive long-term cognitive and behavioral sequelae than had previously been recognized. These general intellectual, language, memory, and psychosocial deficits can be expected to interfere significantly with academic functioning; nevertheless, there are few reports of the effects of head injury on school performance. The need for further research in this area and for appropriate rehabilitation and special education programs for these children is clearly implied.

Chapter 1

Pathophysiologic Correlates of Neurobehavioral Syndromes Following Closed Head Injury

Dachling Pang, MD

The subject of the pathophysiology of traumatic brain syndromes must begin with an understanding of the physics of head injury. This is the biomechanical basis for the type, location, and magnitude of traumatically induced tissue damage. The opening section of this chapter is therefore devoted to this important topic. The clinical sequelae of such tissue damage constitute the neurobehavioral syndromes so familiar to clinicians and rehabilitation specialists. These syndromes, described later in the chapter, are the following: (1) concussion and disturbance of consciousness, (2) motor system disorders, (3) disorders of memory and learning, (4) disorders of emotion and behavior, and (5) hypothalamic-pituitary disorders. Under each subheading, the functional anatomy of the respective neuroanatomic system, incorporating recent research concerning normal and abnormal physiology, is discussed first, followed by a description of pathophysiology. In some cases, the clinical symptoms can be predicted from physiology (as in the pathogenesis of spasticity); in other cases, normal functions are deduced from the pathologic features of lesions (as with the mechanism of memory).

In any case, although the issues presented are complex and often controversial, an attempt has not been made to simplify the discussion for purposes of easy reading. An accurate understanding of the mechanisms of traumatic brain injury and the physiologic basis for consequent impairments is essential for rehabilitation professionals to appreciate more fully their task in helping head injured children regain maximum functioning. Although the physics of head injury is applicable to both adults and children, the immediate biologic response of young children may differ in some respects from that of older children and adults. These differences are also discussed.

PHYSICS OF CLOSED HEAD INJURY

Closed trauma to the head results in two categories of brain injury, primary and secondary. Primary injury occurs immediately following impact and is related to instantaneous events directly caused by the blow. The resultant tissue disruption is usually permanent, does not respond to pharmacologic and physiologic manipulations, and frequently constitutes the limiting factor for the most ideal recovery. Extensive primary injury therefore presupposes a poor outcome, regardless of medical and rehabilitative therapy.

Secondary injury occurs as a result of epiphenomena causally related to the primary injury. Thus, impact disruption of large dural or cortical vessels leads to epidural or subdural hematomas, respectively. Disruption of capillaries or disturbance of vascular endothelial membranes during the original impact leads to vasogenic cerebral edema. Both hematomas and edema constitute mass effect, raise the intracranial pressure, and result in brain shift (herniation) and cerebral hypoperfusion. Herniation and hypoperfusion in turn lead to further brain damage in the form of pressure necrosis and infarction, often remote from the site of the primary injury. These secondary lesions, unlike the primary ones, are potentially avoidable if the epiphenomena themselves are amenable to treatment. Thus, both brain shift and cerebral hypoperfusion may be alleviated by surgical evacuation of hematomas and edema therapy. It follows that the modern management of head injury consists mainly of measures to minimize these secondary lesions.

MECHANISMS OF PRIMARY IMPACT INJURY

Primary brain injuries can be caused by both acceleration dependent and nonacceleration dependent factors.

Acceleration Dependent Factors

Acceleration dependent factors have traditionally received biased attention as the dominant mechanisms in the production of closed brain injuries, partly because the overwhelming majority of clinical head injuries involve acceleration, and partly because of the landmark experiments of Denny-Brown and Russell in 1941.[12] These workers have shown that a blow of moderate intensity to a movable head often produces devastating brain damage, whereas a blow with 20 times the intensity delivered to the rigidly fixed head produces remarkably little brain injury. In the primate model, a fixed skull can literally be crushed to pieces by opposing forces with the animal remaining completely conscious and free of neurologic deficits. It is only necessary to compare the unhappy boxer rendered unconscious by a judiciously aimed left hook with the badly disfigured but neurologically intact automechanic whose entire craniofacial complex has been crushed beneath a faultily propped up car in the grease pit to realize that accelerating injuries are much more deleterious to the brain than nonaccelerating injuries. Moreover, clinical situations involving a fixed head are exceedingly rare, and the contribution of nonaccelerating mechanisms must be small within the overall spectrum of pathologic lesions encountered in head injury.

Two types of acceleration are pertinent to this discussion: translational and angular. If the resultant vector of a force applied to a rigid body passes through the center of gravity (CG) of the body, the body will assume linear acceleration along the direction of the force. This is called translational acceleration (Fig. 1-1A). In this setting, all individual particles within this body will travel at the same acceleration and in the same direction, and hence will sustain no intermolecular stress.

If, however, the resultant force vector does not pass through the CG of the body, the body will assume an angular acceleration and rotate around its own CG. Pure angular acceleration (i.e., without linear motion) exists only if the body is simultaneously acted on by two opposing forces of equal magnitude directed at opposite sides of the CG (i.e., a force-couple) (Fig. 1-1B). A single linear force not passing through the CG will instead resolve into two component vectors: one passing through the CG, causing translational acceleration, and one perpendicular to the CG, causing angular acceleration. In other words, a single eccentric force always produces combined rotational and translational motions, with the body spinning around its own CG while traveling linearly along the path of the translational vector (Fig. 1-1C).

In reality, most impact injuries are produced by unpaired forces not passing through the CG of the head. The observed cranial movement is therefore always a combination of both translation and rotation. Moreover, since the head is attached to the cervical spine, some degree of rotation always occurs around the foramen magnum regardless of the direction of the impact vector. Thus, although translational motion and rotational motion each causes its own brand of tissue damage with unique features of type and location, the authentic histopathology of a traumatized brain always includes inseparable markings of both types of trauma. For the purpose of discussion, translational trauma and rotational trauma will be considered separately.

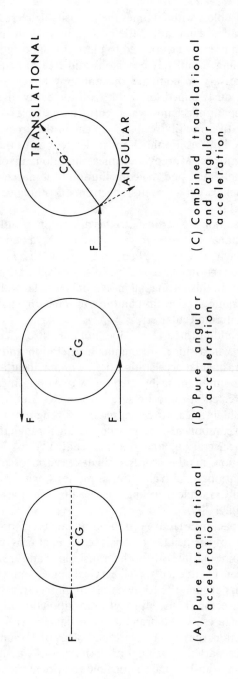

(A) Pure translational
    acceleration

(B) Pure angular
    acceleration

(C) Combined translational
    and angular
    acceleration

Figure 1-1. The effects of different forces acting on a rigid spherical body. *A*, A single force (*F*) passing through the center of gravity (*CG*) of the body produces pure translational acceleration. *B*, Pure angular acceleration results from two simultaneous opposing forces of equal magnitude directed at opposite sides of the CG. *C*, A single force not passing through the CG will produce combined translational and angular motions with both types of acceleration.

Translational Trauma

Brain-Skull Differential Movements and Surface Lacerations. Pure translational trauma is exemplified by a sharply dealt blow to the occiput of an initially stationary but movable head. Assuming no influence from the neck, the head will rapidly accelerate forward. Because of inertia, the brain will lag behind until it is pushed forward by the advancing skull. This lagging results in differential movements between brain and skull, which implies a "rubbing" of the friable cortex against certain rough surfaces of the dura-lined skull base.[43] As the accelerating head finally hits the ground or other unyielding surface (as when the victim falls forward), the skull decelerates to a sudden halt, but the brain continues to plunge forward at its accustomed velocity until it too is stopped by the frontal calvarium. The exact sequence of events remains the same but reverses direction, the brain-skull differential movement and cortical "rubbing" now occurring in the opposite direction. In actual fact, the deceleration process often takes several oscillations before the skull achieves zero velocity; the brain-skull differential movements therefore also undergo several pendular swings, during which the cortex slams repeatedly against sharp dural edges of the falx, the tentorial incisura, the sphenoid ridge, and the jagged floor of the anterior cranial fossa. Lindenberg and Freytag[43] thought this to be the reason for the particularly severe laceration seen on the orbital frontal cortices and the tips of the frontal and temporal lobes. This brain-skull differential movement also readily explains the pathogenesis of chronic subdural hematomas since the fragile bridging veins between the cortex and dura traversing the subdural space are exceedingly vulnerable to shearing strains (discussed later in this chapter).

This mechanism does not, however, explain the presence of contusions in the convexity, where the cortex lies against the smooth calvarium. Lindenberg and Freytag[43] attribute these contusions to the effect of a positive pressure zone immediately underneath the impact site where the brain crowds toward the skull. These contusions were called coup lesions since they occur at the impact pole, as opposed to contrecoup lesions, which are found directly opposite the impact pole (the antipole). This explanation received severe criticism because it was later found that brain cells can withstand very high positive pressure as long as it is uniformly applied— that is, so long as it does not causes tissue displacement. This important discovery shifted interest from the positive pressure effect toward the effects of the negative pressure zone at the antipole, where the brain pulls away from the skull. Spatz[79] and Sellier and Unterharnscheidt[75] argued for the importance of negative pressure by

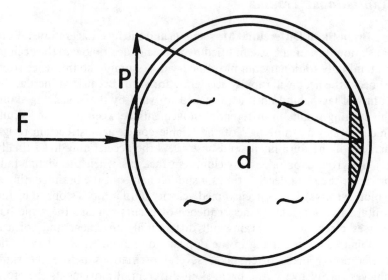

Figure 1-2. In translational motion produced by a force (*F*) passing through the CG of a fluid-filled spherical shell, a pressure gradient (*P*) develops from pole to antipole. P is proportional to the density of the fluid, the linear acceleration, and the diameter of the shell (*d*). The higher the acceleration, the greater the value of P.

showing that contrecoup lesions far outnumbered coup lesions in translational impact trauma. This led to the formulation of the cavitation theory as the causative mechanism for contrecoup injuries.

Cavitation Theory. Under certain conditions, the head may be thought of as an inextensible spherical shell filled with an incompressible inviscid fluid. When a force vector passes through the CG of the system, the shell assumes a translational acceleration. Since the shell is accelerated, the fluid must also be accelerated. If the entire fluid content could be broken into component cubes of fluid, the effective forces causing the fluid to accelerate will be acting on the surfaces of the cubes. A pressure gradient therefore exists across the plane between impact pole and antipole, with the pressure varying linearly from a maximum at the side where the force is applied to a minimum at the diametrically opposite side. It is easy to see how this pressure gradient is set up within the human skull when the brain crowds towards the impact pole and pulls away from the antipole. This pressure gradient P is given by

$$P = \rho \cdot a \cdot d$$

where ρ is the density of the fluid, a is the acceleration, and d is the diameter of the skull (Fig. 1-2). The greater the violence, and the higher the acceleration, the greater will be the pressure gradient.

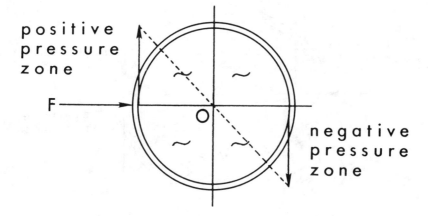

Figure 1–3. As in Figure 1–2, increasing acceleration causes fluid molecules to crowd toward the pole and to draw away from the antipole. This sets up positive pressure at the impact pole equal in magnitude to the absolute value of the negative pressure developed at the antipole, with the zero atmospheric point at the center of gravity. F = Force.

If the shell is completely filled with fluid and the effect of shell bending is disregarded, the maximum positive pressure at the impact pole will be as high above atmospheric pressure as the minimum pressure at the antipole is below, with the zero atmospheric point somewhere near the CG of the shell (Fig. 1–3). With increasing acceleration, the positive pressure on the left becomes more positive, and the negative pressure on the right more negative, until the absolute pressure on the right drops below the vapor pressure (P_V) of the liquid. At this point, the liquid begins to boil and changes rapidly to the gaseous state, causing instantaneous formation of gas bubbles within the zone of negative pressure below P_V— that is, on the extreme right side. When the shell decelerates, the negative pressure once again rises above P_V as it returns toward zero, at which point the gas condenses to liquid and the gas bubbles disappear. If acceleration and deceleration occur in rapid succession, the bubbles will form and collapse with great violence, analogous to the sudden pressure changes in the center of an explosion. This process is known as cavitation[88] and was observed by Gross[23] in 1958 using high speed photography on water-filled dummy skulls.

It is readily seen that if the foregoing principle is applied to the impacted frontal skull, formation and collapse of bubbles near the antipole (the occiput) will produce the so-called contrecoup lesions in the occipital lobe (Fig. 1–4). The positive pressure zone at the impact pole remains relatively innocuous, and this is consistent with the frequent absence of coup lesions in translational trauma. The situation is identical, only in

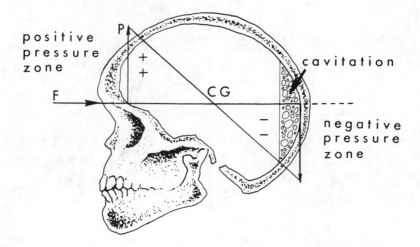

Figure 1-4. If the fluid-filled shell model is transcribed to the human skull-brain system, the negative pressure zone where cavitation takes place is in the antipole— that is, within the occipital lobes with a frontally directed force (contrecoup lesion).

reverse, if the head initially traveling at a constant velocity suddenly hits a rigid wall, as in a backward fall. The occipital skull is stopped instantaneously at a time when the brain is still plunging backward. Similar pressure gradients are set up with the negative zone now in the frontal region. This will result in contrecoup cavitation in the frontal lobes.

The vapor pressure P_V is constant for a given fluid at a set temperature. From Figure 1-5, it can be seen that whereever the pressure gradient line intersects P_V, the segment of fluid thus defined to the right of the intersection will have a pressure below P_V and hence will be uniformly affected by cavitation. The vertical line passing through the intersection that defines the segment is called a pressure isobar. As the pressure gradient widens with greater impact, and the negative pressure to the right becomes more negative, the pressure isobar moves progressively closer to the center to define a correspondingly larger and larger segment. Thus, a mild blow to the head will affect only the summits of gyri, whereas a stronger blow will affect the sulci or even the subjacent white matter. Cavitation within brain tissue produces diffuse heterogeneous tearing of axons and neurons. When small foci of damage coalesce, larger and more homogeneous appearing areas emerge. Rapid pressure changes in regions surrounding capillaries set up ripping forces across the endothelium that result in focal hemorrhages (Fig. 1-6). Also affected are the perpendicularly arranged perforating arteries that normally supply a wedge-shaped area of gyrus with the apex extending deep toward the center of the brain. This

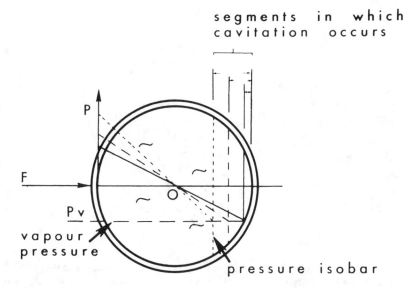

Figure 1-5. The relationship between acceleration (determined by the force of violence) and the depth of the segments at the negative pressure antipole in which cavitation occurs. The pressure isobar, which defines the depth of the segment, is the vertical line that passes through the intersection of the pressure gradient line and the vapor pressure P_v. F = Force; P = pressure gradient.

explains why old contusions are often wedge-shaped and not flat-based, as would be predicted by the theoretical isobars.

The extent of brain surface affected also depends on the radius of curvature of the gyrus involved. With a given degree of violence, the resulting pressure isobar defines a specified depth of the segment. Any gyral surface within this segment will be affected. Therefore, a gyrus with a larger radius of curvature— that is, a "flatter" gyrus— will have a larger surface area of involvement than a pointed gyrus with a small radius of curvature, even though the "depth" of the segment is the same for both (Fig. 1-7). This may explain the extensive lesions seen at the base of the "flatter" frontal lobes compared with the more pointed gyri on the convexity.

Although the cavitation theory provides an elegant explanation for the distribution, geometry, and morphology of cortical and subcortical lesions, it fails to account for a multitude of traumatic lesions scattered among deep brain structures. The topography of pressure changes dictates a constant zone of zero pressure at the center of the skull irrespective of the force of impact. This means that gas bubbles can never form in the central portions of the brain. Some other mechanism would have to

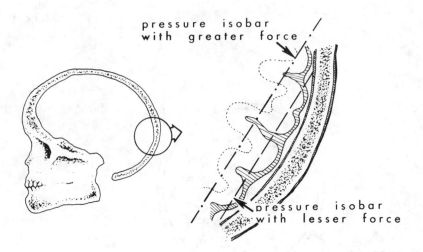

Figure 1-6. The relationship between the depth of the cavitating segment and the depth of brain involvement. A pressure isobar close to the surface of the brain defines a shallow segment and produces superficial damage to the tops of the gyri, whereas a pressure isobar closer to the center of the head *(CG)* defines a deeper segment, which leads to damage deeper around the sulci and in the white matter.

account for the small foci of petechial hemorrhages and white matter degeneration commonly found in the subependymal tissues surrounding the third ventricle, the corpus callosum, and the hypothalamus.

Rotational Trauma

As mentioned earlier, pure translational (linear) trauma is rare in clinical practice. Most impact forces do not pass through the CG of the head and hence will produce a combination of translational and angular accelerations. Whereas translational mechanisms depend on the effect of cavitation and slamming of the brain against body structures, rotational mechanisms emphasize the important concept of shearing strain. In engineering terminology, stress is force per unit area and strain is the displacement of one point relative to another caused by the stress. Shearing occurs when parallel or diverging stresses impel displacement along an intermediate plane.

The most common example of rotation-induced shearing occurs near the brain surface and would conveniently account for some surface contusions and lacerations. An impact on the skull results in a direct application of force that accelerates the skull. For the brain to accelerate

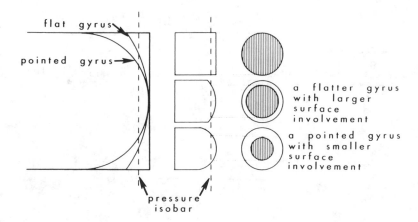

Figure 1-7. The relationship between the radius of curvature of the gyrus involved and the surface extent of damage. With any given depth of segment, a flatter gyrus suffers larger surface damage than a more pointed gyrus, in which the area included within the segment is much smaller.

with the skull, force must be applied to it by the skull. For pure translation, the force is applied by the simple process of the skull pushing against the brain, with the force, in most cases, being distributed over an appreciable area of the brain. During angular acceleration of the head, the brain will initially tend to remain stationary while the skull rotates. Eventually, the brain is dragged along by frictional forces exerted by bony prominences on the rough anterior and middle fossa floor, the crista galli, the petrous bone, the tentorial notch, and the sphenoid ridge. The brain adjacent to these prominences is subjected to parallel shearing, which may be expected to cause cortical contusions (Fig. 1-8). The theoretical locations of these surface shearing sites correspond remarkably well with the distribution of contusive lesions in the basal frontal and temporal lobes (against jagged floors), the cingulate gyri (against the edge of the falx), the temporal poles (against the sphenoid ridges), and the frontal poles (against crista galli). It also explains why the inferior surface of the occipital lobes often escapes injury, being cushioned by the smooth tentorium.

The importance of cortical contusion in producing serious neurologic deficits has been overemphasized in the past.[9,43,88] It is now known that deep lesions play an equal if not more essential part in determining outcome, and it remains to be shown that rotational trauma can set up shearing within the interior of the brain. Angular acceleration of a rigid sphere results in a linear acceleration of its parts in a direction perpendicular to the radius. The linear acceleration a is given by

$$a = r\alpha$$

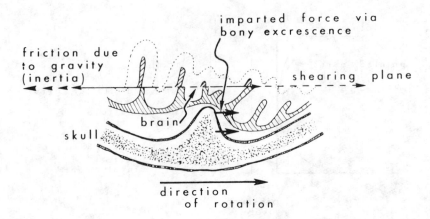

Figure 1-8. Surface shearing occurs when forces propelling the rotation of the brain are imparted by bony prominences in the inner table of the skull.

where *a* is angular acceleration and r is the distance of the part from the CG of the sphere (r = radius if a surface particle is considered) (Fig. 1-9). Thus, the linear acceleration of any component part undergoing angular acceleration is directly proportional to its distance from the CG, and always in a direction perpendicular to the radius. If the CG is also accelerated linearly, as in combined translational and rotational motions, the acceleration of the CG will be added to this linear acceleration. Two adjacent parts within a rotating body with unequal distances from the CG (r_1 and r_2) and located on different radii will therefore travel away from each other in different linear accelerations (a_1 and a_2) and along slightly different paths (Fig. 1-10). This sets up a shearing plane defined by the magnitude and direction of the respective linear accelerations of the two adjacent parts. (This is in contrast to translation acceleration, for which all particles in the body share the same acceleration and direction of motion.) In a rigid body, component parts are held together by physicochemical bonds strong enough to withstand such shearing. In the brain, however, the neurons, glia, and axons are held together loosely. Brain tissue has a small modulus of rigidity and will suffer damage with even slight distortion of shape.[29] Shearing strains resulting from angular acceleration in the cell to cell and cell to axon interphases therefore lead to multiple tearing of neural elements (Fig. 1-10) throughout the deep portions of the brain.

The clinical correlation of diffuse shearing injuries was first described by Strich[80] in 1956. She documented a traumatic brain syndrome in which surface contusion seems to play a negligible role. A typical patient is usually

$$a = r \cdot a$$

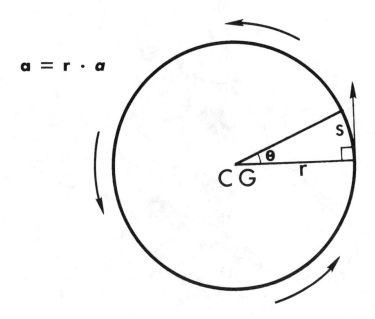

Figure 1-9. The linear acceleration (a) of a surface particle on a rigid sphere undergoing angular motion. r = Radius of the sphere and is the distance between the surface particle and the CG; S = distance on the surface arc traveled by the particle; θ = angle in radian traveled by the particle; a = angular acceleration.

unconscious from the time of the accident but will improve over weeks or months to a definite waking state during which he or she opens eyes, rouses to stimulation, coughs, chews, and swallows, and may even follow loud sound or bright light with his or her eyes. However, there is no content to the patient's consciousness. There may be attacks of decerebrate spasm, hyperventilation, diaphoresis, and tachycardia. This syndrome has variously been called akinetic mutism, protracted posttraumatic encephalopathy,[33] and persistent vegetative state.[35] In autopsy studies, Strich[81,82,83] and others[1,33,61] have consistently noted a conspicuous absence of cortical lesions, intracranial hemorrhages, and evidence of raised intracranial pressure. Instead they found diffuse white matter lesions consisting of axon retraction balls indicative of widespread axonal transection mechanistically compatible with multiple shearing insults (Fig. 1-11). In long-term survivors, the degree of white matter degeneration was so severe as to render the brain grossly atrophic. Strich[80] concluded

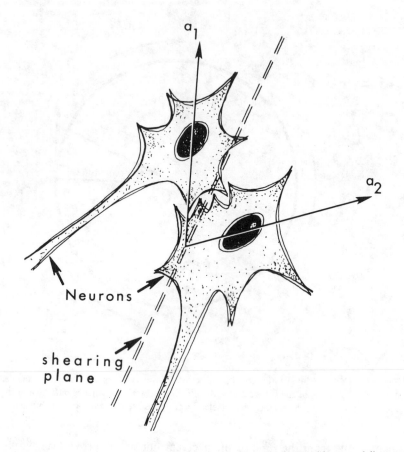

Figure 1-10. The linear accelerations a_1 and a_2 of two adjacent neurons with unequal distances from the center of the brain undergoing angular acceleration. Since a_1 differs from a_2 in magnitude and direction, shearing strain is set up along a plane in between the a_1 and a_2 vectors. This shearing strain will tear neural elements.

that the clinical picture was due to the widespread axonal disruption and generalized disconnection between cortex and subcortical structures.

Although diffuse, these shearing lesions have a predilection for the gray-white matter junctions around the basal ganglia, the periventricular zone of the hypothalamus, the superior cerebellar peduncles, the fornices, the corpus callosum, and fiber tracts of the brain stem. This is not surprising if one recalls that, unlike the perfect sphere, for which shearing strains are mathematically predictable, the human brain is a heterogeneous structure with uneven contours and constituent parts with varying configurations and densities. Shearing strains are exaggerated along

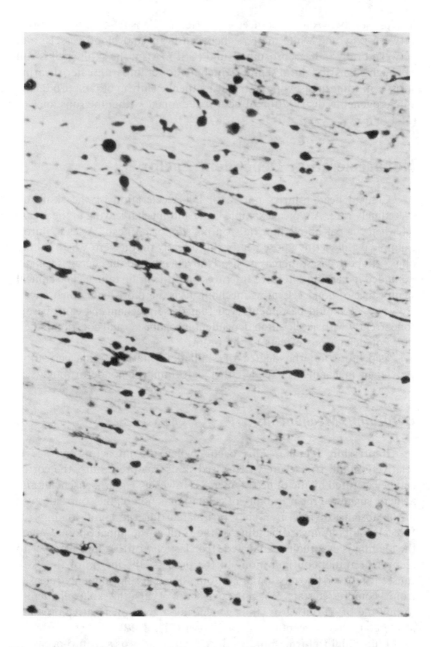

Figure 1-11. Photomicrograph of white matter that had suffered severe shearing strains, stained with silver impregnation technique to show the axons. Multiple axon retraction balls are seen, indicative of diffuse axonal rupture and outward leakage of axoplasm.

interphases between substances of different densities— for example, between gray and white matters, between brain and blood vessels, and between brain and cerebrospinal fluid (CSF). Also, the skull shell is full of rough edges and dural septae, which no doubt impart greater shearing stresses in some areas while distributing them evenly in others, producing a heterogeneous distribution of neuronal damage within the substance of the brain.

Nonacceleration Dependent Factors

Clinical head injuries not involving acceleration of the skull are exceedingly rare. A typical example is the automechanic lying in the grease pit when the car above him falls on his supported head. A less "pure" example is the victim whose head is hit directly on the vertex by a falling object. In both cases, there is no head movement, and the energy is usually expanded in causing extensive fractures but little brain injury. The clinical significance of nonaccelerating mechanisms is therefore highly theoretical. However, it should be remembered that these mechanisms can operate concurrently with acceleration dependent mechanisms and contribute their share of deleterious effects to the brain.

Depending on the degree of skull deformation, nonacceleration dependent mechanisms can be either deforming or nondeforming.

Deforming Mechanisms

Impression Trauma. This occurs when the impacting surface is relatively small. If a severely depressed skull fracture results, the cortex can be lacerated by the bone fragments. However, Unterharnscheidt and Sellier[88] suggested the possibility of cavitation action on the coup side even in the absence of fracture. They postulated that the initial loading (of forces) results in inward bending of the skull at the impact point. When the loading is eventually exhausted, the elasticity of the skull forces it to recover its initial configuration. In the process, the inertia of the skull causes it to overshoot its initial contour, like a spring suddenly released from a compressed state. When the overshoot occurs, the skull will attempt to pull the brain outwards, thus generating a zone of negative pressure at the coup side susceptible to cavitation (Fig. 1–12).

Ellipsoidal Deformation. In the circumstances of a fronto-occipital impact to the supported head, the impact axis will be in line with the sagittal diameter of the skull, with the effect that with subsequent deformation,

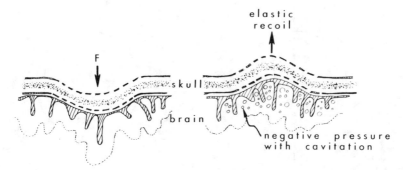

Figure 1-12. Impression trauma without acceleration. The elastic recoil of the indented skull creates a negative pressure zone in the subjacent brain where cavitation at the pole can take place. F = Impact force.

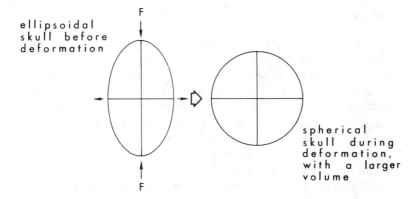

Figure 1-13. Deformation of an ellipsoidal skull to give a more spherical skull under opposing fronto-occipital forces. The sphere has a larger enclosed volume than the original ellipsoid.

the bitemporal axis is lengthened and the fronto-occipital axis shortened. This momentarily converts the ellipsoidal skull into a sphere (Fig. 1–13). The volume confined by a given surface area enclosing any three dimensional ellipsoidal body reaches maximum value when the ellipsoid becomes a sphere. The volume of the deformed skull, which now is approaching a sphere, must therefore be increased. Assuming that the impact is too short-lived for CSF to fill the suddenly enlarged ventricles, a negative pressure zone will be set up in the center.[88] Portions of the brain located along the collision axis will move to the center because of the shortening of the axis; those portions parallel to the vertical axis will move away from center (Fig. 1–14). Thus, destructive shearing strains will occur in and around the center of the brain. The ventricular walls and part of

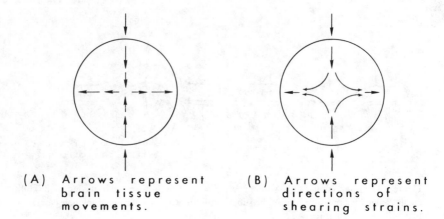

Figure 1-14. The skull deformation and volume changes depicted in Figure 1-13 lead to brain tissue movements (arrows in *A*) prompted by internal shearing strains (arrows in *B*).

the corpus callosum abutting against the lateral ventricles may be particularly vulnerable to this type of central shearing.

Skull Vibration. Marcal and Nickell[48] postulate that a blow to the skull sets up skull vibrations that can create pressure fronts across the cranial cavity. The vibrational characteristics of the skull, which determine the mode of vibration, depend on the regional thickness and curvatures of the bone. The authors have computed some of the modal shapes and frequencies and found that local deformations in these modes are concentrated in the subfrontal region near the zygoma. One mode shows a straightening of the subfrontal curvature, whereas another shows an increased curvature. A frontal or occipital impact with a force application that would excite these modes could presumably produce large intracranial pressure changes capable of setting up alternating pole-antipole pressure gradients along the fronto-occipital axis through which shearing injury might occur.

Nondeforming Mechanism

Stress Waves. The stress wave theory proposed by Engins presumes that shock waves set up by the impact will travel from the point of impact to the antipole. This creates zones of differential pressures where shearing strains may be generated.

In practice, however, the stress wave hypothesis breaks down in most cases of closed head injury. Physical laws dictate that a shock wave may be expected only if the collision time (time of contact between the head and the impacting object) is less than the traveling time of an acoustic wave in the head. For a sagittal collision, the traveling time (t_0) of this wave from one end of the head to the other is given by

$$t_0 = \frac{S}{V} = 0.13 \text{ millisecond}$$

where S equals the sagittal diameter of the skull and V equals the velocity of sound in water. The measured collision times are in no case shorter than 2 milliseconds. They depend on the impacting mass: the smaller the mass, the shorter the collision time. A strong blow with a hammer has a t_0 of 2 ms, and hence it will not set up a stress wave. A bullet of small mass and high velocity, however, has a small collision time and sets up tremendous shock waves as it penetrates the brain.

PATHOPHYSIOLOGY OF SECONDARY BRAIN INJURY

Primary impact injury generates a cascade of secondary pathologic events (epiphenomena) that are themselves harmful to the central nervous system (Fig. 1–15). The pathogeneses of hematomas and cerebral edema are well known, but not that of "acute cerebral swelling" and traumatic vasospasm. Left unchecked, these pathologic entities often result in the familiar cycle of increased intracranial pressure (ICP)→cerebral hypoperfusion→further increase in ICP. The inevitable end result is brain herniation, multiple cerebral infarctions, and permanent brain stem necrosis, the hallmark of irreversible coma. The main factors in the final fatal scenario of serious head trauma are in fact these secondary brain injuries, not the primary impact lesions.

For the sake of clarity, the paradigm in Figure 1–15 left out complex interactions between these epiphenomena. For example, local pressure effect exerted by an expanding blood clot breaks down the blood-brain barrier in the surrounding brain and leads to further vasogenic edema, which in turn aggravates the ICP. Fluctuations of ICP may further weaken the integrity of already injured vessels and cause them to undergo delayed rupture. Several types of brain herniation can compress strategically located blood vessels to cause tissue ischemia. Also, the local or generalized brain ischemia secondary to vasospasm no doubt will accentuate the cerebral edema.

Finally, it must be remembered that in cases of multiple trauma, the brain is only one of many organs injured. Cerebral function and metabolism are exquisitely sensitive to changes in internal milieu normally maintained in perfect homeostasis by the other organs. Encephalopathy

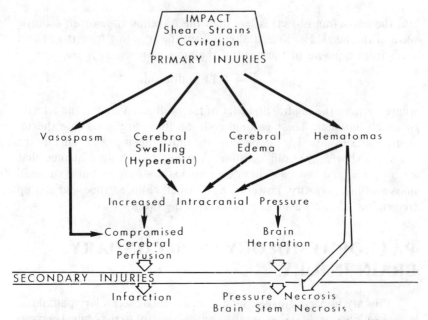

Figure 1-15. Paradigm of head injury lesions. Primary impact injuries result in epiphenomena (edema, hematoma, cerebral swelling, vasospasm) that lead to increased intracranial pressure and brain herniation. The end results are the secondary lesions of cerebral infarction and pressure necrosis, which usually dictate the outcome of the patient.

rapidly supervenes during end-stage hepatic and renal failure. Electrolyte imbalance due to blood loss and fluid restoration aggravates cerebral edema. Hypotension due to blood loss from splenic or skeletal injuries further compromises cerebral perfusion, which is already rendered precarious by vasospasm and high ICP. Hypoxia from pulmonary contusion or infection profoundly affects brain metabolism and can negate vigorous treatment directed at the brain. Thus, the plethora of neuropathologic lesions met at the autopsy table represents the results of hopelessly complex permutations of some or all of the aforementioned insults.

Traumatic Hematomas

Epidural Hematoma

Bleeding from the middle meningeal artery, vein, or venous sinus into the epidural space is an event related principally to the extent of skull fracture or skull bending that occurs at the time of impact. An adjacent skull fracture is found in approximately 90 per cent of patients with epidural hematomas, but the incidence of fractures is much lower in young children because of the resilience of the developing skull.[59] At the point of impact, the in-bending skull pushes the dura inward. As the elastic recoil of the skull causes the indented portion to spring back to resume the normal contour, the less elastic dura is left behind, in essence stripped away from the inner skull table. This leaves a large potential space, which may fill up with blood if dural or diploic vessels were also damaged during the in-bending.[19,30] The rapidity of clot expansion depends on whether the bleeding is from an arterial or venous source. This is the most important factor determining the time course of neurologic deterioration and outcome, for a rapidly enlarging hematoma can be fatal within hours, whereas a slowly accumulating clot from venous oozing may be entirely subclinical.[59] The location of the clot is also important: a temporal or posterior fossa clot causes early brain shift and brain stem compression, whereas a frontoparietal clot may spread out widely and is better tolerated.

Because the pathogenesis of epidural hematoma is related to bony rather than brain injuries, the result of management is excellent so long as irreversible brain stem damage has not taken place. A subacute or chronic epidural hematoma not producing neurologic deficit can often be treated conservatively without surgery,[59] for spontaneous resolution invariably takes place. For those clots causing neurologic deterioration, the mortality and morbidity are almost exclusively dependent on the timing of surgery.[51]

Acute Subdural Hematoma

Acute subdural hematoma is at least twice as common as epidural hematoma, and the mortality rate is at least twice as high.[74] Unlike the latter, most acute subdural hematomas result from massive cortical disruption and lacerated cortical vessels. The underlying damaged brain undergoes rapid edema formation that generates additional mass effect. In most cases, the enlarging edema of the "pulped" brain is far more lethal than the subdural clot itself. Surgical treatment of acute subdural hematoma therefore involves not only simple evacuation of the clot, but also extensive resection of the swollen, "pulped" brain, as well as vigorous means to limit the concomitant edema.

Since the pathogenesis of most acute subdural hematomas involves the same mechanisms that cause brain contusion and shearing, the outcome for the patient depends not only on the expediency of surgical removal, but also on the extent of the primary lesions underlying the subdural bleeding. In contrast, a rare type of acute subdural hematoma results from rupture of a single cortical artery without parenchymal brain disruption. Prompt evacuation of this lesion is associated with normal recovery.

Intracerebral Hematoma

Intracerebral hematomas are uncommon lesions in blunt head trauma. Most cases result from penetrating injuries involving missiles and low velocity objects. The prognosis of this type of intracerebral clot depends on the extent of brain devastation by the projectile. Another type of intracerebral clot results from severely depressed skull fractures with in-driven bone fragments. This type is usually small and superficial and often does not require surgical intervention.

A third type of intracerebral bleeding occurs 24 to 72 hours after the initial head injury.[24] These are rare lesions, found only in 1.8 per cent of a large series of patients with closed head injury.[13] Most of these delayed clots are discovered after surgical decompression of an unrelated mass lesion elsewhere, and they are invariably found in areas of intrinsic tissue damage previously shown on computed tomography (CT).[28] The source of bleeding is thought to be already injured blood vessels (e.g., due to shearing) that were tamponaded by brain swelling or by a contralateral mass. Removal of the tamponading factor and vasomotor changes in the diseased vessels subsequently lead to delayed extravasation. Delayed clots can be treacherous, since they often escape detection after the original CT showed no hematoma. This emphasizes the importance of repeat radiographic studies in severe head injury.

Cerebral Edema

Cerebral edema is best defined as an increase in brain volume that is due to an increase in its water content. It is the nonspecific response of the brain to a great variety of insults, including trauma and ischemia. Klatzo and Seitelberger's[38] original classification of brain edema mentioned three types, but only the first two are relevant to a discussion of head injury.

Vasogenic Edema

Vasogenic edema, the most common form of brain edema, is characterized by increased permeability of brain capillaries. The increase in permeability is due to a breakdown of the blood-brain barrier (BBB). Normal extracerebral capillaries are permeable to both lipid and water soluble substances because of large fenestrations between plasma membranes of neighboring endothelial cells. Water soluble particles leak through these fenestrations or are carried through the endothelial cells by a process of pinocytosis (a series of transport vacuoles containing the particles), whereas lipid soluble molecules go through the cells directly. Brain capillaries are made of endothelial cells closely bound together at numerous locations on the cell membranes by tight, occluding junctional complexes that preclude the existence of fenestrations. These cells also do not normally show pinocytotic activity. Each capillary is surrounded by a basement membrane outside which lies a continuous ring of astrocytic cytoplasm formed from fusion of investing astrocytic foot plates. Thus, water soluble substances cannot easily leak through to the brain extracellular space (ECS) except by specialized carrier transport systems available for specific sugars, amino acids, and ions.[64]

In vasogenic edema, there is abnormal opening of the tight junctions through which water, proteins, and other solutes rapidly exude out into the ECS. It is easy to imagine how shearing or cavitation can generate ripping forces across the vessel wall and damage the integrity of the endothelial barrier. Tissue ischemia and cytotoxins can likewise damage BBB by paralyzing endothelial metabolism. The capillary wall now behaves like a semipermeable membrane. The osmotic forces exerted by the extravasated proteins and solutes perpetuate the efflux of water into the ECS and sustain the edema formation.[17]

Since fluid leakage is a slow process, traumatic brain edema usually becomes clinically significant 4 to 6 hours after injury. Assuming no continuous insult, the edema peaks in 24 to 36 hours, following which repair of the endothelial tight junction takes place. Clearance of the existing edema fluid is by bulk flow through the network of ECS channels from the cortical surface through white matter to the subependymal zone. It then enters the ventricles through breaks in the ependyma and is ultimately absorbed back into the blood stream along with CSF, or it is resorbed by subependymal and cortical capillaries.

Reduction in extracellular brain water content is the basis for the treatment of raised ICP by hyperosmolar agents and corticosteroids. Hyperosmolar agents such as mannitol and glycerol depend for their action on an intact BBB, across which an osmotic gradient can be developed, so that water can be preferentially removed from the brain.[40,96] In essence, they hasten the resolution of edema fluid. In a severely injured brain with extensively damaged BBB, however, mannitol molecules leak across the sieve-like BBB, where they gradually set up a reverse gradient that draws water back into the brain. This explains why indiscriminate use of hyperosmolar agents in head injury can induce a paradoxic rise in ICP. The action of steroids is less well understood. They may hasten the repair of endothelial membranes.

Cytotoxic Edema

In cytotoxic edema, all the cellular elements (astroglia, neurons, and endothelial cells) undergo swelling due to entry of water into the cells through a damaged cell membrane. Normally, the ionic contents within an astrocyte (or neuron) are meticulously maintained by energy dependent Na^+, K^+, and H^+ pumps within the cell membrane. Ischemia or metabolic toxins (such as cyanide) cause a rapid depletion of adenosine triphosphate (ATP, high energy compound serving as energy store) and paralysis of the ATP-dependent Na^+ pump. Sodium rapidly accumulates within the cell, and water follows to maintain osmotic equilibrium. Ischemia also causes an abnormal increase in carbonic anhydrase activity, an enzyme system that enhances a Cl^- carrier transport system. The net effect is an intracellular accumulation of Cl^- and water.[37]

The endothelial cells may also undergo cytotoxic swelling. In extreme cases, the capillary lumens are swollen shut and tissue ischemia may be compounded. Swelling of the astrocytic foot plates also damages the integrity of the BBB and causes secondary vasogenic edema.[36] The combined effect is an invariable vicious cycle of edema-ischemia-edema.

Unlike vasogenic edema, cytoxic edema is not usually responsive to hyperosmolar therapy. The hyperosmolar particles stay on the capillary side of an intact BBB to draw water from an already drastically reduced ECS without affecting the intracellular water volume. Loop diuretics (Lasix and ethacrynic acid), on the other hand, block the carrier transport mechanism that facilitates chloride influx and may reduce cytotoxic edema.[5]

Intracranial Pressure and Head Injury

Since the early development of the so-called Monro-Kellie doctrine, the concept has been established that any increase in the four intracranial constituents within the noncompliant skull—namely, brain, CSF, cerebral blood, and extracellular fluid — will cause an increase in intracranial pressure.[41] As an approximate guide, glial and neural tissues account for about 70 per cent of the contents, with CSF, cerebral blood, and extracellular fluid each accounting for 10 per cent of the total volume.

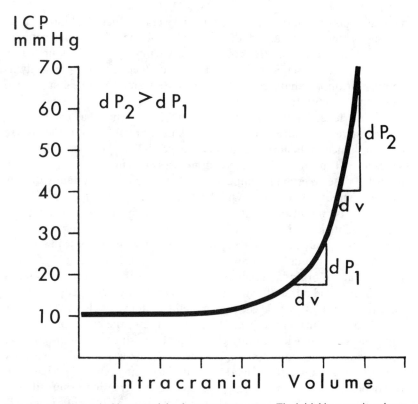

Figure 1-16. Theoretical intracranial volume-pressure curve. The initial increase in volume causes only a negligible rise in pressure due to compensatory capacity of the intracranial system. As progressively more volume is added, the change in pressure (dP) per change in unit volume (dV) gradually rises. The intracranial elastance (dP/dV) thus rises with the intracranial pressure.

The presence of a hematoma and edema implies an increase in the blood (extravasated) and extracellular fluid compartments. This would induce an increase in ICP, just as a brain tumor or hydrocephalus would cause high ICP through an increase in the other two compartments.

As can be seen in a plot between intracranial volume (V) and pressure (P) (the volume-pressure curve) (Fig. 1-16), the relationship between intracranial volume and ICP is not linear. When fluid is injected into the intracranial cavity, the initial rise in volume causes very little rise in ICP, because two of the four constituents may be expelled from the cranial cavity to accommodate an expanding mass. Cerebrospinal fluid may be squeezed from the cranial subarachnoid space and ventricles into the spinal subarachnoid space, and cerebral venous blood may be expelled into the jugular veins or into the scalp via emissary veins.[45] Increased intracranial pressure results from any addition to the volume of these intracranial constituents in excess of this compensatory capacity. The pressure curve then rises exponentially, a little at first, but steepening progressively as compensation is exhausted, until an infinitely small increase in volume causes an asymptotic rise in pressure.

The critical factor here is the increase in pressure that results from a given increase in intracranial volume. This expression, $\frac{dP}{dV}$, is the inverse of compliance and can be termed elastance.[53] The elastance is in effect a measure of the gradient of the volume-pressure curve at any point, and it predicts the reserve of compensatory capacity of the system with any further increase in volume. On the left of the curve (Fig. 1-16), the elastance is small, so that a large increment of volume can be accommodated, whereas on the steep part of the curve, the high elastance predicts a very large increase in ICP with only a slight increase in volume.

A single volume-pressure curve describes the intracranial system in a given state of brain "stiffness." Brain stiffness is related to the amount of ECS fluid and intracellular water, the amount of vascular engorgement, and the compliance of the brain cells (extensive gliosis decreases compliance). Thus, for a given state of stiffness, the curve predicts the compensatory capacity for any given ICP by noting the rise in pressure with changes in volume; the higher the ICP, the less the compensatory capacity. But brain stiffness increases with increasing cerebral edema. This is independent of compensatory capacity. The increasing brain stiffness when the extracellular space is engorged with edema fluid results in a much steeper rise in pressure for the same increment in volume that normally would cause only a small rise in pressure if the brain is less stiff; that is, it induces a change in the *shape* of the volume-pressure curve. Figure 1-17 shows three brain systems with different degrees of stiffness. The brain described by Curve 1 is much stiffer than that described by Curve 3, for, given the same ICP of 30 mm Hg, the elastance ($\frac{dP}{dV}$) of Curve 1 is much higher than that of Curve 3. Thus, for any given ICP, the elastance is a measure of the stiffness of the intracranial system. Herein lies the most important clinical use of elastance. If the three curves in Figure 1-17 represent three patients having different degrees of brain stiffness, the reading of an ICP of 20 mm Hg in all three patients at any given time may give the false impression that they are in approximately the same clinical state. A determination of elastance (by noting the rise in pressure after injecting a given small amount of saline into the ventricular catheter), however, will immediately reveal that patient 1 has a stiffer brain, has a much lower compensatory reserve, and is in a much more critical state than the other two patients.

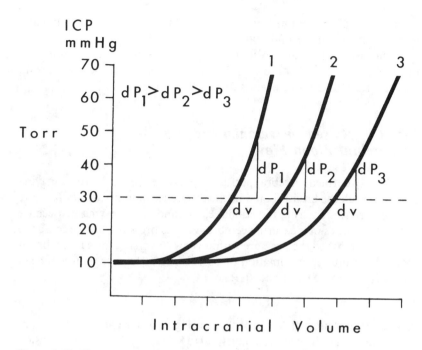

Figure 1-17. The theoretical volume-pressure curves of three patients. For the same intracranial pressure (*ICP*) of 30 mm Hg, Patient 1 has a much greater elastance (dP/dV) than do Patients 2 and 3. This implies that Patient 1 has a "stiffer" brain and a much lower intracranial compensatory reserve, and is in a much more critical state than the other two patients. The elastance therefore predicts the changes in ICP with additional increments in volume before such changes actually occur.

Since mannitol and steroids reduce brain stiffness by lessening the brain edema, they lower elastance and alter the configuration of the volume curve by changing it from a steep curve (Curve 1 in Fig. 1-17) to a flatter one (Curve 3 in Fig. 1-17). Now, for the same ICP, the brain whose elastance has been lowered has more compensatory reserve and is less liable to show troublesome ICP rises.[54] Hyperventilation, on the other hand, does not reduce edema and therefore does not alter the elastance. It induces hypocapnia and vasoconstriction, which lowers the ICP by reducing the intravascular blood volume. Hyperventilation, as it were, operates merely along the points of a *single* volume-pressure curve without changing the configuration of that curve. The cessation of hyperventilation causes a rise in cerebral blood flow and immediately returns the ICP to its former, higher value. This underscores the folly of prolonged vigorous "bagging" of a patient who is having a sudden, sustained climb in ICP. Bagging per se does not lower the brain elastance; it merely lowers the ICP temporarily so that more permanent measures, such as administration of mannitol and loop diuretics, can be undertaken.

The two factors that explain impairment of brain function are (1) the effect of high ICP on cerebral blood flow, and (2) the relationship between raised ICP and brain shift.

Effect of Raised Intracranial Pressure on Cerebral Blood Flow

Strictly defined, cerebral perfusion pressure (CPP, the force driving blood through the brain) should be the difference in intravascular pressure between arteries entering the cranial cavity and veins leaving it. Because of the difficulties in measuring cerebral venous pressure, and because the ICP is very close to the pressure within veins traversing the subarachnoid space,[53] a useful approximation of CPP is the difference between mean arterial pressure (MAP) and ICP, or

$$CPP = MAP - ICP$$

(Considering a normal MAP of 90 mm Hg and normal ICP of 10 mm Hg, the normal CPP is approximately 70 to 80 mm Hg.) Cerebral perfusion pressure can, therefore, be reduced by one of two mechanisms: (1) by a reduction in arterial pressure, or (2) by an increase in ICP.

The relationship between CPP and cerebral blood flow (CBF) is far more complicated. Cerebral blood flow remains relatively constant if CPP falls between 50 mm Hg and 180 mm Hg (Fig. 1-18). Below 50 mm Hg, CBF will fall according to the drop in CPP. This ability of the brain to maintain a constant blood flow within a wide range of driving pressures is due to the intrinsic capacity of the cerebral vessels to constrict when the transmural pressure (CPP) rises, and to dilate when it falls. The brain in effect maintains its own fuel supply in spite of changes in cardiovascular dynamics. This process is called autoregulation, and it is peculiar to cerebral vessels. Thus, for a normal person with a mean arterial pressure of 90 mm Hg, the ICP will have to increase to above 40 mm Hg (much higher than normal) before any change in CBF will occur.

The mechanism of autoregulation, however, is abolished by a variety of insults, including trauma and ischemia.[42] In severe trauma, cerebral blood flow becomes completely pressure-passive and will therefore show a significant fall proportional to the fall in CPP. Much smaller increases in ICP (e.g., above 25 mm Hg) will now induce a sufficient reduction in cerebral blood flow to produce neurologic dysfunction. In multiple trauma, hypotension from other organ injuries may further narrow the difference between MAP and ICP. Thus, since raised ICP is common in brain trauma

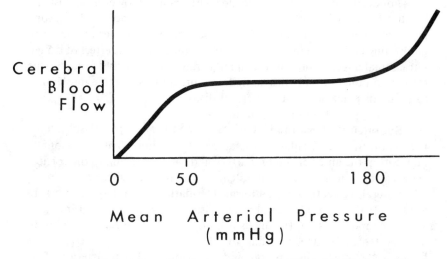

Figure 1-18. Autoregulation of cerebral vasculature to changes in mean arterial blood pressure. Cerebral blood flow (CBF) remains relatively constant between blood pressures of 50 mm Hg and 180 mm Hg due to locally integrated vasodilatation and vasoconstriction: a higher blood pressure causes vasoconstriction, and conversely, a lower blood pressure causes vasodilatation. CBF changes passively with blood pressures outside this physiologic range or if autoregulation is damaged.

and trauma impairs autoregulation,[68] it should not be surprising that ischemic brain damage is found in up to 80 per cent of patients who die of head injury.[22]

When cerebral ischemia associated with intracranial hypertension is encountered in clinical practice, it is tempting for the clinician to attempt to improve CBF by increasing arterial pressure. In practice, this maneuver is both futile and dangerous. When autoregulation is completely lost, an increase in MAP causes the cerebral vessels to dilate passively (because the pressure across vessel walls is increased). This induces a rise in ICP pari passu with the arterial pressure; the CPP has not changed and CBF remains the same. Due to the passive vasodilation, however, the cerebral blood *volume* has increased: The cerebral blood pool has enlarged without more blood passing through the brain. This sudden rise in ICP thus sets the stage for brain herniation.

Raised Intracranial Pressure and Brain Shift

In certain cases of generalized increase in ICP from diffuse cerebral processes, such as in benign intracranial hypertension, brain herniation does not occur. Mass lesions associated with trauma, however, are usually localized and will initially generate a pressure gradient from one intracranial compartment to another to cause brain herniation. The devastating effect of herniation compared to the innocuous effect of benign intracranial hypertension once again illustrates the capacity of brain tissue to function under evenly distributed pressure and its extreme intolerance to tissue displacement and structural distortion.

Four types of herniation occur.

Subfalcine Herniation. The most common type is subfalcine herniation of one cingulate gyrus across the midline. This occasionally may entrap the anterior cerebral artery and cause ischemia to the cortical leg area, but most cases of subfalcine herniation are silent.

Lateral (Uncal) Transtentorial Herniation. The largest pressure gradient from a supratentorial mass exists across the tentorial incisura. With a temporal lesion, the uncus insinuates itself between the midbrain and the tentorial edge, catching the third cranial nerve as it runs out between the posterior cerebral and superior cerebellar arteries. This produces ipsilateral pupillary dilatation, since the pupillary fibers are the most superficially located within the third nerve. The pressure cone also pushes the brain stem downward. Since the basilar artery is fixed to the circle of Willis and cannot move caudally with the brain stem, the ventral perforating arteries to the brain stem are stretched, elongated, and narrowed. This process is worsened when side-to-side compression of the brain stem increases its anteroposterior diameter, aggravating the brain stem ischemia and causing progressively deeper coma. If this ischemia is prolonged, and the integrity of the vessel walls is weakened, intermittent reperfusion of this region will lead to hemorrhages in the central portion of the pons (Duret hemorrhages).[39] This is the pathologic substrate of irreversible coma and underscores the importance of prompt intervention in cases of transtentorial herniation.

Central Transtentorial Herniation. If the mass effect is from the frontal region or is bilateral, the brain stem will more likely be symmetrically displaced caudally without injuring the third nerve. The same mechanism for brain stem ischemia as in uncal herniation causes coma early, but the backward pressure on the midbrain crushes the tectorial plate (containing the third nerve nuclei) against the posterior edge of the incisura to cause bilateral pupillary dilatation.[35]

Transforamenal (Tonsillar) Herniation. This results from a posterior fossa mass forcing the tonsils downward between the rim of the foramen magnum and the medulla. The patient loses cardiorespiratory drive and goes into apnea and bradycardia as coma rapidly supervenes.

Syndrome of "Acute Cerebral Swelling"

Recently, Zimmerman and co-workers[98] reported a group of children with moderate and severe head injuries whose initial CT scan showed evidence of increased brain mass. No focal lesions were noted, but the ventricular system and cisternal spaces were symmetrically and severely narrowed, indicating generalized compression. Because the CT attenuation number of the brain is consistently increased in these patients, Zimmerman and colleagues postulated that the increased brain mass is due to generalized cerebral hyperemia (blood has a higher attenuation number than brain, and water [edema] lower than brain). This was subsequently proved by direct measurement of cerebral blood flow on children with acute head injuries using intravenous xenon-133.[57] Zimmerman and co-workers called this phenomenon "acute cerebral swelling" to distinguish it from edema, for the water content of the brain is not increased in these children.

This process of acute vasodilatation can be demonstrated as early as 6 hours after injury, but usually it is self-limiting and subsides from 2 to 4 days after injury.[98] The patient may initially be awake and verbalizing but with the onset of vascular engorgement, the ICP rises progressively and stupor, coma, and brain herniation can occur within several hours. This phenomenon appears to be peculiar to children and young adults: The incidence of such swelling has been known to be as high as 45 per cent in children under the age of 18 years with moderate to severe head injury, but is less than 10 per cent in adults.[99]

The pathogenesis for the generalized vasodilatation is unknown, but it is likely related to diffuse shearing injuries to the blood vessels, or to the brain stem vasomotor center. In patients with less severe injuries, the process subsides in 1 to 2 days, the CT scan normalizes accordingly, and clinical improvement occurs. In more severely impaired children, the subsidence of vasodilatation is followed by formation of diffuse edema, confirmed by a shift of the CT number from higher to lower than normal, and by clinical deterioration.[98]

Traumatic Vasospasm

Yet another factor that may influence cerebral perfusion is cerebral vasospasm noted after acute head injury. Arteriography performed by Suwanwela and Suwanwela[84] in 350 patients with moderate to severe head injury revealed spasm in 18.6 per cent of patients. In these patients the spasm was usually bilateral, but it may be primarily unilateral on the side of a focal contusion. It may be delayed in onset, and it usually lasts for 2 to 3 weeks once it develops.[94] Four categories of spasm are noted: Narrowing of the distal internal carotid and proximal anterior and middle cerebral arteries; narrowing of cerebral arteries at the site of contusion; diffuse narrowing of all the intracranial arteries; and narrowing of an artery adjoining a torn vessel.[84]

Three mechanisms may be responsible for the spasm.

1. Data from studies of vasospasm in subarachnoid hemorrhage caused by ruptured aneurysms suggest that traumatic vasospasm is related to subarachnoid blood surrounding the involved arteries. McCullough, Nelson, and Ommaga[50] in fact found a direct correlation between the magnitude of subarachnoid hemorrhage in the basal cisterns and the degree of vertebrobasilar spasm noted on angiogram.

2. Since some patients with posttraumatic vasospasm show no evidence of subarachnoid hemorrhage, it has been suggested that serotonin released into the CSF as a result of injury to the brain itself may exert a direct chemical effect on the arteries.[58]

3. The last mechanism involves the possibility that injury to an area of the brain important to the maintenance of cerebral arterial tone may be responsible for the spasm. For example, destruction of portions of the canine brain stem can diminish CBF volume,[77] and electrical stimulation of the brain stem of monkeys resulted in vasodilatation.[52] Molnar[55] hypothesized that under normal conditions, impulses from the pontobulbar and hypothalamic pressor centers produce vasoconstriction in the brain. The cerebral cortex normally inhibits such impulses. In decerebrate and decorticate animals, the vasoconstrictor response becomes manifest. Whether this theory is applicable to human head injuries remains to be elucidated.

PATHOPHYSIOLOGIC CORRELATION OF NEUROBEHAVIORAL SYNDROMES

CONCUSSION

Concussion has classically been defined as an essentially reversible syndrome involving transient loss of consciousness without detectable pathology.[12] Later this first definition was expanded slightly to include associated traumatic amnesia, but again the absence of physical damage to the brain was emphasized.[92] This emphasis was based on the earlier observation that patients rendered temporarily unconscious from relatively minor injury appeared to show no lasting neurologic deficit. Because of Magoun's original work on the reticular activating system (RAS),[47] the brain stem has been recognized as the source of cortical arousal in the maintenance of consciousness. Thus, concussion was thought to result from reversible, nonstructural (?biochemical) changes confined to the brain stem.

Results from recent investigations question the validity of this assumption. An enlarging body of evidence now suggests the presence of actual morphologic damage to certain brain stem nuclei in experimental models of concussion. Furthermore, similar or more severe structural damage has also been found elsewhere in the brain. These two issues deserve closer examination.

The Morphopathologic Substrate of Concussion

That the brain stem-diencephalic reticular activating system is responsible for the maintenance of consciousness is beyond question.[47] The changes of consciousness associated with concussion should then be mediated through these brain stem mechanisms. Foltz and Schmidt[18] showed that the evoked potentials in the reticular formation were completely abolished following a concussive blow to the head of a monkey. Changes in cortical and subcortical activity were minimal and transient. Later, Sharpless and Jasper[78] and Jenkner[34] found a sudden rise in CSF acetylcholine following experimental concussion, and they postulated that the cessation of neural transmission reflected by the depression in evoked potential was due to postsynaptic depolarization by acetylcholine.[92] Recovery was thought to be due to degradation of acetylcholine. The crucial question, therefore, is whether the functional alteration in the brain stem is caused by completely reversible biochemical inhibition, or whether concussion produces structural changes in the brain stem neurons.

In 1979, Povlishock and colleagues[65] showed that following mild percussion injury causing temporary loss of consciousness, the endothelial cell membrane in the brain stem raphe nuclei (part of the RAS) of monkeys manifested a dramatic increase in permeability. The tracer protein horseradish peroxidase (HRP) freely crosses the endothelial membrane through luminal pits, cytoplasmic vacuoles, and tubules that are clearly visible by electron microscopy and are apparently induced by the impact. The HRP then inundates the raphe neurons and is subsequently taken up through the neuronal cytoplasm into the nuclei and nucleoli, where nuclear rodlets are formed. These rodlets are thought to reflect an abnormal metabolic and functional state of the neurons related to the traumatically altered function of the brain stem raphe nuclei. This abnormal vascular permeability may also explain the observation of Takahashi and co-workers[86] that mild concussive trauma induces massive leakage of potassium ions (K+) from brain stem neurons of the mouse. The elevated extracellular K+ concentration then causes a depolarization block that suppresses normal neuronal activity. Thus, for the first time, structural changes have been demonstrated in crucial neural tissues following seemingly trivial trauma.

Clinical Implications of Minor Concussive Trauma

Is the structural damage in mild concussive injuries limited to the brain stem, and are there more lasting effects than the transient disturbance of consciousness? Further studies by Povlishock and Kontos[66] led to the discovery that the endothelial membrane leakage also existed in the pial vessels diffusely located over the brain. Other neuronal structures, possibly those related to memory and other higher cortical functions, are therefore affected simultaneously by the concussive blow. In 1981, Rimel and associates[69] furnished unequivocal clinical evidence that long-term disability can be found in patients who had sustained minor head trauma. They studied 538 head injured patients who had suffered a period of unconsciousness of less than 20 minutes and whose Glasgow coma scores were 13 to 15. At 3 months' follow-up, the majority showed problems with attention, concentration, memory, and judgment. Over 70 per cent of patients complained of persistent headaches, and 59 per cent described memory disturbance. The emotional stress caused by these persistent symptoms was a significant factor in the long-term disability of these patients. This high rate of morbidity and unemployment 3 months after a seemingly insignificant head injury strongly suggests that many of these patients had, in fact, suffered lasting organic brain damage. The memory and personality disturbances imply that neuronal structures other than the brain stem were involved. This was later confirmed by the presence of degenerated axons in the brain stem reticular formation, colliculi, pons, and cerebral hemispheres found by the same group of workers in monkeys with mild concussion.[32] It therefore appears that "minor" concussive injury is physiologically and psychosocially a much more disabling syndrome than previously deemed.

MOTOR SYSTEM DISORDERS

Traumatic brain lesions affecting the motor system can be located anywhere from the motor-premotor cortex to the brain stem corticospinal pathways. Cortical and subcortical lesions do not usually cause extensive paralysis because of the broad cortical representation of the motor area. In the posterior limb of the internal capsule, however, the corticospinal and corticobulbar fibers are tightly crowded into a small area measuring less than 1.5 cm in its long axis. Thus, a strategically located lesion in this region of the internal capsule will likely result in profound paresis involving the face, arm, and leg. More detailed information on the somatotopic arrangement of the motor and premotor cortices can be obtained from standard textbooks of neuroanatomy and will not be given here.

Motor weakness following cortical contusions or subcortical shearing almost always improves to some extent with time. With physical therapy and the help of prosthetic devices, the patient can often overcome the difficulties due to weakness alone. However, two aspects of traumatic paralysis are more disabling than weakness per se and will likely pose serious problems in motor rehabilitation. These are spasticity and involuntary movements arising from lesions in the basal ganglia and related extrapyramidal structures.

Spasticity

In the intensive care unit, spasticity interferes with proper patient positioning and postural drainage and predisposes the patient to the development of decubitus ulcers and atelectasis. In the chronic stage, it prevents passive and active joint motions and induces periarticular fibrosis and contractures. When the patient becomes ambulatory, spasticity also precludes execution of fine movements, hinders efficient locomotion, and often nullifies the beneficial effects of regained voluntary strength. It is, therefore, a major obstacle to motor rehabilitation.

Physiology of the Muscle Spindle

The tonic and dynamic state of a skeletal muscle depends on the function of structures called muscle spindles found in all muscles of locomotion and in muscles of mastication, phonation, and extraocular movements. Each muscle spindle consists of a spindle-shaped connective tissue capsule containing three to eight slender muscle fibers. These so-called intrafusal fibers are arranged in parallel with the ordinary, extrafusal muscle fibers that make up the true contractile portion of the skeletal muscle. Both are ultimately attached to the tendon by way of inelastic collagen fibers. When the extrafusal fibers contract, the intrafusal fibers will be subjected to a reduced tension, whereas stretching of the muscle as a whole will increase the length and tension of the intrafusal fibers (Fig. 1-19).

The central equatorial parts of the intrafusal fibers are not contractile and harbor many nuclei arranged in two different patterns: the one containing nmuclei in a central clump is called the nuclear bag fiber, and the one containing nuclei in a single file is called the nuclear chain fiber. The central nuclear portion of the intrafusal fibers is endowed with two types of afferent sensory endings: The primary sensory or annulospiral endings are found in both nuclear bag and chain fibers, and the secondary sensory or flower-spray endings are found only in the nuclear chain fibers. The spindles also receive motor innervation from fine gamma (γ) fibers arising from motor neurons in the ventral horn. There appear to be two types of γ fibers: γ_1 supply the nuclear bag muscle fibers, and γ_2 supply the nuclear chain fibers. The extrafusal muscle fibers are supplied by α motor neurons. It follows from this arragement that a contraction of the intrafusal fibers in response to γ motor activity will result in stretching of the central "sensory" part of the intrafusal fibers with a consequent stimulation of the sensory endings, just as will stretching of the entire muscle.

The nuclear chain intrafusal fibers are sensitive to changes in the length of the muscle, whereas the nuclear bag fibers are sensitive to the velocity of stretching. When a tendon is suddenly tapped, the primary sensory endings from the bag fibers are preferentially activated and convey impulses into the spinal cord. These impulses in turn stimulate an α motor neuron through a monosynaptic connection to cause contraction of the agonist muscle (tapped). At the same time, collaterals activate inhibitory internuncial neurons to inhibit the antagonist muscle so that more efficient contraction of the agonist can take place. Contraction of these extrafusal fibers shortens the spindles and the spindle sensory endings stop firing, which in turn extinguishes the α motor neuron activity and terminates the extrafusal muscle contraction. The sensitivity of this phasic sensory response can be heightened by increased activity of the γ_1 motor neurons so that the nuclear bag fibers are put on a stretch, resulting in a decreased response threshold in the annulospiral endings on the nuclear bag. This

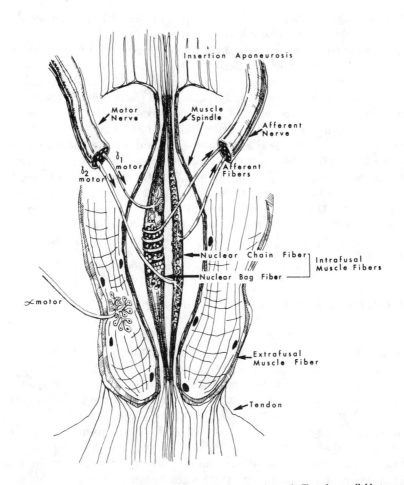

Figure 1-19. Drawing of the muscle spindle and the extrafusal muscle fibers in parallel between the tendon and the insertion aponeurosis. The two types of intrafusal muscle fibers, nuclear bag and nuclear chain, are supplied by the γ_1 and γ_2 motor fibers, respectively. Contraction of these fibers activates the afferent nerves, which then send impulses through the spinal cord to activate the motor fibers that supply the extrafusal muscle fibers, leading to contraction of the entire muscle. Shortening of the muscle spindle relaxes the intrafusal fibers, and afferent signals are deactivated.

is the basis for the hyperactive tendon reflexes seen in spasticity when γ_1 motor activity is abnormally increased.

In daily life, sudden stretching of a muscle is an uncommon event. It is, however, essential that the lengths of the various muscles taking part in a movement be mutually adjusted at all times; that is, the muscle must be maintained in a certain tone. This tone is set by activity of the γ_2 motor fiber through its ability to alter the length of the nuclear chain spindle fibers. A change in the spindle length proportionately tunes the spindle afferent signals to the α motor neurons and indirectly sets the basal length (and tone) of the whole muscle.

Both the α and γ motor systems are under supraspinal control. The vestibulospinal, rubrospinal, and reticulospinal tracts facilitate the action of both types of motor neurons, and inputs from the dentate nucleus of the cerebellum, the premotor cortex, and the basal ganglia inhibit these motor neurons. All three systems—the α, γ_1, and γ_2—are under separate supraspinal influences. Thus, the brain can produce movements by using either the α system (e.g., in rapid and forceful contractions) or the γ system, which then activates the α system (e.g., in "ordinary" muscular contraction). These systems are also influenced by general exteroceptive and interoceptive sensory inputs, which explains how mood, excitement, and the state of general sensory excitation can affect muscle tone and reflex activity.

Pathophysiology of Spasticity and Rigidity

In spasticity, the deep tendon reflexes are exaggerated, but the palpated rest tone is either normal or only slightly increased. Resistance sets in when the muscle is passively stretched. Thus, it appears that the activity of the γ_1 phasic system is heightened, but not that of the γ_2 tonic system. This is almost always due to release from supraspinal inhibitory influence of the nuclear bag system, with only moderate release of the nuclear chain system. With a cortical or internal capsule lesion, the corticospinal and corticorubral inhibitory inputs to the leg extensors are interrupted while the vestibulospinal facilitatory influence of the leg extensors is preserved. The situation with the arm flexors and extensors is opposite to that of the legs. This results in the characteristic posture of arm-in-flexion and leg-in-extension in the type of spasticity seen with a capsular lesion. It must also be remembered that spasticity may just as likely be caused by release of the α motor system as by release of the γ system. Both systems probably are involved in most cases.

The two drugs commonly used in the treatment of spasticity are dantrolene sodium (Dantrium) and baclofen (Lioresal). Dantrolene sodium acts directly on the myoneural junction of the muscle; it prevents calcium release from the sarcoplasmic reticulum necessary for the contractile response to membrane depolarization. Baclofen inhibits monosynaptic and polysynaptic activities in the cord and decreases facilitatory tone to the α and γ motor neurons.

In rigidity, the tendon reflexes are not exaggerated, but the rest tone of both the flexors and extensors is greatly increased. Thus, in rigidity there is predominantly an increased activity in the nuclear chain γ_2 motor system, which augments only the static tone of the muscles.

Basal Ganglia Disorders

Anatomy

The basal ganglia comprise a collective group of subcortical nuclei functionally involved in the execution of movements. These include the striatum (formed by the caudate nucleus and the putamen), the globus pallidus (pallidum), the substantia nigra, the subthalamic nucleus, the nucleus accumbens, septi and the olfactory tubercle, the latter two being ventral extensions of the caudate nucleus.

The striatum is the major receptive portion of the basal ganglia (Fig. 1-20). It receives (1) cortical inputs from all areas of the neocortex but especially the motor and premotor fields and the association sensory cortex; (2) exteroceptive and interoceptive inputs from the centromedian nucleus of the thalamus so that sensorimotor signals from the cortex can be integrated with moment-to-moment information from the outside world; and (3) important inputs from the substantia nigra containing the nigrostriatal dopamine fibers. Other dopamine neurons from the ventromedial brain stem tegmental nuclei project to the nucleus accumbens and the olfactory tubercle in the "mesolimbic dopamine system." From the same tegmental nuclei, dopamine fibers also project to the frontal cortex in the "mesocortical dopamine system."

The striatum projects solely on the two output nuclei of the group, the pallidum and the substantia nigra (SN). Both the pallidum and SN project to the ventrolateral (VL) and ventroanterior (VA) nuclei of the thalamus (Fig. 2-20). The pallidum also projects to the centromedian nucleus, thus closing the feedback loop pallidum→centromedian nucleus→putamen→pallidum. There are also reciprocal projections with the limbic system to suggest that emotions can influence motor performance. The pallidum and SN also project downward to certain brain stem structures so that the basal ganglia can bypass the feedback loop to the cortex and influence brain stem and spinal cord motor neurons directly.

The significance of the major termination of basal ganglia output in the thalamic nuclei (VL and VA) lies in the subsequent projections of these nuclei upon the premotor cortex and wide areas of the frontal lobe, thus

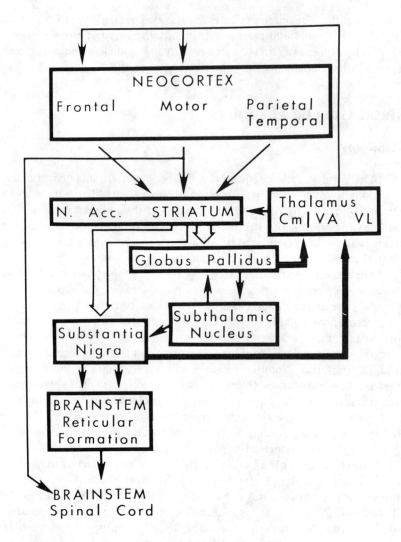

Figure 1-20. Schematic diagram of the principal connections of the basal ganglia. *N. Acc*, Nucleus accumbens; *CM*, centromedian nucleus; *VA*, ventroanterior nucleus; *VL*, ventrolateral nucleus. The striatum, the major receptive portion, receives inputs from the motor, premotor, prefrontal, and parietotemporal cortices. The striatum projects mainly to the major efferent portions, the pallidum (globus pallidus) and substantia nigra. From these two nuclei, basal ganglia outputs return to the neocortex via the thalamus, completing the loop circuit whereby cortical motor outflows can be modified by the basal ganglia. The side loop involving the subthalamic nucleus and the descending projections from the substantia nigra to the brainstem reticular nuclei are also shown.

closing the most important functional loop: premotor and other neocortices→basal ganglia→thalamus→premotor frontal cortex. After receiving and integrating motor inputs from the cortex, the basal ganglia can influence motor functions by means of projections back to the precentral motor fields (via the thalamus) as well as by descending projections to certain brain stem structures.[11]

The subthalamic nucleus receives inputs from the pallidum and projects back to the pallidum and the SN. It is thus positioned to directly modulate the output of the basal ganglia (Fig. 1-20).

Functions

From animal and human data, the following characteristics are thought to be true of the basal ganglia:

1. It does not appear that the basal ganglia directly influence the regions of motor cortex controlling fine movements of the distal musculature. Rather, their influence on the premotor and prefrontal areas suggests a role in exerting proximal and axial muscle control in the maintenance of posture, as well as in fixation of the limbs so that distal movements can be appropriately executed.

2. The basal ganglia help to coordinate complex motor behaviors by focusing attention on one motor pattern at a time while inhibiting all others, so that one main "set" of movement sequence can be performed smoothly without disruptive adventitious movements from other "sets."[25]

3. Once a movement pattern is begun by the motor and premotor cortex, the basal ganglia modulate different aspects of the movement pattern, such as the direction, velocity, and acceleration of motion, the force and amplitude of movements, and the frequency of self-paced alternating movements.

4. The mesolimbic dopamine system is thought to be responsible for the initiation of movements. Once the movement is initiated, this system also "energizes" and "facilitates" the motion.[11]

5. The mesolimbic system is also thought to provide an essential element for the performance of the large variety of semi-automatic actions that make up the full repertoire of natural human activity.

Basal Ganglia Syndromes

In general, human diseases of the basal ganglia are characterized pathologically not by total destruction of a nucleus but by a gradual or partial alteration in cell structure and function. It is the abnormal function of diseased neurons, such as overactivity, unbalanced activity, or underactivity, rather than the complete loss of neurons that is responsible for the unique signs of disease. This explains why experimentally placed destructive lesions of various nuclei do not produce malfunctions that mimic natural diseases.

Since the pallidum and SN are the major output nuclei, abnormal activities often result from loss of inhibitory or modulating inputs from their upstream nuclei, the striatum and subthalamic nucleus. Abnormal output from the pallidum predominantly affects limb movements, whereas abnormal output from the SN more likely affects orolingual and head movements. Also, the mesolimbic and nigrostriatal dopamine systems are independent of each other and individual malfunction leads to totally different symptoms.

Rigidity. The activity of the pallidum is normally harnassed by the subthalamic nucleus and the striatum through separate projections. Lesions in either of these nuclei or their outflow fibers release the pallidum and lead to distinguishable patterns of abnormal pallidal activity. Rigidity results from deranged and overactive outputs from the pallidum secondary to failure of striatal control. This in turn is most commonly caused by destruction of the nigrostrial dopamine fibers.[49] (The best example is parkinsonism with degeneration of the SN dopamine neuron.) Pallidal overactivity causes increased descending facilitatory influence to the α and γ_2 (tonic) motor neurons to both flexor and extensor muscles.[8] This produces sustained and rigid contractions of both agonist and antagonist so that the muscles are taut to palpation and the limbs are stiff to passive motions in all directions. Since the γ_1 (phasic) system is not involved, the deep tendon reflexes are not exaggerated.

In support of the hypothesis of pallidal overactivity, rigidity can be improved by stereotactic lesioning of the pallidum or the ventrolateral nucleus of the thalamus, the main output target of the pallidum.

Dyskinesias. The dyskinesias are a group of related involuntary movement disorders. Chorea refers to involuntary arrhythmic, forcible, rapid, and jerky movements of a limb or of the facial musculature. If the chorea is unusually violent and flinging in nature, it is called hemiballismus. Athetosis consists of slow, sinuous, purposeless movements that have a tendency to flow into one another. Dystonia is an exaggerated form of athetosis in which different body musculatures are asymmetrically contracting, resulting in peculiar contortions and deformities. Buccolingual dyskinesia is choreiform movements involving the tongue and facial muscles.

Dyskinesia may be an uncontrolled and exaggerated form of stereotypic behavior. The latter is seen in primitive form as the continuous sniffing, licking, or gnawing of rodents[15] and may be mediated by the pallidum.[16] Thus, dyskinesia, like rigidity, results from excessive pallidal outflows following release from normal inhibition exerted by the striatum or the subthalamic nucleus. If the striatal control is lost (as in caudate degeneration in Huntington's disease), the pallidal overactivity is manifested as chorea and athetosis. If the subthalamic nucleus–pallidum–subthalamic nucleus loop is interrupted by subthalamic necrosis, the pallidal overactivity results in hemiballismus. Both chorea and hemiballismus can be abolished by stereotactic lesioning of the pallidum.

Akinesia. Akinesia refers to the disinclination to engage an affected part in any of the natural activities of the body. The patient shows a severe poverty of movement; the frequent automatic habitual movements observed in the normal state, such as putting the hand to the face, folding the arms, or crossing the legs, are absent. The face lacks expressive motility. There is also great difficulty in initiating a movement: the patient takes a long time to get up from a chair.

Akinesia is not due to rigidity of muscles. Although both conditions may coexist, pallidal lesioning eliminates rigidity but not akinesia. In contrast to the rigidity that occurs with failure of the nigrostriatal dopamine system, akinesia is due to failure of the mesolimbic dopamine inputs into the nucleus accumbens, which is normally responsible for automatic behaviors and the initiation of movements.[31]

Resting Tremor. In monkeys, experimental lesions confined to the SN or to the striatopallidal connections do not cause tremor. Resting tremor can be produced only by a combined disturbance of the nigrostriatal dopamine pathways and the cerebellar–red nucleus–olive–cerebellar loop.[63] It appears that excessive pallidal activity requires coexisting alterations in the cerebellar influence on movements to cause rest tremor. This is not unreasonable, since outflows from both the pallidum and the dentate nucleus (from the cerebellum) converge on the VA and VL nuclei before ascending to the motor cortex. This combined disturbance permits a lower brain stem or thalamic center to oscillate, presumably involving the limb innervation via the reticulospinal pathway. This results in tremor. Clinically, interruption of the cerebellar contribution is usually due to lesions in the dentate nucleus, the red nucleus, or the branchium conjunctivum of the midbrain.

AFFECTIVE DISORDERS — THE LIMBIC SYSTEM

Affective disorders are common in head injury and are among the most difficult posttraumatic disorders to understand and to treat.

Pathogenetically, they are probably related to malfunction of the limbic system, but because of this system's diverse connections and the many unsettled controversies concerning its functional anatomy, the mechanisms proposed later in this chapter no more than hypotheses gleaned from a broad survey of the pioneering work of Papez,[60] Yakovlev,[97] MacLean,[46] and White.[93] Because of the extreme complexity of the structures involved in emotion, it will be helpful to outline the *functions* of the system before describing its anatomy.

The Physiology of Emotion

There are two components to emotion: the subjective and the objective. Put in a different way, a stimulus with emotional significance generates two different sets of responses: (1) the internal or subjective feeling related to the stimulus and known only to the organism (i.e., affects); and (2) the external response, or efferent behaviors related to the original stimulus or to the subjective response to the stimulus. These include visceral, humoral (neuroendocrine), and motor responses that can be measured objectively.

Subjective Feelings

1. Among the subjective affects, some are vital to the survival and procreational functions of the organism— that is, they are primitive affects that are phylogenetically old (Fig. 1-21). For example, the feelings of hunger and thirst and the complex but primal feeling known as the sex drive are both evoked in the lower mammals by olfactory stimuli. Subprimates, therefore, possess a well-developed rhinencephalon and related primitive structures, such as the medial septal area, the entorhinal cortex, the dorsomedial amygdala, and the pyriform lobe. In humans, the olfactory afferents and their extensive central connections are reduced, but the primitive rhinencephalon (composed of phylogenetically old cortex, allocortex) still retains these functions previously activated only by smell. This may explain the observation, relevant to rehabilitation efforts, that olfactory stimulation often increases motor responsiveness in head injured patients.

2. The feelings of fear, anxiety, and rage provoke protective behaviors of flight or fight and are therefore related to survival. These affects are probably integrated in the phylogenetically intermediate cortex or mesocortex, such as the subcallosal, cingulate, insular, and hippocampal gyri.

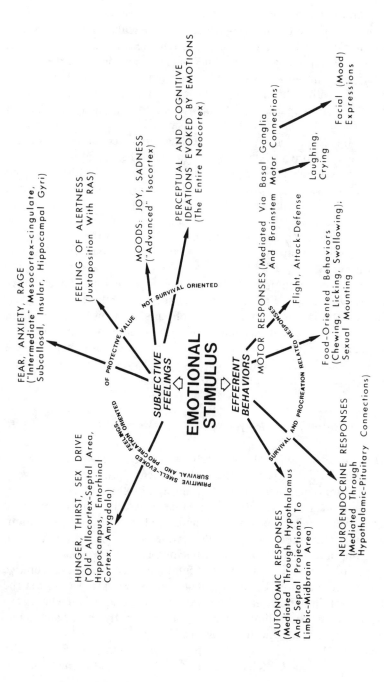

Figure 1–21. The two components of emotion: the subjective affects and efferent (objective) behaviors generated by an emotional stimulus.

3. Another "feeling" vital to survival is alertness. This is primarily the function of the brain stem–diencephalic reticular activating system (RAS), but deeper limbic structures, such as the fornix, the septal area, and posterior hypothalamus, have intimate connections with the ventral midbrain tegmentum known as Nauta's "limbic-midbrain area." This juxtaposition with the RAS explains the many clinical syndromes associated with limbic lesions characterized by psychomotor hypoactivity, the most extreme form of which is akinetic mutism.[44]

4. "Higher" and more complex feelings not essential to survival but descriptive of the private internal environment of the individual are known as moods; examples are joy and sadness and their infinite shades and variations. These feelings are integrated by the phylogenetically advanced cortex, the isocortex (neocortex): namely, the lateral temporal, frontal, and parietal cortices that are directly and indirectly connected to the mesocortex via the dorsomedial and anterior nuclei of the thalamus, the uncinate fasciculus, and the posterior portion of the superior and middle temporal gyri.

5. Even more complex than moods are perceptual and cognitive ideations evoked by the primitive affects and the subtler feelings. These are important in the formation of concepts, judgment, motivation, prediction, and anticipation compatible with the emotional experience of the original stimulus. The entire neocortex probably takes part in these activities, and malfunction is characterized by perceptual distortion, illusion, delusion, and hallucination.

Efferent Behavioral Patterns

Emotional stimuli evoke three groups of efferent behaviors mediated through the major outputs of the limbic system. In order of phylogeny they are autonomic, neuroendocrine, and motor (Fig. 1–21).

Autonomic responses to a stimulus that elicits fright, anger, or sexual desire are very similar, consisting of increased heart rate and respiration, pupillary dilatation, perspiration, piloerection, salivation, shiver reaction, and lacrimation. The increase in cardiac output and oxygenation primes the organism for fight, hunting, or mounting behaviors. These primitive responses are mediated by hypothalamic and septal projections via the medial forebrain bundle, mamillotegmental tract, and stria medullaris to the midbrain–tegmental limbic area, which in turn activates the autonomic centers of the brain stem and spinal cord.

Neuroendocrine (humoral) responses important to survival and procreational functions include increased output of antidiuretic hormone, corticosteroids, epinephrine, growth hormone, and thyroid hormone. The elevated blood sugar levels, plasma volume, blood pressure, and basal metabolic rate prepare the organism for hunting, fighting, fleeing, or mounting. These primitive responses are mediated through hypothalamic control of the pituitary gland (see pages 59 to 66).

Motor responses to emotions can be primitive or sophisticated. The most primitive are the instinctive behaviors concerned with eating (such as food-oriented behaviors of oral grasping, chewing, lip smacking, swallowing, and pouting) and procreation (sexual mounting). Equally important for survival are flight and attack-defense behaviors, which utilize axial and appendicular musculature. These are present in all mammals and can be elicited by medial temporal lobe stimulation; and they also occur as automatism in temporal lobe seizures. Phylogenetically more recent motor responses are those expressing moods (e.g., smiling, laughing, crying, and facial expression). These more sophisticated motor patterns, present only in humans and perhaps some primates (a dog does not smile or cry), are mediated through limbic connections with the basal ganglia and their descending projections to the brain stem and spinal motor neurons. More primitive activities such as chewing and swallowing may be integrated directly in the brain stem.

The Anatomy of Emotion

The anatomy of emotion conforms roughly to the phylogeny of the physiologic responses already listed. The complex structures of the limbic system can readily be divided into two mutually interconnected concentric rings, each encircling the diencephalon and the midbrain. The *inner limbic ring* consists of the hippocampus, fornix, septal area, diagonal band of Broca, dorsomedial amygdala, and stria terminalis. Its relationship with the brain stem and hypothalamus allows direct autonomic and neuroendocrine effector action via the efferent projection system, which comprises the fornix, medial forebrain bundle, and stria medullaris. Because the inner ring is the most primitive limbic structure, its cortical structure is the phylogenetically old allocortex. It is likely that the inner limbic ring is responsible mainly for the outward expression of emotion vital to survival and procreation, such as the endocrine and visceral changes associated with hunger, fear, and sex and the primitive motor patterns of chewing, licking, and swallowing.

The *outer limbic ring* is made up of the subcallosal, cingulate, and hippocampal gyri, the uncus, the insula, the association bundles of uncinate and cingulum fasciculi, and projection pathways with the anterior and dorsomedial thalamic nuclei. Because the outer ring is organizationally more advanced than the inner ring, its cortical structure is the phylogenetically intermediate mesocortex. It is probably responsible for the subjective feelings of fear, rage, hunger, and sex. These affects are important for survival and require no memory or judgment, although there is obviously restraint from higher cortical centers (from the extralimbic cortex). The outer ring also has descending connections with the extrapyramidal motor system. Through interactions with the striatum, pallidum, substantia nigra, ventral thalamic nuclei, and the cerebellorubroreticularis circuits, the motor patterns of flight, attack, mounting, gesticulation, facial expression, laughing, and crying are integrated.

The *extralimbic cortex* consists of the lateral hemispheres, in which the cortex is fully differentiated isocortex and is related to receptive and associative function. Strictly speaking, this is not part of the limbic system, but through connections with the outer ring it monitors the finer shades of mood and integrates incoming stimuli with past memories to formulate higher cognitive-affective activity, such as judgment, morality, motivation, prediction, and anticipation. However, the most important function of the extralimbic cortex is to exert volitional control over the primal and instinctive behaviors mediated by the outer and inner rings. Thus, satisfaction of sexual urges may be curtailed or postponed for reasons of moral propriety; excessive indulgence in food intake may be restrained by vanity (dieting); and aggression may be sublimated for fear of legal retribution. The most common affects of sadness and happiness depend on a proper balance of drives and satisfaction of such drives. Ultimately, the organism achieves ''emotional maturity'' when its extralimbic cortex, through thought, judgment, memory, and intellect, modifies behaviors related to sex, hunger, anger, and fright to suitable levels compatible with social graces, ethics, and ethnicity.

Disorders of Emotion

In general, disturbances of emotion can be viewed as release of the activity of the phylogenetically oldest and most primitive inner limbic ring from the phylogenetically intermediate and more advanced outer ring due to lesions of the latter, or release of the outer ring from extralimbic control due to neocortical lesions. In both cases, the more primal being is revealed and behaviors contrary to societal norms emerge, to be interpreted as abnormal.

Aggressive Behaviors — Pathologic Rage

Aggressive behavior in animals is biologically important in securing food and repelling sexual rivals. In humans, it has a sublimated but equally important survival role. Pathologic rage is differentiated from aggressive behavior by the following: it is elicited by nonspecific stimuli; it is of excessive proportions; and its course is both aimless and cannot be interrupted. Pathologic rage is best known as a component of temporal lobe seizures, but in certain cases of damage to the temporal lobe and septal nuclei, increased emotional excitability gradually builds up to severe rage attacks and paranoid ideas without other aspects of seizures.[62] In rare cases, human rage may be so acute, elementary, and stereotyped in its course and brought about by such nonspecific stimuli that it seems to resemble the "sham rage" of experimental animals.

Electrical stimulation of the ventromedial nucleus of the simian hypothalamus provokes rage ("sham rage"), whereas stimulation of the rostral and caudal hypothalamus provokes flight and attack-defense behaviors, respectively. In humans, mild electrical stimulation of the medial hypothalamus gives rise to feelings of restlessness, anxiety, fright, terror, and extreme anger. Similar stimulation experiments show that the dorsomedial nucleus of the amygdala (in the medial temporal lobe) inhibits the ventromedial hypothalamic "rage center" whereas the ventrolateral amygdaloid nucleus facilitates rage reactions.[7] Thus, the defense reaction akin to aggressive behaviors is a survival-oriented primitive emotion functionally organized within the hypothalamus, but is normally harnessed by descending inhibition by the amygdala. Pathologic rage can then be looked upon as release of the "rage center" from inhibition by the amygdala. This explains the rage attacks seen in medial temporal lobe seizures and in medial temporal necrosis in rabies. Temporal lobe contusion being such a common traumatic lesion, it is understandable that agitated and combative behaviors are commonly observed following head injury. Indeed, it is surprising that true rage reactions are not seen more often.

Placidity–Abulia

On occasion, the posttraumatic patient may become indifferent toward his or her environment. Affective reactions level out, facial expression decreases, speech becomes monotonous, and the patient may seem dull and apathetic. Placidity is not the psychopathologic mirror image of rage. In the latter, the loss of inhibition pertains only to aggressive behaviors, not to other affective reactions, such as joy or anxiety. In placidity, however, there is a decrease or loss not only of aggressive behaviors but also of affective responses in general.[62]

Since placidity cannot be biologically advantageous, it is not likely to be a result of simple release phenomenon. It probably results from removal of an "energizing center" that normally sets the level of affect. This is not inconceivable if one recalls the intimate anatomic relationship between the limbic system and the RAS.[44] Pathologic studies revealed that placidity is associated with lesions in widely separated areas of the brain. For example, it commonly occurs after bilateral temporal lobectomy. In addition, bilateral lesions in the anterior cingulate gyrus or interruptions of anterior cingulate projections to the prefrontal lobes (frontal leukotomy) can decrease drive and affective reactions to the point of akinetic mutism.[27,91] Moreover, it has recently been shown that deep anterior forebrain nuclei (nucleus basalis of Meynert, nucleus of the diagonal band of Broca) have widespread projections to the entire cerebral cortex[26] and that destruction of these nuclei can lead to a syndrome consisting of decreases in impulsivity, initiative, and general drive (abulia). It must be emphasized that the relationship between lesions and symptoms is by no means strict. The individual emotional makeup of the patient prior to injury, etiology, and the presence or absence of additional diffuse brain damage all influence the clinical picture.

Anxiety and Depression

Anxiety and depression following head injury are usually due to psychological reaction to the stress and disability incurred by the injury rather than to organic lesions. When they are related to organic pathology, anxiety and fear usually occur in the context of temporal lobe epilepsy. The patient often experiences "unnatural" anxiety of a quality not familiar to him or her. The anxiety is often nonspecific, and it is accompanied by unpleasant visceral sensations. A state of sadness very rarely can be an epileptic phenomenon. Severe depression has also been seen with tumors in the temporal lobe, septal region, and the anteromedial thalamus.[62] Although pleasure sensation, a feeling of happiness or elation, has been described in medial temporal lesions, more unpleasant feelings usually predominate. This is probably related to the accompanying disturbances in visceral sensations and autonomic activity, which are generally experienced as unpleasant.

These observations show that limbic lesions do not always uncover extreme behaviors from the primal brain, such as rage and mutism. Loss of a coherent balance between primal emotions and rational thought can also lead to more subtle alterations of mood and affective reaction patterns. Thus, depression may be considered as "normal sadness" gone unchecked, and mania and euphoria as "normal joy" released from the restraints of reality.

The Klüver–Bucy Syndrome

In humans, bilateral resection of the temporal lobe results in a dramatic syndrome characterized by the following features[62]:

Increased Oral Tendency. The patient grasps and puts into his or her mouth all types of objects, including inedible and dangerous items. This behavior is likened to the stage of development when the human infant automatically puts objects into his or her mouth. Thus, it can be interpreted as a release of the primitive and instinctive food-finding practice, a sort of oral grasping, that is normally coordinated by the limbic system.

Placidity. See discussion earlier in this chapter.

Abnormal Sexual Behaviors. Abnormal behaviors may be manifested as uninhibited conversation concerning sexual topics, verbal and physical sexual advances toward the nurse, increased masturbation, increased libido, and even homosexual choice of partners.

Severe Disturbance of Memory. See subsection on memory disorders later in this chapter.

Hypermetamorphosis. The patient can easily be distracted by any type of external stimulus, especially visual (extremely common following head injury).

Visual Agnosia. The patient has difficulty interpreting the meanings of visual inputs.

The most consistent lesion causing this syndrome involves the phylogenetically old medial temporal lobe (including hippocampus and amygdala) on both sides. It can be easily imagined that interruption of outer limbic ring control over the inner (more primal) ring will lead to release of primitive survival (oral grasping, docility) and procreational (hypersexuality) functions.

Pathologic Laughing and Crying

In the disorder termed pathologic laughing and crying, the patient goes into sudden uncontrollable laughing or crying, sometimes beginning with one and then merging into the other. The facial expressions are inappropriate to the situation and are unprovoked. The motor pattern is monotonous and stereotypic, and its onset is paroxysmal rather than gradual.

These pathologic facial expressions do not correspond to an analogous emotional change. Thus, this is not so much a disorder of affect as a disorder of the motor concomitants of affective expression. Wilson[95] postulated that a pontobulbar faciorespiratory center integrates the necessary musculature for both crying and laughing. This center is in turn under the control of two separate supranuclear pathways: one, from the motor cortex, deals with voluntary facial movements; and the other, from the limbic system, deals with involuntary facial expressions such that crying and laughing can be appropriately coupled with the correct emotions. These two pathways can be damaged separately. If only the voluntary pathway is lost, laughing and smiling can occur normally even though the patient may have no voluntary facial movements. If the involuntary pathway is damaged selectively, voluntary facial movements are retained, but the patient no longer shows the subconscious grimaces and the innumerable patterns of facial expressions reflecting internal mood changes. The unbridled laughing and crying centers now appear overactive and the patient bursts out laughing or crying without the appropriate underlying mood. Pathologic laughter and crying can therefore be looked upon as a release phenomenon when the higher limbic emotions are uncoupled from the effector that mediates the motor concomitants of these emotions. Indeed, the most frequently found lesions are located bilaterally in the internal capsule, thalamus, and the basal ganglia, where the involuntary pathway passes through.

Recent evidence reveals that the laughing and crying centers are not in the same location in the brain stem.[62] Ontogenetically, facial expressions of displeasure, a need for help, and defense are apparently of greater importance to survival and thus may be elaborated at a lower and more early maturing level of the brain stem. The movements of smiling and laughing, which have primarily social significance, probably mature later at a higher level of the brain stem.

MEMORY DEFICITS

Memory deficits are probably the most common cognitive disorders following head injury. The mechanism of memory is far from clear. Most current hypotheses are derived from the study of lesioned animals and from charting human behaviors following specific diseases. It is well known that extensive ablation of the neocortex neither causes learning disability nor erases well-established memory. However, disturbance of new learning can be produced by certain discrete lesions. In this method of study, the search is not for the site in the brain where learning and memory take place or for the location of memory traces (engrams). Instead the investigator is tracking the anatomy of memory disorders, not that of memory. Tracking memory itself would require some method of recognizing what memory "looks like." Although the identification of certain brain lesions correlates fairly well with a number of consistent amnestic patterns, the complete inability to recognize the structural image of memory makes any hypothesis of memory mechanism no more than bold conjectures attempting to bridge the immeasurable gulf between pathology and physiology.

Lesions of Amnestic Syndromes

Hippocampus and Hippocampal Gyrus

Some of the very first descriptions of memory deficits came from observations following bilateral infarction or resection of the medial temporal lobe.[73] Subsequent ablation studies on animals revealed that the key structures within the medial temporal lobe responsible for the memory disturbance were the hippocampus and hippocampal gyrus. The most prominent feature of the memory deficits is a complete and permanent loss of the ability to recall numbers, events, and names several minutes after learning them, although immediate recall is possible. This means that new information, although correctly perceived, cannot be stored beyond immediate use unless the hippocampi are intact. There is always an associated retrograde amnesia of variable duration, which implies an obligatory erasure of memory engrams that had been recently stored. This raises the question whether the medial temporal lobe is also involved with the stabilization of recently stored engrams before they become permanently filed. Long-term (remote) memories are not disturbed following these lesions. In summary, these findings suggest that the medial temporal lobe is involved in learning new information and in stabilizing recently acquired memory, but not in storing or retrieving old memory.

Fornix

Whether bilateral destruction of the fornices will produce permanent memory deficits remains unsettled. Some writers claimed no memory problems,[2,14,21] whereas others found marked changes in recent memory.[85] Since the fornices are the major efferent tracts of the hippocampi, their bilateral interruption must compromise recent memory function to some extent. This learning disability is, however, transient and can be offset by concentrated efforts and by association maneuvers, suggesting that the other hippocampal efferents can compensate for the loss of the fornices.

Dorsomedial Nucleus of the Thalamus — Korsakoff Syndrome

In 1887, Korsakoff described a syndrome commonly seen in chronic alcoholics characterized by, among other features, profound deficits in recent memory very similar to those seen with bilateral hippocampal lesions. In an extensive autopsy study of this syndrome, Victor and Adams[90] concluded that the most consistent lesions in patients with Korsakoff syndrome are found not in the hippocampus but in the dorsomedial thalamic nuclei (DMN). This suggests that the hippocampus and the DMN are part of one functional circuit that is involved in embedding new information. The DMN has reciprocal connections with the prefrontal, frontal, cingulate, and parietal cortices; with the basal ganglia, where information regarding body movements is integrated; with the hippocampus, amygdala, and septal area of the limbic (emotion) system; with the hypothalamus, where visceral inputs converge; and with the intralaminar and other nonspecific thalamic nuclei, where exteroceptive sensory inputs converge. These extensive connections make the DMN an ideal clearinghouse for new information processed by the hippocampus before "delocalizing" it to widespread areas of the cortex.

How Does the Hippocampus–Dorsomedial Nucleus Circuit Subserve Memory Functions?

The hippocampus–dorsomedial nucleus circuit probably performs two memory functions:

1. It selects from the myriad of sensory inputs bombarding the nervous system useful information to be stored as short-term memory engrams. These short-term engrams are then ready to be processed and filed as permanent (long-term) memory engrams. Hippocampal damage therefore prevents incorporation of new information into short-term (and subsequently permanent) memory traces.

2. This circuit also maintains constant access to and temporary control over the recently acquired short-term engrams. It appears that these recently acquired engrams need to be "stamped-in" by the hippocampus–DMN circuit over a variable period of time before they can become stored as permanent engrams. Thus, damage to this circuit would result in extinction of those engrams that have not completed their "stamp-in" process because they were the most recent engrams acquired shortly before the brain lesion. This would explain the variable period of retrograde amnesia present in all patients with Korsakoff syndrome. Once permanent engrams are stored, they are beyond control by this circuit, and bilateral hippocampal–DMN destruction does not disturb old memory.

How does this circuit perform the selection and "stamping-in" functions?

The hippocampus and DMN are major components of the limbic system and have long been implicated as the anatomic substratum for emotions.[46,60,97] It would seem logical that the same structures subserve both memory and emotion functions if it is assumed that the strength of a particular memory trace depends on the emotional significance of the information for the organism.[71] It is therefore possible that the hippocampus–DMN circuit normally assigns each incoming input a relative emotional weight so as to signal to the organism some measure of the importance of the data. This weighting function is obtained by coupling the input to immediately preceding events and to remote emotional associations. Comparison of the input with the moment-to-moment status of the organism's exteroceptive and interoceptive worlds is made possible through connections with olfactory, auditory, visual, and somatosensory substations and with the hypothalamic-septal visceral sensory areas. Comparison with past emotional experiences is by way of the extensive connection of the DMN with the neocortex. A low weight given to emotionally neutral data may serve to keep such material only within very short-term memory. For example, a pseudorandom list of numbers (e.g., a telephone number) is held in temporary memory only until the completion of an immediate task (dialing) and then discharged. Vivid events vital to survival (such as those associated with fright or anger) are given heavy emotional weight and are strongly embedded as short-term engrams, quickly "stamped," and permanently stored as long-term memory. Thus, emotional experiences heavily influence the embedding of memory engrams.

A similar interaction between memory and emotional circuits may explain how memory can affect emotional responses to incoming stimuli. A normally innocuous input, such as the screeching sound of a braking car, will ordinarily not be given much emotional significance. However, for a trauma victim, this otherwise neutral random input may trigger highly poignant memory engrams of the recent accident and will generate strong emotional responses.

Once short-term engrams are properly stamped, they are ready to be filed as long-term memory. The transitional process between short- and long-term memories remains a mystery. Whatever the hypothesis, it must explain the extraordinary resistance of long-term memory against permanent erasure by even the most extensive destruction of the cortex. Its retrieval is also independent of the hippocampus–DMN circuit because patients with bilateral medial temporal lobe contusion have no problems with remote memory. This must mean that long-term engrams do not "reside" in fixed sites but are somehow scattered, or "delocalized," to widespread areas of the cortex once sanctioned by the hippocampus–DMN unit. But how are long-term engrams delocalized and where are they stored?

The Hologram Theory of Memory Delocalization

Pribram[67] postulates that memory storage utilizes the principle of the hologram. In a hologram the information in a scene is recorded on a photographic plate in the form of a complex interference pattern that appears meaningless. When the pattern is illuminated by coherent light, however, the original image is reconstructed. What makes the hologram unique as a storage device is that every element in the original image is distributed over the entire photographic plate. This hypothesis is attractive because remembering literally implies a reconstructive process—the assembly of dismembered mnemonic events. The neutral events producing the interference pattern necessary to create the "memory hologram" are set up by complex interacting wave fronts of impulses generated by the original input. The electrical events of these mutually interfering wave fronts somehow produce lasting effects on protein molecules and perhaps other macromolecules at the synaptic junctions and can serve as a neural hologram from which, given the appropriate input, an image can be reconstructed. The attractive feature of this hypothesis is that the information is distributed throughout the stored hologram (cortex) and thus is resistant to insult. Moreover, if even a small corner of a hologram is illuminated by the appropriate input (e.g., a related object or fragments of a familiar scene), the entire original scene reappears.

Given the fact that mnemonic events become distributed in the brain, some organizing process analogous to the triggering coherent beam in the hologram must be required for remembering. The anatomic substrate for this function is not known, but it does not appear to involve the hippocampus–DMN since long-term memory is intact in their absence.

HYPOTHALAMIC-HYPOPHYSEAL INJURIES

Anatomy and Physiology

The hypothlamus has a functional importance quite out of proportion to its size. Its two sides bound the lower portion of the third ventricle and occupy the interval between the thalami above and the subthalamus and midbrain below. The optic chiasm attaches to its anteroinferior corner, and behind the chiasm, the lowest portion of the hypothalamus, the median eminence, narrows to an infundibular process (pituitary stalk), which goes through a shelf of dura called the diaphragm sella to enter the pituitary fossa. Here the infundibular process expands into the neurohypophysis (posterior pituitary lobe), which is embryologically fused with the anterior pituitary lobe derived from the mucosa of the oral pharynx.

The hypothalamus receives inputs from four major sources. Visceral sensory inputs carry pain and other sensations from the gut and bladder. These inputs, together with data concerning blood osmolarity, temperature, glucose content, and hormone levels, apprise the hypothalamus of the internal environment of the body. At the same time, pain and temperature sensations from the paleospinothalamic pathways supply information from the external environment. Both the internal and external sensory information is then integrated with past emotional experiences coming through connections with the limbic system.

Thus informed, the hypothalamus can now respond to metabolic, sexual, nutritional, and emotional needs through its various output systems. Blood osmolarity, glucose content, and hormonal levels are finely adjusted to achieve internal homeostasis through neuroendocrinologic connections with the pituitary gland. Blood temperature and pressure and other vegetative functions, gastrointestinal secretory and motility states, and emotional reactions can be adjusted and affected through projections to the brain stem and spinal autonomic centers, as well as through outputs to the skeletal motor nuclei involved in eating, drinking, and running-hunting behavioral patterns. Also, through projections back to the limbic system, visceral sensations (such as nausea, hunger, thirst, and sexual feelings), somatic sensations (such as pain, cold, and extreme heat), and blood chemistry (such as blood sugar and steroid contents) will all be woven into the complex fabric of emotion. Finally, through projections to the frontal and prefrontal cortex via the medial thalamic nuclei, the experiences of fear and anger, sexual and hunger drives, and fatigue will be added to the higher cerebral machinery that generates judgment, inhibition, anticipation, frustration, and other subtle mood changes.

Mechanisms of Hypothalamus-Pituitary Injury

Hypothalamic-hypophyseal injuries are uncommon but important complications of head injury. Mechanical shearing is the major culprit, commonly causing petechial hemorrhages in the periventricular zone and subsequent cell loss and focal degeneration. The supraoptic nucleus (located just above the chiasm) is particularly vulnerable because the optic nerves are tethered rostrally at the optic foramen by the investing dural sleeves, and any rotational shearing motion of the brain will cause tearing where the optic chiasm is attached to the brain (i.e., at the supraoptic nuclei) (Fig. 1–22).[87] A similar mechanism explains how the infundibular stalk can be sheared from its lower fixation point where it penetrates the diaphragma if the brain above shows rotatory movement (Fig. 1–22).[10]

Hypothalamic disorders can also be due to vascular insufficiency. Infarction can result from shearing disruption of arterial feeders from the anterior communicating and superior hypophyseal arteries or from posttraumatic vasospasm induced by subarachnoid blood. Rarely, severe hypovolemic shock may cause total pituitary infarction by inducing relative ischemia in a highly active gland with heavy metabolic demand.[10] Finally, extensive basal fractures with in-driven fragments through the sella floor occasionally injure the pituitary gland.

Hypothalamic-Pituitary Syndromes

Syndrome of Inappropriate Secretion of Antidiuretic Hormone (SIADH)

The syndrome of inappropriate secretion of antidiuretic hormone is by far the most common posttraumatic hypothalamic disorder. Normally, serum osmolarity and electrolyte concentrations are adjusted through antidiuretic hormone (ADH) manufactured within the supraoptic (SON) and paraventricular nuclei (PVN) of the hypothalamus. ADH binds to the contraluminal side of the renal collecting tubule cells, induces phosphorylation of the luminal membrane protein, and causes increased permeability to water, which is quickly reabsorbed from the tubular

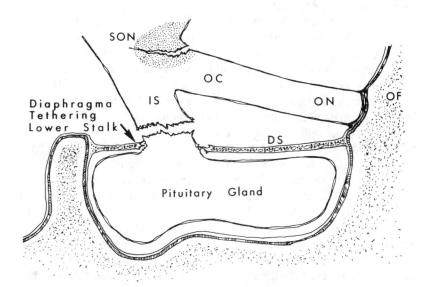

Figure 1-22. Injury to the supraoptic nucleus (*SON*) due to rotational shearing occurring at the attachment of the anterior hypothalamus to the optic chiasm (*OC*) when both optic nerves (*ON*) are fixed to the investing dura at the optic foramina (*OF*). Shearing transection of the infundibular stalk (*IS*) likewise occurs when the stalk is tethered at the point where it penetrates the diaphragma sella (*DS*).

filtrate. Physiologic output of ADH is controlled by plasma osmolarity and volume through a feedback servomechanism. High blood osmolarity and low volume augment ADH secretion to increase water reabsorption in the renal tubules, and hyposmolarity and hypervolemia shut off ADH to allow excretion of free water. Nonspecific hypothalamic shearing or vascular injuries, pulmonary sepsis, and prolonged positive pressure ventilation can upset this physiologic control mechanism and cause inappropriate secretion of ADH in the face of hyposmolarity and a high plasma volume. This is manifested as hyponatremia, reduced urine output, and signs of water intoxication. Mild to moderate degrees of SIADH may respond to simple fluid restriction, but seizures or cardiac arrhythmia requires 3 per cent hypertonic saline and diuretics to restore normal serum sodium concentration and facilitate excretion of free water.

Diabetes Insipidus

ADH normally is produced by modified neurosecretory neurons of the SON and PVN and is transported as secretion granules along with axoplasmic flow within axons that extend from the median eminence to the neurohypophysis. Within the neurohypophysis, the axon terminals form intimate contacts with capillary units. Impulses generated within the soma of these neurons liberate ADH into the capillary blood traversing the neurohypophysis. The SON and PVN are therefore the factory, and the neurohypophysis is merely a temporary storage site, for ADH.

Traumatic diabetes insipidus (DI) is rarely seen except with very severe injuries. Permanent DI is due to destruction of the SON and PVN.[87] More commonly, posttraumatic DI is transient and is due to transection of the infundibular stalk. The abrupt cessation of ADH supply from disconnection of the SON and PVN axons leads to immediate diuresis. However, since the neuronal bodies of the SON and PVN are spared, regeneration of their axons frequently reestablishes new contact units with capillaries supplying the basal hypothalamus.[3] Thus, ADH granules once again find their way to the blood stream, and DI spontaneously abates. Severe DI and intractable hypernatremia in a deeply comatose patient with high ICP usually means complete hypothalamic necrosis secondary to caudal herniation of the diencephalon into the tight incisural ring. This usually signals a fatal outcome.

Hypopituitarism

Hypopituitarism is an exceedingly rare occurrence following trauma. The hypothalamus controls anterior pituitary secretions through releasing factors transported down to the adenohypophysis via long portal vessels serving as vascular conduits from the median eminence to the adenohypophysis. These long portal vessels lie on the surface of the infundibular stalk and are also the sole blood supply to most of the adenohypophysis.[10] A low stalk transection eliminates this vascular supply and leads to massive infarction of the adenohypophysis and permanent panhypopituitarism. A high stalk section spares these vessels, and although partial hypopituitarism may result from loss of the conduits for the releasing factors, physiologic rejoining of the stalk and establishment of new conduits will improve the hyposecretory state (Fig. 1–23).[10]

Disorders of Thermal Regulation

Neuronal sensors of heat change are located in the anterior hypothalamus. Heat-sensitive receptors are norepinephrinergic and cold-sensitive receptors are serotoninergic. These sensors activate heat

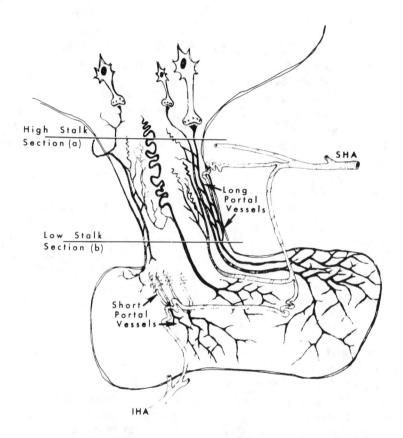

Figure 1-23. Infundibular stalk transections. A high transection (a) spares the long portal vessels and the blood supply to the adenohypophysis but destroys the axon-capillary units through which releasing factors are transported to the adenohypophysis via the long portal vascular conduits. A low transection (b) severs the long portal vessels and the blood supply to the adenohypophysis, causing anterior pituitary infarction and permanent panhypopituitarism. *SHA* = Superior hypophyseal artery; *IHA* = inferior hypophyseal artery.

production or heat loss effector mechanisms in the posterior hypothalamus to cause either heat production through shivering, metabolic increase, or vasoconstriction or heat loss through vasodilatation and sweating. Appropriate response is set by a separate thermostat coordinating the sensor and effector units through linking negative feedback loops.[9]

Hyperthermia occasionally follows lesions of the anterior hypothalamus. The heat sensor unit appears to be more vulnerable than cold sensors to trauma and other insults, and unbalanced heat production results. Alternatively, the feedback loop may be interrupted from a lesion intermediate between the anterior sensors and the posterior effectors, so that the effector mechanisms are not properly controlled. Posttraumatic hyperthermia is usually transient and spontaneously subsides in 2 to 3 weeks. It is important to distinguish "central" hyperthermia (resulting from hypothalamic damage) from "normal" fever of infectious origin since infections are common in the severely traumatized patient. Infection releases pyrogens from the bacterial cell wall and leukocytes, which in turn mediate fever through prostaglandins. Aspirin inhibits prostaglandin synthesis and is effective for infective fever, but since prostaglandins are not involved in fever from hypothalamic lesions, aspirin is ineffective in central hyperthermia.[89]

A more common disorder than hyperthermia is poikilothermia. Patients with poikilothermia adjust poorly to changes in ambient temperatures and have difficulty maintaining body temperature, which rises and falls with the environment. Whether this is due to loss of the integrating thermostat mechanism or to destruction of effectors is unclear. Thermal discomfort, which is an integrated autonomic response also mediated by the hypothalamus, disappears as well.[6]

Generalized Dysautonomia

In the occasional patient with severe hypothalamic injury, spikes of high fever are only a component part of a generalized autonomic mass reaction consisting of shivering, diaphoresis, piloerection, flushing, tachycardia, and hypertension. These mass responses may be precipitated by a full bladder or by gastric distention. They probably represent uncoordinated and indiscriminate discharges from autonomic centers. If the patient survives, hypertension may persist for months and will require medication.

Another abnormal hypothalamic response results from nonspecific biasing of the descending central autonomic pathways.[76] Increased parasympathetic discharge to the vagus may increase the volume, acidity, and pepsin content of gastric juices enough to cause gastric erosion and ulcers (neurogenic ulcers). This often causes fatal hemorrhages and emphasizes the need for vigorous antacid therapy in head injury patients.

Disturbance of Caloric Balance

A small group of neurons in the periventricular zone above the median eminence, the ventromedial nucleus (VMN), acts as a "satiety center" concerned in the set point regulation for caloric intake. This satiety center is counterbalanced by a "feeding center" in the lateral hypothalamic area, which causes eating on stimulation. Fiber tracts linking these two centers project to the basal ganglia and brain stem motor nuclei, which in turn coordinate the complex motor patterns involved in masticating, swallowing, chewing, and hunting. In addition, glucoreceptors have been found within the lateral hypothalamus that influence caloric activity and growth hormone release, such that hypoglycemia can initiate the sensation of hunger, food finding behaviors, eating, and appropriate endocrine changes.

Bilateral lesions of the VMN cause hyperphagia, gross obesity, sustained hyperglycemia, and aggressive behavior.[9] Lesions in the tuberal region involving the feeding center result in anorexia and weight loss. These are rare syndromes encountered in children and adults with severe hypothalamic trauma. In marked contrast are the infants or young children with an anterior hypothalamic tumor who become emaciated despite normal eating behaviors.[70] Endocrine studies in these infants have been remarkably normal. It is not understood why the immature hypothalamus of infants and younger children responds in a different fashion than that of adults with similar lesions.

Drinking behaviors also appear to be coordinated through a "drinking center" in the lateral hypothalamus. There are complex interactions among thirst, drinking behavior, blood pressure control, and ADH release mechanisms. Moreover, both the feeding and drinking centers are strongly influenced by limbic and telencephalic inputs, so that eating, drinking, and other oral behaviors are very much subject to the melange of psychoaffective tones of ordinary living. This is illustrated by the extreme cases of the hyperphagic and obese, depressive patient with poor self-image and the hyperactive, passive-aggressive patient with anorexia nervosa. The posttraumatic patient with his or her heavy burden of psychosocial maladjustment and physical disability may easily display disturbances in feeding behavior and caloric imbalance without true hypothalamic injury.

Disturbance of Sleep

Wakefulness depends upon a functionally intact brain stem reticular activating system. Normal waking behavior is, however, heavily modified by an anterior hypothalamic "sleep center," which appears to function by inhibiting the reticular formation, thereby inducing electroencephalographic synchronization and producing the behavioral phenomenon characteristic of sleep.[56] Destruction of this area leads to insomnia. The posterior hypothalamus contains the most rostral component of the diencephalic–brain stem reticular activating system, and a large lesion here will induce hypersomnia.

Changes in Affective Behavior

The general affective functions of the hypothalamus have been discussed earlier in the context of limbic system disorders. Specific lesions confined to the hypothalamus can profoundly alter affective behaviors. Sham rage in animals has been produced by posterior hypothalamic stimulation.[4] Stimulation of the medial posterior hypothalamus or the lateral posterior hypothalamus in humans elicits fear and horror responses.[72] These findings suggest that the motor and autonomic effector systems for pseudoaffective rage behavior lie in the posterior hypothalamus. Lesions in these areas result in apathy and inactivity. This posterior effector locus appears to be normally inhibited by telencephalic (forebrain) pathways, which exert indirect control through the VMN. Lesions in the VMN therefore release the rage effectors and produce aggressive behaviors as well as hyperphagia. Interestingly, destruction of the anterior hypothalamus by tumor in infants under the age of 2 years results in inappropriately cheerful behavior, as in the diencephalic emaciation syndrome of infancy.[70] The cheerful behavior is usually associated with hyperactivity and often evolves into a more aggressive behavior pattern as the child advances in age.[20]

REFERENCES

1. Adams JH: The neuropathology of head injury. In Vinken PJ, Bruyn GW (Eds), Handbook of Clinical Neurology. Vol. 23, Injuries of the Brain and Skull, (Part I) Amsterdam, North-Holland Publishing Company, 1975, pp. 35–65.
2. Akelaitis AJ: Studies on the corpus callosum. VII. Study of language functions (tactile and visual lexia and graphia) unilaterally following section of the corpus callosum. J Neuropathol Exp Neurol 2:226–262, 1943.
3. Antunes JL, Carmel PW, Zimmerman EA, Ferin M: Regeneration of the magnocellular system of the rhesus monkey following hypothalamic lesions. Ann Neurol 5:462–469, 1972.
4. Bard PA: Diencephalic mechanism for the expression of rage with special reference to the sympathetic nervous system. Am J Physiol 84:490–515, 1928.
5. Bourke RS, Kimelberg HK, Daze MA, Popp AJ: Studies on the formation of astroglial swelling and its inhibition by clinically useful agents. In Popp AJ, Bourke RS, Nelson LR, Kimelberg HK (Eds), Neural Trauma. New York, Raven Press, 1979, pp 95–113.
6. Branch EF, Burger PC, Brewer DL: Hypothermia in a case of hypothalamic infarction and sarcoidosis. Arch Neurol 25:245–255, 1971.

7. Breathnach CS: The limbic system. J Irish Med Assoc *73*(9):331–339, 1980.
8. Burke DE, Hagbarth E, Wallin BG: Reflex mechanisms in Parkinsonian rigidity. Scand J Rehabil Med *9*:15–23, 1977.
9. Carmel PW: Surgical syndromes of the hypothalamus. Clin Neurosurg *22*:133–159, 1979.
10. Daniel PM, Treip CS: Lesions of the pituitary gland associated with head injuries. In Harris GW, Donovan BT (Eds), The Pituitary Gland. London, Butterworth, 1966, Vol 2, pp 519–534.
11. Delong MR, Georgopoulos AP: Motor functions of the basal ganglia. In Brookhart JM, Mountcastle VB (Eds), Handbook of Physiology. Section I. Nervous System. Bethesda, MD, American Physiologic Society, 1981, pp 1017–1061.
12. Denny-Brown DE, Russell WR: Experimental cerebral concussion. Brain *64*:93–164, 1941.
13. Diaz FG, Yock DH Jr, Larson D, Rockswold GL: Early diagnosis of delayed post-traumatic intracerebral hematomas. J. Neurosurg *50*:217–223, 1979.
14. Dott NM: Surgical aspects of the hypothalamus. In Clark WE, Legros A, Beattie J, Riddoch G, Dott NM (Eds), The Hypothalamus: Morphological, Functional, Clinical and Surgical Aspects. Edinburgh, Oliver and Boyd, 1938, p 131.
15. Ellinwood EH: Effect of chronic methamphetamine intoxication in rhesus monkeys. Biol Psychiatry *3*:25–32, 1971.
16. Ernst AM, Smelik PG: Site of action of dopamine and apomorphine on compulsive gnawing behavior in rats. Experientia *22*:837–838, 1966.
17. Fishman RA: Brain edema. N Engl J Med *293*:706–711, 1975.
18. Foltz EL, Schmidt RP: The role of the reticular formation in the coma of head injury. J Neurosurg *13*:145–154, 1956.
19. Ford LE, McLaurin RL: Mechanisms of extradural hematomas. J Neurosurg *20*:760–769, 1963.
20. Gamstorp I, Kjellman B, Palmgren B: Diencephalic syndromes of infancy. J Pediatr *70*:383–390, 1967.
21. Garcia-Bengochea F, De La Torre O, Esquivel O, Vieta R, Fernandez C: The section of the fornix in the surgical treatment of certain epilepsies. A preliminary report. Trans Am Neurol Assoc *79*:176–178, 1954.
22. Graham DI, Adams JH, Doyle D: Ischemic brain damage in fatal non-missile head injuries. J Neurol Sci *39*:213–234, 1978.
23. Gross AG: A new theory on the dynamics of brain concussion and brain injury. J Neurosurg *15*:548, 1958.
24. Gudeman SK, Kishore PRS, Miller JD, Girevendulis AK, Lipper M, Becker DP: The genesis and significance of delayed traumatic intracerebral hematoma. Neurosurgery *5*(3):309–313, 1979.
25. Hassler R: Striatal control of locomotion intentional actions and of integrating and perceptive activity. J Neurol Sci *36*:187–224, 1978.
26. Hedreen JC, Struble RG, Whitehouse PJ, Price DL: Topography of the magnocellular basal forebrain system in human brain. J Neuropathol Exp Neurol *43*(1):1–21, 1984.
27. Heppner F: Eingriffe am limbischen System. Zentralbl Neurochir *17*:140–151, 1957.
28. Hirsch LF: Delayed traumatic intracerebral hematomas after surgical decompression. Neurosurgery *5*(6):653–655, 1979.
29. Holbourn AHS: Mechanisms of head injuries. Lancet *2*:438–441, 1943.
30. Hooper R: Observations on extradural hemorrhage. Br J Surg *47*:71–87, 1959.
31. Jackson DM, Anden NE, Dahlstrom A: A functional effect of dopamine in the nucleus accumbens and in some other dopamine-rich parts of the rat brain. Psychopharmacologia *45*:139–149, 1975.
32. Jane JA, Rimel RW: Prognosis in head injury. Clin Neurosurg, *29*:346–352, 1982.

33. Jellinger K, Seitelberger F: Protracted post-traumatic encephalopathy—pathology, pathogenesis and clinical implications. J Neurol Sci *10*:51–94, 1970.
34. Jenkner FL: Treating and preventing cerebral edema. Acta Neurol Lat Am *4*:184–189, 1958.
35. Jennett WB, Stern WE: Tentorial herniation, the midbrain, and the pupil. Experimental studies in brain compression. J Neurosurg *17*:598–609, 1960.
36. Kimelberg HK: Glial enzymes and iron transport in brain swelling. In Popp AJ, Bourke RS, Nelson LR, Kimelberg HK (Eds), Seminars in Neurological Surgery: Neural Trauma. New York, Raven Press, 1979, pp 137–153.
37. Kimelberg HK, Burke RS, Stieg PE, Barron KD, Hirata H, Pelton EW, Nelson LR: Swelling of astroglia after injury to the central nervous system: Mechanisms and consequences. In Grossman RG, Gildenberg PL (Eds), Head Injury: Basic and Clinical Aspects. New York, Raven Press, 1982, pp 31–44.
38. Klatzo I, Seitelberger F: Brain Edema. New York, Springer-Verlag, 1967.
39. Klintworth GK: Evaluation of the role of neurosurgical procedures in the pathogenesis of secondary brainstem hemorrhages. J Neurol Neurosurg Psychiatry *29*:423–425, 1966.
40. Langfitt TW: Possible mechanisms of action of hypertonic urea in reducting intracranial pressure. Neurology (Minneap) *11*:196–209, 1961.
41. Langfitt TW: Increased intracranial pressure. Clin Neurosurg *16*:436–471, 1969.
42. Lewelt W, Jenkins LW, Miller JD: Autoregulation of cerebral blood flow after experimental fluid percussion injury of the brain. J Neurosurg *53*:500–511, 1980.
43. Lindenberg R, Freytag E: The mechanism of cerebral contusions. Arch Pathol *69*:440–469, 1960.
44. Livingston KE: Anatomical bias of the limbic system concept. Arch Neurol *24*:17–21, 1971.
45. Lofgren J, Zwetnow NN: Cranial and spinal components of the cerebrospinal fluid pressure volume curve. Acta Neurol Scand *49*:575–585, 1973.
46. MacLean PD: Contrasting functions of limbic and neocortical systems of the brain and their relevance to psychophysiological aspects of medicine. Seminar on the brain. Am J Med *25*:611–626, 1958.
47. Magoun HW: The Waking Brain. Springfield, IL: Charles C Thomas, 1958.
48. Marcal PV, Nickell RE: In-vacuo modal dynamic response of the human skull. Am Soc Mech Engr J Engr Industry 73-DET-*112*:1–5, 1973.
49. Martin JD: The Basal Ganglia and Posture. Philadelphia, JB Lippincott, 1967.
50. McCullough D, Nelson KM, Ommaya AK: The acute effects of experimental head injury on the vertebral basillar circulation: Angiographic observations. J Trauma *11*:422–428, 1971.
51. Mendelow AD, Karmi MZ, Paul KS, Fuller GAG, Gillingham FJ: Extradural hematoma: Effect of delayed treatment. Br Med J *1*:1240–1242, 1979.
52. Meyer JS, Teraura T, Sakamoto K, Kondo A: Central neurogenic control and cerebral blood flow. Neurology (Minneap) *21*:247–262, 1971.
53. Miller JD: The physiology of trauma. Clin Neurosurg *7*:103–130, 1975.
54. Miller JD, Leech PJ: Assessing the effects of mannitol and steroid therapy on intracranial volume pressure relationships. J Neurosurg *42*:274–281, 1975.
55. Molnar L: Role of brainstem in CBF regulation. Scan J Clin Lab Investigations *22* (Suppl 102):6D, 1968.
56. Nauta WJH: Hypothalamic regulation of sleep in rats: Experimental study. J Neurophysiology *9*:285–316, 1946.
57. Obrist WD, Gennarelli, TA, Segawa H, Dolinskas CA, Langfitt TW: Relation of cerebral blood flow to neurological status and outcome in head injury of the patients. J Neurosurg *51*:292–300, 1979.

58. Osterholm JL, Bell J , Meyer R, Pyenson J: Experimental effects of free serotonin on the brain and its relation to brain injury. J Neurosurg *31*:408–421, 1969.
59. Pang D, Horton JA, Herron JM, Wilberger JE, Vries JK: Nonsurgical management of extradural hematomas in children. J Neurosurg *59*:958–971, 1983.
60. Papez JW: A proposed mechanism of emotion. Arch Neurol Psych *38*:725–743, 1937.
61. Peerless SJ, Rewcastle NB: Shear injury of the brain. Can Med Assoc J *96*:577–582, 1967.
62. Poeck K: Pathophysiology of emotional disorders associated with brain damage. In Vinken PJ, Bruyn GW (Eds), Handbook of Clinical Neurology. Amsterdam, North-Holland, 1969, pp 343–367.
63. Poirier LJ, Lafleur J, de Lean J, Guiot G, Larochelle L, Boucher R: Physiopathology of the cerebellum in the monkey. 2. Motor disturbances associated with partial and complete destruction of cerebellar structures. J Neurol Sci *22*:491–501, 1974.
64. Pollay M, Roberts PA: Blood brain barrier: A definition of normal and altered function. Neurosurgery *6*(6):675–685, 1980.
65. Povlishock JT, Becker DP, Miller JD, Jenkins LW, Dietrich WD: The morphopathologic substrates of concussion. Acta Neuropathol (Berlin) *47*:1–11, 1979.
66. Povlishock JT, Kontos HA: The pathophysiology of pial and intraparenchymal vascular dysfunction. In Grossman RG, Gildenberg PL (Eds), Head Injury: Basic and Clinical aspects. New York, Raven Press, 1982, pp 15–29.
67. Pribram KH: The neurophysiology of remembering. Sci Am *220*:73–86, 1969.
68. Reivich M, Marshall WJS, Kassell N: Loss of autoregulation produced by cerebral trauma. In Brock M, Fieschi C, Ingvar DH, Larson NA, Schurmann K (Eds), Cerebral Blood Flow. Berlin, Springer-Verlag, 1969, pp 205–208.
69. Rimel RW, Giordini B, Barth JT, Bollt J, Jane JA: Disability caused by minor head injury. Neurosurgery *9*:221–228, 1981.
70. Russel A: A diencephalic syndrome of emaciation in infancy and childhood. Arch Dis Child *26*:274, 1951.
71. Salcman M: A hypophysis concerning the structural relationship between memory and emotion. Med Hypotheses *4*:581–590, 1978.
72. Sano K, Mayanagi Y, Sekino H, Ogashiwa M, Ishijima B: Results of stimulation and destruction of the posterior hypothalamus in man. J Neurosurg *33*:689–707, 1970.
73. Scoville WB, Milner B: Loss of recent memory after bilateral hippocampal lesions. J Neurol Neurosurg Psychiatry *20*:11–21, 1957.
74. Seelig JM, Becker DP, Miller JD, Greenberg RP, Ward JD, Choi SC: Traumatic acute subdural hematoma: Major mortality reduction in comatose patients treated within 4 hours. N Engl J Med *304*:1511–1518, 1981.
75. Sellier K, Unterharnscheidt F: The mechanics of the impact of violence on the skull. Proc Third International Congress of Neurological Surgery, 1965, pp 87–92.
76. Senn RN, Anand DK: Effective electrical stimulation of the hypothalamus on gastric secretory activity and ulceration. Ind J Med Res *45*:507, 1957.
77. Sharlit MN: On the regulation of cerebral blood flow and metabolic activity in coma, clinical and experimental studies. Progr Brain Res *35*:229–243, 1972.
78. Sharpless S, Jasper HH: Habituation of the arousal reaction. Brain *79*:655–680, 1956.
79. Spatz H: Brain injuries in aviation in German aviation medicine World War II. Department of the Air Force *1*:616–640, 1950.
80. Strich SJ: Diffuse degeneration of the cerebral white matter in severe dementia following head injury. J Neurol Neurosurg Psychiatry *19*:163–185, 1956.
81. Strich SJ: Shearing of nerve fibers as a cause of brain damage due to head injury. Lancet *2*:443–448, 1961.
82. Strich SJ: The pathology of brain damage due to blunt head injury. In Walker AE, Caveness WF, Crichley M (Eds): The Late Effects of Head Injury. Springfield, IL, Charles C Thomas, 1969, pp 501–524.

83. Strich SJ: Lesions in the cerebral hemispheres after blunt head injury. J Clin Pathol (Suppl) 4:166–171, 1970.
84. Suwanwela C, Suwanwela N: Intracranial arterial narrowing and spasm in acute head injury. J Neurosurg 36:314–322, 1972.
85. Sweet WH, Talland GA, Ervin FR: Loss of recent memory following section of fornix. Trans Am Neurol Assoc 84:76–82, 1959.
86. Takahashi H, Manaka S, Sano K: Changes in extracellular potassium concentration in cortex and brainstem during the acute phase of experimental closed head injury. J Neurosurg 55:708–717, 1981.
87. Treip CS: Hypothalamic and pituitary injury. J Clin Pathol (Suppl) 23(4):178–186, 1970.
88. Unterharnscheidt F, Sellier K: Mechanics and pathomorphology of closed brain injuries. Conference Proceedings. In Caveness WF, Walker AE (Eds), Head Injury. Philadelphia, JB Lippincott, 1966, pp 321–341.
89. Veale WL, Cooper KE: Evidence for the involvement of prostaglandins in fever. In Lederis K, Cooper KE (Eds), Recent Studies of Hypothalamic Function. Basel, S Karger, 1973, pp 359–364.
90. Victor M, Adams RD: Wernicke-Korsakoff syndrome. Philadelphia, F A Davis, 1971, pp 164–174.
91. Ward AA Jr: The anterior cingular gyrus and personality. Res Nerv Ment Dis Proc 27:438–445, 1948.
92. Ward AA Jr: The physiology of concussion. Conference proceedings. In Caveness WF, Walker AE (Eds), Head Injury. Philadelphia, JB Lippincott, 1966, pp 203–208.
93. White LE Jr: A morphologic concept of the limbic lobe. Int Rev Neurobiol 8:1–34, 1965.
94. Wilkins RH: Intracranial vascular spasm in head injuries. In Vinken PJ, Bruyn GW (Eds), Handbook of Clinical Neurology. Vol. 23, Injuries of the Brain and Skull (Part I). Amsterdam, North-Holland, 1975, pp 163–197.
95. Wilson SAK: Some problems in neurology. II. Pathological laughing and crying. J Neurol Psychopathol 16:299–333, 1924.
96. Wise BL, Çhater N: The value of hypertonic mannitol solution in decreasing brain mass and lowering cerebrospinal fluid pressure. J Neurosurg 19:1038–1043, 1962.
97. Yakovlev PI: Motility, behavior and the brain. J Nerv Ment Dis 107:313–335, 1948.
98. Zimmerman RA, Bilaniuk LT, Bruce D, Dolinskas C, Obrist WD, Kuhl D: Computed tomography of pediatric head trauma: acute general cerebral swelling. Radiology 126:403–408, 1978.
99. Zimmerman RA, Bilaniuk LT, Gennarelli T, Bruce D, Dolinskas C, Uzell B: Cranial computed tomography in diagnosis and management of acute head injury. Am J Roentgenol 131:27–34, 1978.

Chapter 2

Neuropsychological Sequelae Following Pediatric Head Injury

Linda Ewing-Cobbs, MA,
Jack M. Fletcher, PhD, and
Harvey S. Levin, PhD

It is commonly hypothesized that neurobehavioral recovery following brain injury is better in children than in adults. This hypothesis is based on studies of a variety of brain injury cases, including children with congenital vascular disease, traumatic injury, and hemispherectomy for intractable seizures (Lenneberg, 1967; Smith 1981). More recently, it has become apparent that the extent of recovery observed following pediatric brain injury is determined by a variety of factors, including etiology, length of recovery interval, size of the lesion, and lesion site. Because of these factors, many investigators have become more cautious in invoking age as an explanatory variable (Isaacson, 1975; St. James-Roberts, 1979). For example, the differences in recovery rates after acquired aphasia in children and adults were once broadly interpreted as a demonstration of better recovery in children (Lenneberg, 1967). Although the rate of spontaneous recovery in children is striking, a significant proportion exhibit persistent aphasic deficits (Satz and Bullard-Bates, 1981). Even when specific linguistic symptoms resolve, cognitive and academic difficulties often remain (Alajouanine and L'hermitte, 1965).

Head injury, a prominent cause in many of the studies of recovery in children and adults, represents an area in which the maxim of better recovery in children has been questioned (Levin, Ewing-Cobbs, and Benton, 1984). Because of the high incidence of head trauma and the risk for long-term cognitive, educational, and motor handicaps in children, head injuries

Acknowledgment. This work was supported in part by NINCDS Grant, IR01 NS *21889-01*, Neurobehavioral Outcome Following Head Injury in Children, and by DHEW Grant, 5P01 NS *077377-11*, Center for the Study of Central Nervous System Injury.

require a multidisciplinary approach to rehabilitation. The purpose of this chapter is to systematically review the nature and sequelae of head injury in children. Our approach to case management is then described, and case studies are provided that illustrate common neuropsychological sequelae.

MECHANISMS AND PATHOPHYSIOLOGY

The primary mechanism producing brain injury following closed head injury (CHI) is diffuse neuronal damage occurring at the time of impact (Adams, Mitchell, Graham, and Doyle, 1977; Strich, 1956). Rotational acceleration of the skull produces shear strains within the intracranial contents. Widespread injury to the cerebral white matter apparently results from shearing and stretching of nerve fibers (Adams et al., 1977). Holbourn (1943) inferred that shear strain was most pronounced in the anterior tip of the temporal lobes and the orbital region of the frontal lobes due to impaction against the bony sphenoid wing.

The types of cognitive alterations observed following CHI appear to be related to the mechanisms producing cerebral injury. Generalized cognitive impairment, as reflected in decreased IQ scores and a reduction in information processing capacity, is commonly associated with severe CHI producing diffuse cerebral involvement (Levin, Benton, and Grossman, 1982a). Posttraumatic amnesia (PTA) and residual memory impairment may result from the vulnerability of the temporal lobes to shearing injuries. Frontal lobe involvement may contribute to the presence of behavioral disturbances, particularly disinhibition.

It is unclear how the mechanics of injury differ in children from those in the adult. Strich (1969) suggested that the shearing strains produced by rotational acceleration were less pronounced in smaller brains. This could result in less microscopic neuronal injury in infants and young children than in adults following comparable blunt trauma. Additionally, it is unclear how the gelatinous consistency of the partially myelinated brain is affected by mechanical distortion (Mealey, 1968). Since children are more likely to be injured by falls or low speed accidents, many pediatric injuries may result in less severe rotational acceleration (Levin et al., 1982a). Injuries sustained by adults in high speed motor vehicle accidents are likely to yield greater diffuse brain injury. For example, Jamison and Kaye (1974) observed that neurologic sequelae were present only in children injured in road traffic accidents.

The pathophysiologic response of the brain to trauma varies with age. The incidence of mass lesions is significantly reduced in children compared with adults (Jennett, 1972). Bruce and colleagues (1979) examined the pathophysiology of head injury in children and adolescents with Glasgow Coma Scale (GCS) scores of 8 or less. The most common computed tomography (CT) scan findings were subarachnoid hemorrhage and general cerebral swelling. Based on regional cerebral blood flow studies, the general cerebral swelling was attributed to vascular congestion produced by increased blood volume and flow. In adults, general swelling is often associated with edema, which involves accumulation of excess water in the brain parenchyma. Cerebral blood flow may be decreased (Zimmerman et al., 1978).

Studies comparing outcome in children and adults must be interpreted cautiously. From the foregoing, it is clear that many factors associated with CHI vary with development. The cause of injury, mechanisms of impact, and the pathophysiologic response of the brain differ in children. The extent to which these variables influence outcome measures is unclear.

EARLY EFFECTS ON BEHAVIOR

Behavioral changes after CHI may be classified according to their time course. "Early" effects appear after termination of coma, whereas "late" effects are manifested after resolution of confusion and may involve relatively permanent changes. Although previous studies suggest that grossly aberrant behavior is frequently transient and confined to the initial phase of recovery, persistent cognitive deficit and behavioral changes are common after severe head injury in children.

Confusion and anterograde amnesia (i.e., inability to consolidate information about ongoing events) usually persist for varying durations after emergence from coma (Russell and Smith, 1961). The duration of PTA may range from a few minutes following mild CHI that produces no coma to several months after severe CHI. The duration of PTA is a good prognostic indicator in both children (Chadwick, Rutter, Shaffer, and Shrout, 1981) and adults (Levin et al., 1982). The behavioral characteristics associated with PTA in children are not established. Although some investigators have described impulsive and restless behavior, others have emphasized withdrawal and mutism (Blau, 1936; Todorow, 1975). Children exhibit lethargy, irritability, and agitation as well as retrograde and anterograde amnesia (Klonoff, Low, and Clark, 1977). The absence of precise instruments for measuring PTA and behavioral alterations in children precludes more specific statements as to the length and characteristics of the initial recovery period.

LONG-TERM NEUROPSYCHOLOGICAL SEQUELAE

Despite the high incidence of pediatric CHI, there are few studies of long-term cognitive recovery. Generalization of findings across various investigations is complicated by the differing criteria used for grading the neurological severity of injury. Additionally, the specific neuropsychological functions examined vary considerably.

Bruce and co-workers (1979) reported that 90 per cent of a series of pediatric CHI patients showed a good recovery or moderate disability after injury that produced coma (GCS score $\leq$ 8) and pervasive neurologic deficit. Although the focus of their studies was on the pathophysiology and clinical management of acute CHI in children, they conveyed the impression of relatively minor residual deficit after severe injury compared with the outcome in head injured adults. Our review of research concerning neuropsychological recovery from CHI in children indicates that cognitive impairment frequently persists after severe injury despite impressive resolution of focal motor and sensory deficits and resumption of daily activities. This disparity in findings suggests that the improved motor function and restoration of childhood activities may lead to an overestimation of the quality of recovery (Levin, Eisenberg, and Miner, 1983.)

Intellectual Sequelae. Persistent intellectual and academic problems are encountered by children following severe head injury. Levin and Eisenberg (1979b) examined intellectual recovery at least 6 months post injury in 23 children and adolescents. Intelligence scores below 85 (which fell below the preinjury level estimated from school records) were common in children rendered comatose for longer than 24 hours. Virtually all of the other children, who either had no loss of consciousness or were comatose for less than one day, recovered to an IQ of at least 85. Chadwick and colleagues (1981a) evaluated intellectual recovery in 25 children following severe head injury that produced PTA persisting for at least 1 week. Compared with matched orthopedic controls, the head injured children were impaired on both the Wechsler Intelligence Scale for Children–Revised (WISC–R) Verbal IQ (VIQ) and Performance IQ (PIQ) scales at 4 months post injury. By one year post injury, impairment was present only on the PIQ. These findings are consistent with patterns of intellectual recovery in adults that indicate a more rapid return of the VIQ than the PIQ to the normal range (Mandleberg and Brooks, 1975). The dissociation between the VIQ and PIQ is likely due to the different response requirements of the two scales. While the VIQ examines retrieval of previously learned information, the PIQ has a significant motor component and evaluates problem-solving skills within a limited time frame (Fletcher, Ewing-Cobbs, McLaughlin, and Levin, in press). As noted by Chadwick and associates (1981a), posttraumatic deficits are most likely on tasks requiring rapid motor responses. Consistent with the above-mentioned findings, Flach and Malmros (1972) reported an intellectual decline in 80 per cent of their sample; the PIQ was most affected.

In general, most studies suggest that intellectual sequelae persist following severe closed head injury (Levin et al., 1982a). Levin and Eisenberg (1979a) compared premorbid estimates of intellectual functioning obtained from academic records to WISC-R scores obtained at least 6 months post injury. Only a partial intellectual recovery was achieved by most children. Similarly, Richardson (1963) reported a 10 to 30 point decrement in IQ scores following severe injury. Despite the significant intellectual sequelae commonly identified, prospective longitudinal evaluations assessing intellectual recovery at yearly intervals have shown progressive increments in IQ up to 5 years post injury following predominantly mild or moderately severe head injury (Black, Blumer, Wellner, and Walker, 1971; Klonoff et al., 1977).

Academic Sequelae. Scholastic achievement is often significantly affected by moderate or severe head injury. Despite the importance of academic skills for the adaptive functioning of the child, few investigators have examined the type and severity of posttraumatic academic difficulties. This is a serious omission since scholastic performance is a major developmental task facing children and adolescents.

Chadwick, Rutter, Thompson, and Shaffer (1981b) examined scholastic achievement in 97 children who sustained a unilateral compound depressed skull fracture with gross damage to the underlying cortex. Age at injury was not associated with substantial differences in IQ scores. By at least 2 years post injury, there was a tendency for cognitive scores to be more impaired if a left hemisphere injury was sustained before the child was 5 years of age. However, the authors stressed that age at injury was not a major variable in determining the extent of persistent cognitive impairment. Similarly, Shaffer, Bijur, Chadwick, and Rutter (1980) evaluated reading ability in 88 children with unilateral depressed skull fractures. Fifty-five per cent of the sample were reading at least 1 year below chronological age; 33 per cent performed at least 2 years below age level. Age at injury was not related to reading impairment. However, the prevalence of reading delays was significantly higher in children injured prior to 8 years of age who were unconscious for longer intervals. Although the duration of coma was significantly related to reading delays in the younger children, no association was observed between coma duration and reading difficulties in children at least 8 years of age at injury.

Klonoff and associates (1977) indicated that 26 per cent of children less than 9 years old had either failed a grade or been placed in resource classes. Twenty-one per cent of the older children received special placements. These rates are striking in view of the generally mild injuries in this sample. Other studies have confirmed that a high proportion of children require special classroom placement (Brink, Garrett, Hale, Woo-Sam, and Nickel, 1970; Flach and Malmros, 1972; Fuld and Fisher, 1977; Heiskanen and Kaste, 1974; Richardson, 1963).

Language Functions. Levin and Eisenberg (1979a) examined posttraumatic language dysfunction following pediatric CHI using the Neurosensory Center Comprehensive Examination for Aphasia (Spreen and Benton, 1969). Sixty-four children and adolescents were evaluated within 6 months of injury. Linguistic deficits were observed in 31 per cent. The most common deficits were dysnomia for objects presented visually (13 per cent) or tactually to the left hand (12 per cent). Auditory comprehension was impaired in 11 per cent of the sample while verbal repetition was affected in only 4 per cent. A higher incidence of linguistic disturbance was identified in head injured adults receiving similar evaluations. One half of the adults exhibited dysnomia or decreased verbal fluency, or both, whereas one third showed impairment on measures of auditory comprehension (Levin and Eisenberg, 1979b). Levin and Eisenberg (1979b) inferred that their findings were consistent with those of previous studies of acquired aphasia that suggest more rapid and complete recovery in children.

We recently completed an examination of subacute linguistic disturbances following resolution of PTA in children and adolescents. Moderate to severe CHI was defined by neurologic deficit, CT scan findings, coma persisting for at least 15 minutes, or a combination of these findings. Moderate to severe injury was associated with deficits in visual confrontation naming, object description, verbal fluency, and writing to dictation. Comparison of the effect of age at injury on linguistic performance revealed no sparing of language functions in children compared with adolescents. Moreover, children were more impaired than adolescents on measures of written language.

Recent findings converge in identifying subtle language processing deficiencies that persist following pediatric head injury. Chadwick and associates (1981a) reported that object naming latency was impaired 1 year post injury. By 2 years post injury, performance was in the normal range. Similarly, Gaidolfi and Vignolo (1980) identified residual impairment of oral expression, which was characterized by a reduction in spontaneous speech, in 4 of 21 children evaluated approximately 10 years following severe head injury.

Memory Functions. While the capacity to consolidate and retrieve information is clearly critical for scholastic performance, relatively few studies have evaluated memory functions in head injured children. Levin and Eisenberg (1979b) indicated that memory impairment was the most common cognitive deficit following pediatric CHI; nearly one half of patients with injuries of varying severity exhibited memory dysfunction. Similarly, other studies suggest that memory impairment persists despite improvement in motor functions and resumption of daily activities (Fuld and Fisher, 1977; Richardson, 1963).

Levin, Eisenberg, Wigg, and Kobayashi (1982b) examined the recovery of verbal and visual memory at least 6 months post injury. Children and adolescents were matched for the severity of injury on the GCS score as well as the presence and lateralization of mass lesions visualized by CT scans. The Selective Reminding Test (Buschke and Fuld, 1974), which permits separation of the storage and retrieval components of memory, was used to evaluate verbal memory. As depicted in Figure 2–1, severe CHI (GCS less than or equal to 8) produced residual impairment in the retrieval of information from long-term storage in both age groups. The severity of memory impairment was comparable in children and adolescents, suggesting no sparing of function in children. Visual recognition memory was evaluated by asking the patients to distinguish between recurring pictures of familiar objects and distractor pictures (Hannay, Levin, and Grossman, 1979). Children, but not adolescents, with severe CHI exhibited residual deficits in recognition memory.

Related Neuropsychological Sequelae. Few studies have examined the recovery of visuospatial, somatosensory, or motor skills. Klonoff and colleagues (1977) administered a comprehensive test battery to a sample composed predominantly of mildly injured children. Initial and 1 year follow-up findings suggested that slow visuomotor performance on the Trail Making Test, reduced finger and foot tapping speed, impaired formboard assembly, and poor maze performance were the most salient deficits. Similar findings were presented by Chadwick and associates (1981a). Deficits in finger tapping and manual dexterity were present at baseline and 1 year follow-up evaluations.

Levin and Eisenberg (1979a,b) indicated that visuospatial impairment, as evaluated by construction of three-dimensional block designs and copying the Bender designs, was present in nearly one third of pediatric CHI patients. Consistent with the reduction in motor speed identified by Klonoff and Chadwick and their co-workers, reaction time was frequently prolonged following CHI in adolescents, whereas thumb-finger opposition was slow in head injured children. Somatosensory performance was

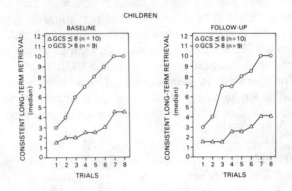

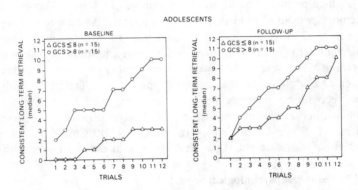

Figure 2-1. Retrieval from long-term storage plotted against trials on the baseline and follow-up selective reminding tests. The graph includes the data from children who were given the children's version of the test in both examinations, whereas the data from children who were older than 12 years at the time of follow-up were analyzed separately. From Levin, H. S., Eisenberg, H. M., Wigg, N. R., and Kobayashi, K. (1982b). Memory and intellectual ability after head injury in children and adolescents. *Neurosurgery, 11*, 668–673. Reprinted with permission.

reduced in approximately one fourth of the pediatric cases on measures of stereognosis, finger localization, and graphesthesia. It appears that children and adults exhibit a comparable range of posttraumatic deficits (Levin et al., 1983).

Psychosocial Recovery. Although the severity of head injury is directly related to residual cognitive difficulties, the relationship with psychosocial adjustment may be more complex (Rutter, 1981). Rutter (1981) found that the severity of brain injury was related to the likelihood of behavioral difficulties. However, other factors, including premorbid characteristics and the post-injury environment, are probably also contributory. The prospective research of Rutter, Chadwick, and associates (Brown, Chadwick, Shaffer, Rutter, and Traub, 1981; Rutter, 1981; Rutter, 1982; Rutter, Chadwick, Shaffer, and Brown, 1980) was based on groups of severe and mild head injury patients that were divided according to the length of PTA. Patients with severe injuries had PTA persisting for at least 1 week, whereas those with mild injuries had PTA from 1 hour to less than 7 days. These children were matched on a variety of social and demographic variables with a group of children who sustained orthopedic injuries. Neuropsychological and intellectual tests, parent and teacher interviews, and personality questionnaires were administered at the time of injury and at 4 months, 1 year, and 2¼ years post injury. The mild injury group had a higher rate of behavioral disturbance at baseline than either the severe injury or control groups. This implies that children who sustained mild injuries were behaviorally different prior to the injury. Such a finding is consistent with the hypothesis that children who are impulsive and active are more likely to take the kinds of risks that lead to head injury. In contrast, the severe injury group did not show a higher frequency of preinjury behavioral disturbances compared with controls.

To evaluate the relationship between head injury and psychiatric disturbance, Brown and co-workers (1981) examined the rates of psychiatric disorder arising after the injury in children without evidence of premorbid disorder. No differences in the rate of new disorders were observed between the mild head injury and control groups on any of the follow-up assessments (Fig. 2–2). Approximately half of the severe head injury group developed new psychiatric disorders. In fact, by 2¼ years, the rate of behavioral disturbance was three times higher in the severe injury group than in controls. Although mild head injury was not associated with an increased incidence of disturbance, severe head injury was clearly associated with a marked increase in the rate of psychiatric disorder. Behavioral problems commonly reflected preinjury behavior such that preexisting difficulties were exacerbated after injury. Similarly, adverse social circumstances in the preinjury environment were also related to the presence of behavioral disturbances after severe head injury. Brown and colleagues (1981) also found that the degree of cognitive disturbance had a weak relationship with post-injury behavioral sequelae.

Statements attributing post-injury behavioral disturbance solely to the cerebral insult are probably simplistic explanations. The impact of trauma on the family must also be considered. One hypothesis is that

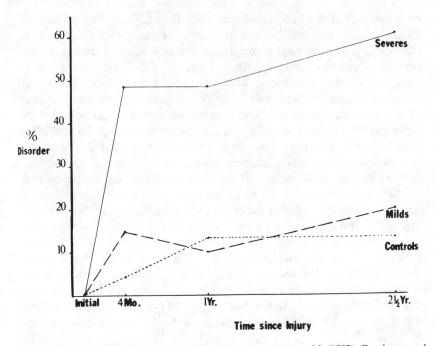

Figure 2-2. Rates of "new" psychiatric disorders. From Rutter, M. (1982). Developmental neuropsychiatry: Concepts, issues and problems. *Journal of Clinical Neuropsychology, 4,* 91-115. Reprinted with permission.

families that are intact and communicative prior to injury are more likely to absorb and cope with trauma than are families with more stress and less cohesiveness. Additional research is needed in this area. However, the view that brain injury leads to a characteristic behavioral syndrome including impulsive, overactive, and hyperkinetic behavior may also be rather simplistic (Strauss and Lehtinen, 1947). In the prospective studies cited, there was no single homogeneous pattern of disrupted behavior following injury with the exception of a tendency toward disinhibited behavior by children in the severe injury group (Brown et al., 1981). The notion of a postconcussive syndrome with specific behavioral features can be questioned in light of these data (Dillon and Leopold, 1961). Children with mild injuries may be more susceptible to injury, so that their post-injury behavior may reflect those behavioral characteristics rather than a direct effect of head injury. Moreover, the expression of behavioral changes after severe injury may also be affected by preinjury personality, psychosocial adversity, and the capacity of the family to cope with the injury.

AGE AT INJURY

Brain injury may preferentially disrupt new learning (Hebb, 1942). Rutter (1981) inferred that young children may be disproportionately affected by cerebral insult since learning is necessary for their acquisition of new skills. Children sustaining CHI may be significantly at risk for cognitive delays since learning and memory are often impaired.

However, no consistent pattern has emerged regarding the effect of age at CHI on cognitive outcome. This may be due partly to the restricted age ranges examined and the relatively few studies that have compared the neurobehavioral outcome of CHI in children at different ages. Several studies have reported that the age at injury was unrelated to either the rate of recovery or the severity of cognitive sequelae (Chadwick et al., 1981a; Klonoff et al., 1977; Levin and Eisenberg, 1979a). With the exception of the study by Klonoff and associates, these studies were restricted to children at least 5 years old at injury. In contrast, studies including infants or preschoolers have documented more severe long-term cognitive deficits in younger children (Brink et al., 1970; Chadwick et al., 1981b; Lange-Cosack, Wider, Schlesner, Grumme, and Kubicki, 1979; Shaffer et al., 1980).

The available data do not permit evaluation of the effect of CHI on cognitive skills at different ages. However, our experience suggests that the type of deficits observed following severe CHI often vary with age. Preschoolers, in whom cognitive skills are developing rapidly, typically exhibit generalized cognitive impairment. Significant attentional, fine and gross motor, intellectual, linguistic, and visuospatial disturbances are common. Children with these deficits may be at risk for developing significant academic delays. The neuropsychological profiles of school-age children and adolescents are fairly similar; memory, visuomotor, and attentional difficulties predominate. In addition, adolescents often exhibit marked difficulties with later-developing functions, such as social judgment, planning, and strategy usage. Additional research on age-related factors is clearly needed.

ASSESSMENT AND MANAGEMENT OF THE SEQUELAE OF HEAD INJURY

The successful rehabilitation of the brain injured child requires systematic follow-up, including repeated neuropsychological assessment, liaison with schools and parents, and careful attention to the child's behavior in the context of the family and school placement. Our approach to case management begins in the hospital immediately after injury. As part of an interdisciplinary team, our role is to evaluate the child's cognitive capacities throughout the recovery period. Since one of the major problems is the quantification of the child's level of PTA, we have developed a scale permitting assessment of the degree of disorientation and amnesia. This scale, the Children's Orientation and Amnesia Test (COAT), is analogous to the Galveston Orientation and Amnesia Test commonly used with adults (Levin, O'Donnell, and Grossman, 1979). The COAT consists of a series of simple questions examining temporal orientation, recall of autobiographic information, and immediate and short-term memory. Norms are available for normal children that permit specification of the child's degree of PTA.

When a sufficient level of orientation and working memory is apparent from the COAT, a baseline neuropsychological evaluation is obtained that supplements ongoing work by speech therapists, occupational therapists, and members of other disciplines. This battery consists of an IQ test (WISC-R) and achievement tests, along with standard measures of language, memory, and tactile, spatial, motor, and construction skills (Taylor, Fletcher, and Satz, 1982). After discharge, children are reevaluated at 6, 12, 24, and 36 months post injury. After each evaluation, an assessment of the child's educational progress is made. Liaisons with schools, private rehabilitation agencies, and members of other disciplines are used to plan and evaluate the child's remediation program. Recommendations for special classes, curricula, and other, similar needs are communicated to the parents and educators responsible for providing treatment to the child.

We assess the child's behavior at home and at school. The need for this careful monitoring of behavior is especially apparent with patients who have preexisting behavioral and family difficulties. However, even families that were intact before injury can show disruptive effects associated with the trauma. These effects can range from guilt over the accident to altered relationships with siblings, as well as general feelings of resentment of the injured child because of the amount of care required. School personnel frequently require explanations not only of the child's strengths and weaknesses, but also of the nature of head injury and its consequences for behavior. When problems arise and short-term solutions are not applicable, referrals for counseling and pharmacologic intervention are considered. School-based interventions emphasize the appropriateness of classroom placement, need for special services, and appropriate expectations for the injured child.

Children with severe head injuries are at risk for cognitive and behavioral difficulties that can persist for several years. Outcomes following injury are heterogeneous, and no single remediation strategy is optimal for every child. Our goal is careful assessment and systematic case management over time. As members of one discipline among many, we provide relatively little direct treatment. However, liaisons with schools, parents, and remediation agents can impact on the child's post-injury behavior. It is hoped this type of systematic long-term follow-up will facilitate the child's readjustment in the family and at school.

To illustrate the types of neuropsychological sequelae we commonly observe, two case studies are presented.

Case 1

A 2 year, 6 month old boy was immediately rendered unconscious when he sustained a diffuse CHI in a motor vehicle accident on June 9, 1982. He was intubated during transport via helicopter ambulance. Examination on hospital admission disclosed no eye opening and localizing responses to pain (GCS = 7). Two days post injury, eye opening to noxious stimulation was observed. Although spontaneous movement was noted in all extremeties, a right hemiparesis was evident. The child began responding to commands 8 days post injury. Despite continuing neurologic improvement, he remained mute for 23 days.

A CT scan obtained on the day of admission was unremarkable. However, 13 days post injury, a repeat scan disclosed ventricular enlargement and enlarged fissures and sulci compatible with widespread atrophy. Focal involvement of the posterior right parietal lobe, possibly attributable to an infarct, was visualized.

Language skills were evaluated 29 days post injury using the Sequenced Inventory of Communication Development (SICD) (Hedrick, Prather, and Tobin, 1975). The majority of receptive language tasks were performed at a 2 to 2½ year level. The child was able to follow two-stage commands and demonstrated comprehension of certain function words. In contrast, expressive language skills were consistent with a 4 to 12 month level. Meaningful single-word utterances were occasionally verbalized. Spontaneous speech consisted largely of several vowels or consonant-vowel combinations. Although this child was able to imitate motor movements with the upper extremities, he was unable to imitate nonspeech sounds or oral movements. These findings were consistent with a severe nonfluent aphasia with moderate receptive language deficits. In addition, a severe oral-verbal apraxia was suspected.

Assessment of intellectual skills using the Stanford-Binet Intelligence Scale (SBIS) (Terman and Merrill, 1973) yielded a mental age of 27 months and an IQ equivalent of 86. Although many of the child's skills approximate age-appropriate levels, the IQ score was depressed owing to the absence of expressive language. Performance on the McCarthy Scales of Children's Abilities (McCarthy, 1972) Motor and Perceptual-Performance Scales was at the 10th percentile, indicating significant impairment. He demonstrated considerable apraxic deficits, as evidenced by difficulties in organizing and sequencing his movements. Following hospital discharge, the child received speech-language and occupational therapies on an outpatient basis.

Considerable improvement was observed by 1 year post injury. An IQ of 92 was obtained on the SBIS, indicating that the child was functioning in the low average range. Neuropsychological evaluation revealed the continued presence of a constructional apraxia in addition to difficulties with both fine and gross motor coordination. Motor development was almost two standard deviations below the average range. Perceptual-motor skills were approximately 1 year behind age-appropriate levels. The greatest improvement was apparent in spontaneous expressive language. The child's mean length of utterance consisted of five words. On the SICD, he received receptive and expressive language ages of 32 months, which were 11 months below his chronological age. These language scores were underestimates of his level of functioning and reflected difficulties in focusing and sustaining his attention. A referral to an Early Childhood Education program was made for provision of general cognitive stimulation in addition to speech-language, occupational, and physical therapy.

Case 2

A 14 year old boy was involved in a high speed motor vehicle accident on March 9, 1983. Neurologic examination on hospital admission revealed an absence of eye opening and verbalization; application of noxious stimulation produced withdrawal of the extremities (GCS = 6). Spontaneous eye opening and vocalization were initially observed 8 days post injury. The boy was able to follow commands 15 days after the injury.

A CT scan obtained on the day of admission was within normal limits. A repeat scan 12 days post injury was consistent with moderate ventriculomegaly, with most prominent enlargement of the right lateral ventricle.

Following discharge from an inpatient rehabilitation facility, a neuropsychological evaluation was completed on July 7, 1983. Performance on estimates of intellectual functioning was in the average range. Memory for verbal and spatial material was well below age level. Receptive language skills were within normal limits. However, expressive language was characterized by decreased fluency accompanied by mild word retrieval difficulties. Visuomotor skills were significantly impaired, and fine motor coordination was reduced bilaterally. Assessment of academic skills revealed age-appropriate reading and spelling. Computational arithmetic was grossly impaired. Referral was made for outpatient cognitive retraining and resource placement upon resumption of school.

Considerable recovery was apparent by 1 year post injury. Performance during the evaluation was reduced by impulsivity, which was characterized by poor planning and organization. Intellectual function recovered to the high average range. Although memory for spatial material was age appropriate, persistent deficits were apparent in the retrieval of verbal information from long-term storage. Performance on linguistic measures was within normal limits except for mild word retrieval difficulties. Visuomotor and fine motor skills recovered to age-appropriate levels. Considerable improvement was observed on measures of academic achievement. Reading and spelling were in the normal range while computational arithmetic was one standard deviation below expected levels. His current academic placement was on the lower track of a tiered system. Parental report disclosed persistent difficulties with concentration, fatigue, feelings of inferiority, social judgment, and school achievement.

Comparison of these findings with premorbid estimates of cognitive abilities suggested that a significant decline in most skill areas was present 1 year following the accident. The Stanford Achievement Test had been administered several weeks prior to the injury. In comparison with national norms, the composite battery total was at the 75th percentile. Even though performance in many skill areas had recovered to the normal range, this represents significant residual impairment when viewed within the context of premorbid capabilities.

SUMMARY AND CONCLUSIONS

Investigations of outcome in children and adolescents after severe closed head injury have documented persistent cognitive, academic, and behavioral sequelae. Owing to the different methods used to grade the neurologic severity of injury and to the scarcity of outcome studies, it is not possible to predict the extent of neuropsychological recovery in patients with injuries of varying severity. Presently, studies suggest that memory and visuomotor skills are most vulnerable to the effects of CHI. In contrast, language functions are comparatively resistant to disruption, as reflected by predominantly mild linguistic disturbances. Behavioral alterations occur frequently following severe CHI in children; however, a consensus has not been reached regarding the most pronounced characteristics of these personality changes. Examination of interactions between brain injury, premorbid characteristics, and the post-injury environment awaits further study.

The traditional view that children are relatively impervious to the effects of acquired brain injury has clearly been overstated. Evidence is accumulating suggesting that children may exhibit more severe cognitive sequelae following diffuse brain insult than either adolescents or adults (Levin et al., 1984). Studies comparing outcome in head injured children and adolescents do not support the view that recovery is enhanced in children (Brink et al., 1970; Lange-Cosack et al., 1979; Levin et al., 1982b). It is possible that the child's developmental stage at the time of injury influences both the type and severity of cognitive sequelae. Skills that are developing rapidly may be more affected by cerebral injury than well-consolidated and automatized skills. Since different abilities are acquired at different points during development, an interaction between age at injury and profiles of impairment may be present. Further research is needed to investigate developmental factors affecting recovery from brain injury. Knowledge of these factors would assist in the development of age-appropriate intervention strategies.

REFERENCES

Adams, J. H., Mitchell, D. C., Graham, D. I., and Doyle, D. (1977). Diffuse brain damage of the immediate impact type. *Brain, 100*, 489–502.

Alajouanine, T. H., and L'hermitte, F. (1965). Acquired aphasia in children. *Brain, 88*, 653–662.

Black, P., Blumer, D., Wellner, A. M., and Walker, A. E. (1971). The head injured child: Time course of recovery, with implications for rehabilitation. *Proceedings of an International Symposium on Head Injuries* (pp. 131–137). Edinburgh: Churchill Livingstone.

Blau, A. (1936). Mental changes following head trauma in children. *Archives of Neurology and Psychiatry, 35*, 733–769.

Brink, J. D., Garrett, A. L., Hale, W. R., Woo-Sam, J., and Nickel, V. L. (1970). Recovery of motor and intellectual function in children sustaining severe head injuries. *Developmental Medicine and Child Neurology, 12*, 565–571.

Brown, G., Chadwick, O., Shaffer, D., Rutter, M., and Traub, M. (1981). A prospective study of children with head injuries. III. Psychiatric sequelae. *Psychological Medicine, 11*, 63–78.

Bruce, D. A., Raphaely, R. C., Goldberg, A. I., Zimmerman, R. A., Bilaniuk, L. T., Schut, L., and Kuhl, D. E. (1979). Pathophysiology, treatment and outcome following severe head injury in children. *Child's Brain, 5*, 174–191.

Buschke, H., and Fuld, P. A. (1974). Evaluating storage, retention, and retrieval in disordered memory and learning. *Neurology, 24,* 1019–1025.

Chadwick, O., Rutter, M., Shaffer, D., and Shrout, P. E. (1981a). A prospective study of children with head injuries. IV. Specific cognitive deficits. *Journal of Clinical Neuropsychology, 3,* 101–120.

Chadwick, O., Rutter, M., Thompson, J., and Shaffer, D. (1981b). Intellectual performance and reading skills after localized head injury in childhood. *Journal of Child Psychology and Psychiatry, 22,* 117–139.

Dillon, H., and Leopold, R. L. (1961). Children and the post-concussion syndrome. *Journal of the American Medical Association, 175,* 86–116.

Flach, J., and Malmros, R. (1972). A long-term follow-up study of children with severe head injury. *Scandinavian Journal of Rehabilitation Medicine, 4,* 9–15.

Fletcher, J. M., Ewing-Cobbs, L., McLaughlin, E. J., and Levin, H. S. (in press). Cognitive and psychosocial sequelae of head injury in children: Implications for assessment and management. In B. Brooks and D. Hoelzer (Eds.), *The injured child.* Austin: University of Texas Press.

Fuld, P. A., and Fisher, P. (1977). Recovery of intellectual ability after closed head injury. *Developmental Medicine and Child Neurology, 19,* 495–502.

Gaidolfi, E., and Vignolo, L. A. (1980). Closed head injuries of school aged children: Neuropsychological sequelae in early adulthood. *Italian Journal of Neurological Sciences, 1,* 65–73.

Hannay, H. J., Levin, H. S., and Grossman, R. G. (1979). Impaired recognition memory after head injury. *Cortex, 15,* 269–283.

Hebb, D. O. (1942). The effect of early and late brain injury upon test scores, and the nature of normal adult intelligence. *Proceedings of the American Philosophical Society, 85,* 275–292.

Hedrick, D. L., Prather, E. M., and Tobin, A. R. (1975). *Sequenced Inventory of Communication Development examiner's manual.* Seattle: University of Washington Press.

Heiskanen, O., and Kaste, M. (1974). Late prognosis of severe brain injury in children. *Developmental Medicine and Child Neurology, 16,* 11–14.

Holbourn, A. H. S. (1943). Mechanics of head injuries. *Lancet, 2,* 438–441.

Isaacson, R. L. (1975). The myth of recovery from early brain damage. In N. Ellis (Ed.), *Aberrant development in infancy.* London: Wiley.

Jamison, D. L., and Kaye, H. H. (1974). Accidental head injury in children. *Archives of Diseases of Childhood, 49,* 376–381.

Jennett, B. (1972). Head injuries in children. *Developmental Medicine and Child Neurology, 14,* 137–147.

Klonoff, H., Low, M. D., and Clark, C. (1977). Head injuries in children: A prospective five year follow-up. *Journal of Neurology, Neurosurgery, and Psychiatry, 40,* 1211–1219.

Lange-Cosack, H., Wider, B., Schlesner, H. J., Grumme, Th., and Kubicki, S. T. (1979). Prognosis of brain injuries in young children (one until five years of age). *Neuropaediatrie, 10,* 105–127.

Lenneberg, E. (1967). *Biological foundations of language.* New York: John Wiley and Sons.

Levin, H. S., Benton, A. L., and Grossman, R. G. (1982a). *Neurobehavioral consequences of closed head injury.* New York: Oxford University Press.

Levin, H. S., and Eisenberg, H. M. (1979a). Neuropsychological impairment after closed head injury in children and adolescents. *Journal of Pediatric Psychology, 4,* 389–402.

Levin, H. S., and Eisenberg, H. M. (1979b). Neuropsychological outcome of closed head injury in children and adolescents. *Child's Brain, 5,* 281–292.

Levin, H. S., Eisenberg, H. M., and Miner, M. E. (1983). Neuropsychological findings in head injured children. In K. Shapiro (Ed.), *Pediatric head injury* (pp. 223–240). Mt. Kisco, NY: Futura Publishing Company.

Levin, H. S., Eisenberg, H. M., Wigg, N. R., and Kobayashi, K. (1982b). Memory and intellectual ability after head injury in children and adolescents. *Neurosurgery, 11,* 668–673.

Levin, H. S., Ewing-Cobbs, L., and Benton, A. L. (1984). Age and recovery from brain damage: A review of clinical studies. In S. W. Scheff (Ed.), *Aging and recovery of function in the central nervous system* (pp. 169–205). New York: Plenum Publishing Corporation.

Levin, H. S., O'Donnell, V. M., and Grossman, R. G. (1979). The Galveston Orientation and Amnesia Test: A practical scale to assess cognition after head Injury. *Journal of Nervous and Mental Disorders, 167,* 675–684.

McCarthy, D. (1972). *McCarthy scales of children's abilities.* New York: Psychological Corporation.

Mandleberg, I. A., and Brooks, D. N. (1975). Cognitive recovery after severe head injury 1. Serial testing on the Wechsler Adult Intelligence Scale. *Journal of Neurology, Neurosurgery, and Psychiatry, 38,* 1121–1126.

Mealey, J., Jr. (1968). *Pediatric head injuries.* Springfield, IL: Charles C Thomas.

Richardson, F. (1963). Some effects of severe head injury. A follow-up study of children and adolescents after protracted coma. *Developmental Medicine and Child Neurology, 5,* 471–482.

Russell, W. R., and Smith, A. (1961). Post-traumatic amnesia in closed head injury. *Archives of Neurology, 5,* 4–17.

Rutter, M. (1981). Psychological sequelae of brain damage in children. *American Journal of Psychiatry, 138,* 1533–1544.

Rutter M. (1982). Developmental neuropsychiatry: Concepts, issues and problems. *Journal of Clinical Neuropsychology, 4,* 91–115.

Rutter, M., Chadwick, O., Shaffer, D., and Brown, G. (1980). A prospective study of children with head injuries: I. Design and methods. *Psychological Medicine, 10,* 633–645.

St. James-Roberts, I. (1979). Neurological plasticity, recovery from brain insult, and child development. In H. W. Reese and L. P. Lipsitt (Eds.), *Advances in child development and behavior* (Vol. 14) (pp. 253–319). New York: Academic Press.

Satz, P., and Bullard-Bates, C. (1981). Acquired aphasia in children. In M. T. Sarno (Ed.), *Acquired aphasia* (pp. 399–426). New York: Academic Press.

Shaffer, D., Bijur, P., Chadwick, O., and Rutter, M. (1980). Head injury and later reading disability. *Journal of the American Academy of Child Psychiatry, 19,* 592–610.

Smith, A. (1981). On the organization, disorganization and resolution of language and other brain functions. In Y. Lebrun and O. L. Zangwill (Eds.), *Lateralization of language in the child.* Lisse, Netherlands: Swets.

Spreen, O., and Benton, A. L. (1969). *Neurosensory center comprehensive examination for aphasia: Manual of directions.* Victoria, BC: Neuropsychology Laboratory, University of Victoria.

Strauss, A. A., and Lehtinen, L. E. (1947). *Psychopathology and education of the brain injured child.* New York: Grune and Stratton.

Strich, S. J. (1956). Diffuse degeneration of the cerebral white matter in severe dementia following head injury. *Journal of Neurology, Neurosurgery, and Psychiatry, 19,* 163–185.

Strich, S. J. (1969). The pathology of brain damage due to blunt injuries. In A. E. Walker, W. F. Caveness, and M. Critchley (Eds.), *The late effects of head injury* (pp. 501–526). Springfield, IL: Charles C Thomas.

Taylor, H. G., Fletcher, J. M., and Satz, P. (1982). Component processes in reading disabilities: Neuropsychological investigation of distinct reading subskill deficits. In R. N. Malatesha and P. G. Aaron (Eds.), *Reading disorders: Varieties and treatments* (pp. 121-147). New York: Academic Press.

Terman, L. M., and Merrill, M. A. (1973). *Stanford-Binet Intelligence Scale manual for the third revision*. Boston: Houghton Mifflin Company.

Todorow, S. (1975). Recovery of children after severe head injury. Psychoreactive superimpositions. *Scandinavian Journal of Rehabilitation Medicine, 4,* 126-132.

Zimmerman, R. A., Bilaniuk, L. T., Bruce, D., Dolinskas, C., Obrist, W., and Kuhl, D. (1978). Computed tomography of pediatric head trauma: Acute general cerebral swelling. *Radiology, 126,* 403-408.

PART II
THE FAMILY

The chapter on family response to head injury has deliberately been made the opening chapter on rehabilitation in this textbook. The impact of a severe head injury on individual family members and on the family as a functional system, and the importance of family members in the process of rehabilitation, cannot be overemphasized. The long-term stress on family members and the disruption of family life, well documented in head injury follow-up studies, are due in part to the many uncertainties in head injury recovery, to the frequently "invisible" cognitive, behavioral, and social deficits that typically result from head injury, and to the major responsibilities given to families to care for their loved ones despite the often poorly understood deficits. The emergence in recent years of active regional chapters of The National Head Injury Foundation has combined with improved professional understanding of families' needs to ease to some degree the devastating impact of a head injury in the family.

In Chapter 3, two social workers— one with experience in an acute-care children's hospital and the other with experience in a rehabilitation setting— a rehabilitation nurse, and a parent of a head injured child combine to describe the common themes in the natural history of a family's reaction to severe head injury and the types of professional intervention that appropriately address the needs of the family and help to make family members effective partners in the rehabilitation process. The authors stress the importance of understanding the stage of the family's emotional reaction, choosing intervention strategies appropriate to that stage, understanding the family as a system and addressing the effects on all elements of the system, including siblings. Finally, they emphasize the necessity that *all* rehabilitation staff interact in an informed and therapeutic way with members of the family.

Chapter 3

Working with the Family

The Acute Phase
Paul R. Polinko, MSW
The Rehabilitation Phase
Judy J. Barin, MSW, and
Daniel Leger, RN,
with Kathleen M. Bachman,
parent of a head injured child

Severe head injury has a devastating impact on the family as well as on the patient. Initially family members face the shock of having the life of their previously healthy child hanging by a thread. Once they know that the child will live, they begin to receive frightening warnings about cognitive impairments and behavioral and personality changes. Always, when they press for definite answers, the replies are uncertain.

Stress is increased by family members' needs to maintain a supportive and therapeutic role with the patient. It is not surprising that researchers have found family members to be highly stressed immediately following the injury and to remain so at least as long as twelve month follow-up (Oddy, Humphrey, and Uttley, 1978).

In this chapter two social workers, a nurse, and a parent will discuss family reactions and needs and will recommend treatment strategies. The primary goals of professional intervention are to help family members to manage their stress and to accomplish the necessary adjustments in a functional way.

THE ACUTE PHASE

ACUTE CARE AND THE NUCLEAR FAMILY

The family's response during the acute care phase of severe pediatric head trauma can critically affect the patient's long-term prognosis and the family's functioning as a social unit. Although the patient bears the physical injury, the family, facing unforeseen challenges, bears the psychological pain of disrupted family life. By studying the family as a system and employing a cognitive approach, the family-oriented professional can help the family to assimilate information, communicate with the medical staff, and keep anxiety at manageable levels.

Although each family reacts to a child's injury uniquely, general responses can be described in two stages: (1) the period from injury to stabilization, and (2) the time between stabilization and awakening from coma. By designing a process of intervention that is compatible with the family's own coping systems, the professional can aid them in surviving their ordeal as a cohesive group.

First Stage: Injury to Stabilization

The first stage is one of shock and denial, with breakthroughs of panic (Ravenscroft, 1982; Rothstein, 1980), as parents must adjust to having a comatose child whose life is in jeopardy. Their feelings of helplessness are intensified by the child's inability to communicate. The natural "caregivers" must relinquish any opportunity to help the patient. The treatment team, composed of total strangers, now assumes control. The parents must watch helplessly as their child is subjected to a bewildering set of sophisticated, high-technology procedures. While being deluged with information about the child's injury, treatment, and prognosis, they wrestle with feelings of loss, fear, denial, and anger (Epperson, 1980). Often they fail to understand the physician, who can spare only limited time for them while the patient is in danger.

> Parent: *Wild, overwhelming, paralyzing fear. . . . I'm feeling out of control. Where's my doctor? Is he the best? Is this hospital good? I need someone to listen to me and honestly tell me what is going on every day. . . . Who and what should I ask? I don't even belong in this "hospital world." . . . please care. . . reassure and comfort me. . . . I HATE this waiting. What is all this freaky looking equipment? Is this my child? Can I touch her? Can I help with ANYTHING? I need to help. . . . Who the HELL are you to tell me no? I'm her mother! 24 hours. . . 72 hours. . . . Dear God, protect her. . . help everyone who's working with her. . . help me. . . . Can't someone make her better?*

Now the helping professional must intervene to prevent a crisis in the family. They must learn ways to ventilate their feelings and use cognitive structures to organize their understanding of the experience. Our main tools at this stage are empathic listening, repetition of information, and reassurance.

The importance of using a cognitive approach cannot be overemphasized. We must repeat and organize information so the overwhelmed family can grasp its significance. In most cases, regardless of their education, family members do not process information well during their conference with the physician. They are upset by such terms as "intracranial pressure monitor." Giving them written definitions of medical terms likely to be used in their child's treatment can reduce this anxiety. It is equally important to reassure parents about the trauma team's effectiveness. Now dependent on the expertise of strangers and cut off from the trusted family doctor, the parents are understandably nervous. The helping professional must candidly address their questions about the trauma system on which the patient's life depends.

The specter of brain damage often arises at this time, although we often hear the "bargaining" phrase—"I can deal with anything as long as my child survives." Parents may have popularized notions of their child as a "vegetable" or "retarded person," not realizing that it is more likely that the child will be labile, lethargic, or prone to inappropriate behavior. Parents can seldom picture the true consequences of brain injury but often ask questions about loss of function in the areas of their child's development that contain the elements of their own hopes, such as going to college or becoming an athlete. The professional must learn to understand the family well enough to offset these fearsome images, for, as the cognitive therapists have found, anxiety is a direct result of visualizing danger-laden images (Beck, 1976). Once the parents have faced these fears, the professional can help them to modify their images to include the processes of rehabilitation and relearning. Research indicates that the family's perception of symptoms can, in itself, be a cause of great stress (Oddy et al., 1978). Some families do not describe their fears until after the child's survival is secure. We can aid the family simply by keeping abreast of the significance they ascribe to the patient's symptoms.

The helping professional should also begin, even in this early stage, to analyze the family system in terms of (1) the stage of the family's life cycle, (2) the role of the patient in the family, and (3) the parents' ability to provide mutual support. Such information can be useful in assessing the family's reactions to crisis and in predicting their response to the particular crisis of having a head injured child.

The family's life cycle stage is significant. For example, the family of a head injured adolescent who was college bound premorbidly focuses on a different set of fears from those envisioned by the family of a four year old child. The adolescent's family had been engaged in the normal developmental task of separating, with long-standing expectations about to be fulfilled. Now that entire task is called into question. The preschooler's family, although suffering the same fears as the teenager's, does not feel that their shared developmental task is itself being threatened. They are still performing their customary tasks—nurturing and teaching a child. Such anxiety about facing developmental tasks is suggested in outcome studies, which purport that parents are better able to withstand the stress of head injury to a child than adults are able to cope with head injury to a spouse (McKinlay, Brooks, Bond, Martinage, and Marshall, 1981; Weddell, Oddy, and Jenkins, 1980).

The child's role in the family and the parents' ability to provide support for each other are related factors in the family's reaction to the injury. The impact of the injury on the parents is compounded by the fact that the child functions as part of each parent's emotional self. The more psychologically incomplete the parent is, the more likely it is that the child has been seen as an extension of the parent's dreams (Herz, 1980). The more the child's performance has been required for the family to be emotionally complete, the more devastating the injury will be for other family members.

> **Case Illustration.** The mother of a 10 year old boy had massive anxiety attacks during his stay in the ICU. Apparently her husband could not console her. In fact, she seemed to find his presence disturbing. As the family systems unfolded, it became clear that the child, a star performer in local entertainment circles, had been the bearer of the family standard. Mother regarded her husband as a failure and the child as "her" only hope for success. The "future" had become head injured.

Second Stage: Return to Consciousness

> Parent: *We made it! Thank God she's better! Better.... What is better? When is better? I know this little girl better than anyone here, and this isn't better! Can I stand to go home more often? My hand shakes and my stomach hurts when I'm not here.... Don't tell me to go back to work and be with my other kids more — I'm NOT your patient! I'm confused and aching inside and need some time to digest this one step at a time...please understand.... Can't I look at this paperwork later? Can you give me something to read? I need to see how my child is doing now, and I can't think of anything else.... How can I help her get better?*

The second stage of acute care begins with the stabilization of the patient. The parents, who usually have had no previous experience with head injuries, begin a period of anxious waiting. The fears, questions, and expectations that had surfaced accompany a sense of relief that the child will live. Struggling to make sense of an incomprehensible situation, they tend to judge head trauma in terms of previously experienced injuries, no matter how unrelated. They may be encouraged or horrified by the "reports" of well-meaning friends and relatives—"My uncle had the same thing, and he's a lawyer now." Such stories do not have a neutral effect; they tend to generate another series of expectations or fears to be dealt with by the family. As Romano (1980) reports, this is a time of fantasy about measurable improvements when none are actually occurring, e.g., perceiving eye opening as recognition of particular persons. Nothing can prepare a family for what they will witness as their child slowly regains consciousness and function. Their feeling of helplessness is rekindled as they watch the struggle to awaken. Often, on staff advice, the parents provide stimulation to help reorient the child, a process that can be quite frustrating when the child does not respond. Parents may need considerable help in recognizing and accepting their feelings as they begin to work with their child, who now seems strange to them.

    Case Illustration. A 10 year old boy slowly regaining consciousness had been in an agitated state of aimless movement, making incoherent sounds. The parents began to spend less time with him, as the mother admitted that "watching that little animal thrash around" was making her extremely anxious. In a reframing exercise, she translated the image of a "little animal" into one of an experimenting newborn infant, a perception that led to more time spent with her son.

As the child makes the dramatic initial gains of returning to consciousness, parents imagine "timetables," as if recovery consisted only of steady progress and had no limits. We hear parents say such things as, "It took her ten days to wake up; at this rate, she'll be back in school in a month." As the patient improves, the family begins to search for distinguishing characteristics of the premorbid child, conjuring up images that color their perceptions of the current situation. They may associate inappropriate behavior with former personality traits. For instance, on seeing a child whose injury has caused lethargy, they might say, "She never would play when adults were around." The nonverbal ballet of family interaction does not change just because a doctor has said that the child may act differently. To minimize future suffering, the professional must help the family to adjust their view of the patient's role in the family by acquainting them with the realities of the recovery process and the dangers of clinging to unrealistic fantasies.

Although parents tend to be hopeful, they are also plagued by legitimate fears about their child's future, fears that can affect their child's future and fears that can affect their own behavior.

    Case Illustration. An 11 year old patient emerged from coma with significant changes in personality and deficits in social consciousness. The formerly reserved boy was now boisterous and lacked awareness of social cues for conversation and bodily contact. As he improved physically but remained confrontive, his mother visited less frequently. In a discussion, she revealed an anxiety-laden fantasy of the boy at home with family and friends. The image moved her away from her son as she anticipated her own embarrassment.

Romano (1980) calls this second recovery stage one of massive denial. In describing the family seemingly out of touch with the reality of posttrauma life, Lezak (1984) describes a struggle in which premorbid perceptions of the patient, mixed with hopes for "recovery," tend to outweigh reality in the short run. Both authors describe the stress reaction of the family, cognitively blinding itself to the new, threatening reality by calling up images of the past or postulating a hopeful future.

Family Interaction

Thus far, we have examined the family response in terms of the parents' view of the patient. It is also important to study the injury's effect on the relationships among siblings and between the parents. After the milestone of survival is reached and improved functioning begins, the normal rhythms of life reestablish themselves. Members of the extended family return to their usual activities; healthy siblings go back to school. One parent, usually the mother, begins to spend more time with the patient. But the family is still in crisis. "[When] evolutionary crises [such as accidents]. . .occur, the family's modes of dealing with these may help to strengthen or weaken functioning or promote or hinder emotional growth in individual members" (Fleck, 1976, p. 114). The most vulnerable marriages are those in which the child has been the bond between the parents. "Rigid" marital relationships can also suffer, as one parent gives up the role at home. Dysfunction can result if one spouse cannot tolerate a broader role definition.

Case Illustration. Two 9 year old patients were regaining consciousness. Both mothers tended to spend more time at the hospital than did their spouses, who were caring for the other children and going to work. Eventually the husbands became resentful of performing their wives' usual duties, complaining that they felt "neglected." One marriage failed to survive the rehabilitation period. The other remained in conflict until the child was placed in a rehabilitation program and the mother returned home.

Familial stress in the indefinite rehabilitation period can cause marital stress, both in troubled marriages and in normally healthy ones. Since this dysfunction, now in its beginning stages, can remain a problem throughout the entire rehabilitation phase, early counseling may be crucial in preserving the marriage.

This stage can challenge a marriage in other ways. Often the spouse who spends more time with the child will complain of the other's "time off" from the hospital, even when it represents working a full day and coming home to other children and the demands of family life. Another problem occurs when the parents develop differing perceptions of the patient. For instance, one spouse may have more contact with the medical staff and more opportunity to observe sporadic improvement. Elated, this spouse is angered by the other's failure to exhibit equal enthusiasm. Alternatively, the spouse who spends more time with the child may become discouraged at a plateau phase in recovery and may resent the other, who, not having seen the child for a day or two, remarks about how much better the patient looks.

The first "victim" of disrupted family life is usually the couple's time to themselves. Other children and the family business are cared for at the expense of the couple's personal needs. The family-oriented professional, stressing the importance of ongoing dialogue that offers mutual support, can show each spouse how to express frustration to the other without fear of being considered a poor parent. The couple must work to prevent one spouse from emerging as the "protector" of the other or one from feeling that he or she is "failing" the other. A session focusing on the rest of the family (not the patient) can also be helpful. Moreover, parents need to hear that it is both necessary and important for them to take care of themselves and to fulfill needs other than simply eating or sleeping. One couple, who would not take even a few hours together, finally relented when presented with a humorous "prescription" on a hospital form, "ordering" a night out.

Siblings

> Parent: *I can't believe what Missy heard in school about her sister...blind...retarded...vegetable...paralyzed!... As if it isn't enough torture to live through this each day. I need to give her an extra hug as soon as I get home. Dear God, protect my child.... What would I do without my friends and family who are constantly praying and taking care of everything? Could I even get out of bed?... Oh, I wish she were better. Thank God for the wonderful nurses who always listen to my words and my heart.*

Helping the other children in the family is as crucial as helping the parents. To do so, we must monitor two ongoing processes: (1) the well siblings' perceptions of the patient, and (2) the effect on the siblings of prolonged disruption in family patterns. Approaches must be keyed to the siblings' developmental stages. The younger the siblings, the more they have been shielded from visiting the patient and from specific information regarding the patient's situation. Therefore, there is more room for fantasy and fear. Rumor, whether it be in the extended family or in the neighborhood, can create enormous anxiety.

Case Illustration. The mother of a hospitalized 10 year old boy found her 6 year old daughter in tears. Her classmates had been taunting her with the idea that her brother was now "retarded" and would be forced into a special school.

It helps to have the parents listen to the child's perception of the patient. Misconceptions can often be discovered in their early stages and cleared away by using age-appropriate terms.

Teenaged siblings also have problems with fantasy, fear, and rumor, these being compounded by their great sensitivity to what others think about the patient and, indirectly, about them.

Case Illustration. A 17 year old boy came to visit his sister, who had marked psychosocial deficits. After spending 15 minutes in her room, he left and refused to return during her hospital stay. When asked by his father, he simply said, "She's not my sister," describing her as "loud, obnoxious, and *embarrassing*." His sister, formerly a popular cheerleader, he now perceived as a social liability.

Teenagers can be more directly involved in family conferences. Their perceptions of the situation are, again, a good place to start. Like the parents, they should be encouraged to express their feelings without fear of being considered insensitive. Only in this way can they learn to modify their picture of life with a head injured sibling.

The healthy children also experience a huge and, to some extent, permanent, disruption in normal family patterns. The parents have less time for them; one parent may even be spending nights at the hospital. The anxiety level is high. The children may be shuffled from one relative to another. Because of these events, we anticipate a variety of responses in siblings.

In younger children, the loss of parental contact can lead to regressive behavior, acting out, or a rejection of the absent parent. In older children, anxiety can cause a change in school performance. Even good students may come to a class unprepared or preoccupied. Teenagers may begin to resent increased household or childcare responsibilities. These and similar reactions can plague not only the acute phase of care but also subsequent family life. The probability and intensity of the disturbances depend upon the severity of the injury, the level of parental adaptation to crisis, the quality of substitute child care, and the amount of time parents must be away.

The family-oriented professional can teach parents to promote discussions that allow the well siblings to vent their anxieties and to receive information and reassurance. Two additional strategies have also proved helpful: (1) parents should be urged to help the healthy siblings preserve as much of their routine as possible, including recreation, and (2) parents should set aside some time, no matter how brief, for interaction with the well children, especially the younger ones, who need contact to "recharge" emotionally and to be assured that they are still important.

Summary

Family response during the acute phase of recovery of a head injured member has a critical effect on both the patient's recovery and the family's immediate and long-term ability to function as a unit. Several studies stress the family's key role in the patient's recovery (Oddy and Humphrey, 1980; Brooks and McKinlay, 1983). The family-oriented professional can aid in the process of family coping in the acute care stage, when the family first encounters the anxiety-laden world of head trauma recovery.

THE REHABILITATION PHASE

REHABILITATION AND THE NUCLEAR FAMILY

Parent: *Why do I have to consider more rehab?... We need to be a family again at home.... Will this never end?! Why can't she receive services as an outpatient? I'm finally feeling like a mom again, and you tell me I have to let go of her again! How can I stand this horrendous pain? Can our family stand more stress? What does my insurance cover when we leave here? Will it pay for rehab? How can we possibly pay for it otherwise?... How will my confused, broken child ever understand that I can't bring her home yet? Will she be afraid she's not going to get better? Will she be afraid I'm leaving her and not coming back? She's doing so many good things now...don't let it stop...I couldn't stand that. Thank God we're finally able to leave this hospital, but how much more?*

The works of Kübler-Ross (1969) and Lezak (1984) provide a helpful framework for understanding parental reactions during the patient's rehabilitation stay. Based on her work with terminally ill patients and their families, Kübler-Ross described a series of emotional reactions: initial denial, bargaining, anger, despair, and depression. She found these reactions to be necessary parts of the process of grieving, which eventually results in acceptance.

Lezak found similar stages and reactions in the families of adult head injured patients. She saw families as remaining hopeful through the early stages of the rehabilitation process, only to become bewildered and anxious as recovery did not meet their expectations. A depressive reaction followed (often after discharge from the rehabilitation facility) as families tried to deal with patients who were changed and often difficult to live with. This reaction includes feelings of self-doubt and guilt, and even of being trapped. Lezak's experience convinced her that with professional help in understanding their patient's injuries and their own responses, families could reach acceptance of the patient's changed state and they could then reorganize their lives around the new circumstances.

In applying this theoretical understanding to the families of head injured children, we need to anticipate that the process of emotional readjustment may require an extensive period of time. Most families are just beginning to face the implications of their patient's injuries at the time of discharge from the rehabilitation center, and many families continue to struggle with these issues 2 or more years later. When we began a lecture series for families of the head injured, we were surprised to find three sets of parents in attendance whose children had incurred their injuries 4 to 8 years previously. These parents were still looking for answers and still dealing with the emotional struggles that precede acceptance.

The uneven, unpredictable, and often long process of recovery from severe head injury by itself interferes with the parents' grieving process. Patients frequently show improvement over the first year or two following the accident. Sometimes the recovery process seems to continue well beyond 2 years, although the rate of progress slows greatly. Families, eagerly looking for reasons to hope, can find them in small signs of improvement and in uncertain prognoses from professionals. Since family members do not know the extent of their loss, the acceptance of residual deficits is a much more gradual and uncertain process than the acceptance of the death of a family member where the extent of the loss can be immediately known. Rosenthal and Muir (1983) use the term "mobile mourning" to describe the extended turmoil that such a partial, uncertain, and lengthy grieving process can create for family members.

Most professionals involved in the treatment of head injured patients agree that family members need information about the nature of head injuries generally and about the specific deficit areas (including behavior and personality changes) that the patient is experiencing (Diehl, 1983; Oddy et al., 1978). However, their anxiety level is often so great in the initial stages of rehabilitation that they cannot process such material and sometimes actively avoid dealing with it. Written material should be available to families to supplement the ongoing education provided by treatment staff in their contacts with individual patients and their families. A regularly repeated lecture series is also helpful. Ross and colleagues stress the importance of family education and recommend a family therapy approach as a vehicle for providing this education (Ross et al., 1983).

Admission Day

> Parent: *More paperwork today. . .interviews. . .procedures. . . . Who gives a damn?! Where's my child? Is she okay? Will they rock her and say prayers with her every day? Will they feed her right? Does anyone here really care about HER?. . . Will she have the right clothes? Will they remember her teddy bear?. . . How can I just leave her?! Can we stand another crisis? Dear God, give us strength to get through this until she's better. Can they make her better? What is better going to be?. . . They don't know how neat she was. . .such a special girl. . . . Do they really know the answers? Will everyone work hard? I just wish I could observe them every day. I hope someone will let me know what's happening in every therapy—PT. . .OT. . .ST. . .CRT. . .psychologists. . .neurologists. . . ophthalmologists. . . physiatrists. . .social service. . . . Sometimes I could just scream!!!*

On admission day into the rehabilitation facility, parents and other family members are generally anxious and emotionally distraught. It is common to find them that first day in tears or with migraine headaches or tense, nervous postures and body movements. Unfortunately, the admission process itself is usually a demanding one. Parents must meet many new people who will be important in their child's care. They are required to recount over and over again their ordeal with the patient's initial trauma and subsequent treatment.

Parents may also have conflicting feelings about rehabilitation, doubts about the caring and competence of the new facility, and fears about the separation from their child. They may be very worried about the patient, who may still be physically ill or severely confused. All of these factors combine to increase their stress.

At our facility the social worker's first contact with the family is a screening, which is built into the admission process through the joint completion of a "Lifeline" report. The Lifeline is a questionnaire designed to gather important information about the patient, which is later distributed to therapists and nursing unit staff to aid in their work with the patient. Gathering descriptive data about the child's pretraumatic personality, hobbies, interests, and other relevant biographical information makes this initial contact less threatening for families since the focus continues to be on the patient. The information about the child is helpful to all treatment staff in learning to know the patient as a person.

The initial contact can also serve the following purposes:

- To assess how the family members are coping with their stresses and to determine whether or not they have a network of support among extended family and friends.

- To determine the family's needs for transportation, financial support, and child care and to explore possible resources.
- To address their "creature comforts" at the rehabilitation facility, including guest house accommodations and the location of cafeterias and recreational facilities.
- To communicate to parents that it is normal and expected for them to express strong feelings and concerns and that it is important for them to care for their own needs.

In our experience, the trauma of separation that occurs when a child is admitted to a rehabilitation facility can be eased by a policy of liberal visiting hours and by guest house accommodations for out-of-town families. Absent parents are also encouraged to telephone frequently for progress reports.

Patterns of Emotional Reaction Over Time

In this section the emotional reactions frequently observed in family members when the progress of their loved one is slow and the rehabilitation phase correspondingly long are discussed briefly. These reactions include anxiety and helplessness, denial, guilt, anger, and despair. As parents begin to settle into the rehabilitation routine, they are often hopeful, although very anxious and unsure. Because they feel helpless, they will seek verification of their hopes. They also become aware of the complexity of head injury treatment.

Families of patients whose recovery is rapid and whose residual deficits are minor adjust emotionally with relative ease. These families, although initially anxious, soon relax and become optimistic about the future. It is almost as though they have received a reprieve from a heavy punishment. These parents know that they are fortunate because the progress of their children has been more rapid than that of other patients on the unit. They are able to mobilize their energies sooner, which we observe in their seeking out and integrating information about their patient's deficits and in their steady cooperation with the rehabilitation staff. They are also able to focus concern on other family members and on other aspects of their lives. Some of these parents, with professional help, are able to use this crisis and interim time to take stock of their lives and to emerge as stronger and more confident individuals.

Anxiety and Helplessness

Parents of children whose progress is not rapid maintain a high level of anxiety. They continue to seek verification of their hopes but at some point become frustrated with "wait and see" answers to their questions.

Parent: *Is this it?! She was making so much progress, and now she's practically going backwards — incredible and appalling — I can hardly swallow my food again. . . . Do I need to change doctors? Change rehab facilities? Oh, what can I do to help her get better? I'm terrified if this is what "better" is supposed to mean. Such a waste to lose that special personality. She's GOT to get better. . . . Missy can't believe this is really her little sister — She can hardly talk or look at her, and everyone's telling me to be patient. Who are they kidding?! I spend half of my day praying and crying and the other half cursing and screaming inside. . . . Maureen prefers the babysitter to me — and just when did that happen? Will we ever be a family again?*

A parent's anxiety can take many forms. Sometimes it takes the form of "doing." One mother may insist that her child receive several hours of physical therapy daily (on the theory that if some therapy is good, more is better), whereas another may persist in preparing special "health foods" for her child despite dietary and medical contraindications. Some family members experience sleeplessness or weight loss. Stress on the relatives of head injured patients often continues over time, even though the specific concerns may change (Bond, 1983; Oddy, Humphrey, and Uttley, 1978). The social worker should acknowledge the parents' fears and feelings of helplessness and attempt to redirect parents' anxious energy into more constructive tasks.

Denial

Denial of a patient's deficits or of their long-term significance is a persistent and pervasive reaction for most family members during the rehabilitation stay (Romano, 1980), particularly in the early phase of rehabilitation. It is a normal response to painful news and a defense mechanism that gives families the time they need to assimilate and to accept the implication of the injury sustained by their loved one. In this respect, it is healthy and necessary. At support group meetings we have heard parents express intense anger about being repeatedly told bad news about their patients' injuries before they could handle such news. Most admit that at a deep level they knew that what they were hearing was true, but they also knew that they were not ready to admit it.

Denial takes many forms. Sometimes it appears as the reporting of changes in the child that no one else can see. Sometimes it appears as concentration on seemingly inconsequential issues, such as a health food diet, for a child who sustained massive brain damage. Sometimes it takes the form of openly disputing the judgment of treatment staff or demanding that they work with the child at a level far beyond the child's current abilities.

Some degree of denial often continues for family members throughout the rehabilitation period. It is pathologic only when it interferes with needed treatment or with the patient's welfare, or when it continues to the point of disrupting family life and harming other family members.

> **Case Illustration.** One mother was still professing hope for a return to normalcy of her very badly damaged child 2 years after the injury. She often saw gains in the child that no one else was able to observe or duplicate. She admitted the child to whatever treatment facilities would accept her, to the neglect of her angry husband and other children at home. So desperate was her need to restore this child that she repeatedly fought with therapists over prescribed treatments until they discharged the child or she withdrew the child from therapy.

In responding to parents' questions and statements that suggest unrealistic beliefs and expectations, it is important to be honest but also to show respect for the parents' feelings and their need to hope. If parents reject information they are given, staff should not argue, but rather respectfully restate the information and then drop the subject. Questions about specific aspects of the patient's program should always be referred to the appropriate staff member.

Confrontational techniques, especially in the early phase of rehabilitation, are ineffective, often serving only to alienate the parents. However, when denial interferes with the patient's welfare, confrontation becomes necessary. The technique is most effective when planned among several key staff members so that support can be combined with confrontation. For example, the treatment team may ask the physician to give the bad news while the social worker prepares to aid the family afterwards.

With education, repetition of information, experience, and support over time, most family members eventually come to accept the patient's deficits. They are then able to integrate their experience of loss, freeing themselves to cope effectively with their patient's changed needs and behaviors. Bond (1983) states that this process occurs for most family members between 1 and 2 years post injury. Our observations suggest that although for most the major adjustments have taken place within a 2 year period, some families require much more time.

Guilt

Guilt is a natural response to any tragic event or loss. It is also a common component of the dynamics of depression. When parents have an injured child, guilt is pervasive since the parents' role includes nurturing and protection. Harm to their child indicates to most parents that they have somehow failed despite the circumstances of the accident.

Early in the rehabilitation phase the parents are told that their feelings of guilt are a normal response to the tragedy so that they can place this feeling into perspective. It is useful to remind parents that harm is the last thing they would have wanted for their child—that despite the circumstances of the accident, their concern was solely for their child's well-being. Parents who have reason to feel responsible for the child's accident (for example, as driver of the car) experience guilt in a particularly acute manner. This may result in chronic depression or denial. Techniques to help these parents reduce the stress of their guilt include the following: reminding the parents that their intentions for the child have been good; demonstrating acceptance, caring, and concern for the parents as individuals; and helping parents to recognize that raising children involves risks and that protection can never be complete.

Later in the rehabilitation period, guilt and feelings of inadequacy can combine to leave parents unsure of their ability to care for and make decisions for their child. We help these parents by giving them information about these feelings and their dynamics and about their child's condition and needs so that the parents can again feel that they are making intelligent and well-informed decisions for their child.

Anger

Many parents feel anger at some point in the rehabilitation process, usually brought about by their growing feelings of frustration and helplessness in the face of their child's slow progress. The anger is sometimes diffuse and sometimes specifically directed. It may be directed at family members or at the person who caused the accident. It may take the form of growing resentment toward a particular staff person or toward the agency as a whole. Occasionally, parents say that they are angry with God. It is deeply moving to watch family members struggle to maintain their faith while they question how they could have sinned so or how any being could allow such a tragedy to happen.

Angry parents require understanding and acceptance in the face of their anger, and they need to understand the source of this anger. Social service staff can provide a setting in which parents freely voice their frustrations and in which they are understood and accepted. With help in exploring their feelings, family members become better able to identify the source of their anger and to learn about the grieving process which they are undergoing.

It is also very important for other rehabilitation professionals to understand the dynamics of the family's grief and to be able to treat angry parents with respect and concern rather than defensiveness. When one staff person becomes the object of a parent's anger, colleagues should recognize this and provide the support needed for that staff member to maintain a therapeutic relationship with the patient and the family.

Despair—A True Depressive Reaction

Despair, which is a true depressive reaction, may recur intermittently during the rehabilitation process. For some, it occurs early, possibly as the result of the loss of another family member in the same accident in which the patient was injured. For others, it occurs when a badly injured child seems to reach a plateau in progress. Still others experience despair during discharge planning because it appears to them that the experts have "given up" on their child and have little hope for future gains. Finally, the loss of hope may occur following discharge when parents experience fully their changed and damaged child.

Parents can face these terribly painful feelings better if forewarned that they will occur and that they are normal responses. Therefore we describe to the parents the symptoms of depression, including the feeling that they are going crazy or that they are the world's worst parents. Having heard these warnings, they are also more likely to seek help and to talk about their feelings when the depression begins. During such periods of despair, the most powerful professional tools are good listening and an empathic concern. It is also helpful to reassure parents regularly that their depression is normal and that it will gradually ease.

Although situational and usually time-limited, these depressions can become dysfunctional and dangerous. It is necessary to warn the other family members of the need to call for help if the depressed member appears suicidal and to seek psychiatric consultation if the depression does not begin to change and lift over a period of a few months.

Parents and Their Personal Needs

Caught up in the crisis of concern for their head injured child, family members, and especially parents, have difficulty disengaging themselves from this level of concern. They seriously neglect other areas of their lives. They may, for instance, indefinitely postpone their own medical appointments and treatments.

> **Case Illustration.** Two years after her daughter's accident, one mother became increasingly concerned about her tiredness and weight loss. She finally discovered that this was due to badly infected teeth, which had been scheduled for extraction just following her daughter's injury and had simply been forgotten. Still fearful of leaving her daughter, she was now able, with urging, to reschedule the needed dental appointments.

It is very important for professionals to assure family members that they do not need to devote all their attention to the injured child. We urge them to attend to their own needs and offer them assistance in doing so when necessary. An afternoon shopping, a day at the beach, or an evening out can help parents to maintain a balanced perspective about their obligations to their child and to themselves. For many parents, however, the first few outings are very painful. One mother likened her pain to physical withdrawal. Professionals must help parents to understand that it is better for their child in the long run if they take care of themselves as well.

Siblings

In head injury rehabilitation, siblings are probably the most overlooked of family members. As mentioned in the discussion of the acute phase, siblings can experience significant adjustment difficulties as a result of the family tragedy. This, in turn, can negatively affect the adjustment of the family unit and the long-term recovery of the patient. Sibling reactions may include feelings of neglect, embarrassment about the patient's disability, guilt about surviving and being normal, resentment toward the patient for monopolizing the parents' attention and focus, and hostility for being burdened by the patient's need for care.

Treatment decisions depend upon the sibling's age and situation. It is helpful to include older siblings in parent conferences or to engage them in volunteer roles among other head injured patients to aid them in gaining perspective. With younger siblings it is preferable to assist parents in forming explanations of the accident and resulting injuries to present to them. Group discussion with preadolescent and adolescent siblings is useful to promote an understanding of head injuries. The group can also address other important issues, such as how to deal with peers who ridicule the injured sibling or what to do when parents will not talk about the problems posed by the injured sibling's behavior. Adolescents are also concerned with the responsibilities that they are given to care for the injured sibling when the parents are gone, and with the fairness of these expectations.

Milestones

On a day-to-day basis, most parents focus narrowly on what needs to be done at the moment. A broader perspective and the devastating pain that accompanies it are pushed aside. There are several milestones, however, in the course of a rehabilitation stay, which crystallize and make more acute their awareness of their child's deficits and their own resulting emotional pain. These include the first weekend home, readmission to an acute care hospital, emerging behavior patterns, discharge from rehabilitation, and community school placement. It is important that helping professionals recognize the effects that these events may have on parents and provide the parents with the understanding and support they will need to cope with them. Parents should be warned of the potential effects these events might have on them and be encouraged to communicate their feelings about them.

Each of the following illustrates one parent's emotional reactions to these milestones.

First Weekend Home

Parent: *I'm ecstatic we're going to be a whole family again! When will someone tell me what to do? I'm afraid she'll "break"... she seems so emotionally fragile. Can I remember the logbook, medications, her helmet, and all the care she needs? There seems so much! If I forget and she has a seizure, I'll feel so guilty. Who can I call if there's trouble? The other kids will just have to wait. I've no more energy! They're feeling so cheated and resentful, but just let's get through this weekend. Don't they understand there's no more to give? Dear God, we can't do this alone. Help us!... We did it! Everyone pulled together, and we made it! She did so well... maybe she will get better! Really better.... We're all exhausted—thought I'd die when she cried and hung on and begged me to stay, but we can do it again until we are finally out of this place!*

Setbacks to Acute Care

Parent: *Not again! Is this necessary? Will this work? Why wasn't this caught earlier? How much more can she take... poking, shoving, pinching.... We're all ready to scream! Was there any more damage this time? If anyone else tells me they don't know for sure I just might punch them! Can someone please tell me what is happening and why? I can't wait until we can go back to rehab and get better.... What we wouldn't give for a break from this constant pressure. WHEN?*

Emerging Behavior Patterns

Parent: *It's so embarrassing for everyone to see her doing such weird things—no one understands. How can I explain? Why do I have to explain?! If anyone else tells me she looks OK, when they don't have any idea what it is like to live here day after day, I'll scream. She doesn't realize people are staring* and laughing, thank God...or is that good? Maybe if she did then we could work on that behavior—but NOT another behavior modification program! Between the logbook and keeping peace at home on weekends, don't add another star chart! Straighten out one behavior, and something else always comes up. I just wish she could be her old self. I die inside when she acts so inappropriately or cries and says she hates herself.... We all love her so much. Will this ache ever go away? Will we ever have confidence that she will be happy as her life goes on? Her old friends don't want to play anymore—such loneliness.... She doesn't interact well, but then she is so upset when they go. Some days go smoothly, and others—CRASH! We start again. Oh, how I desperately wish she were better.... How will she ever get back to school or hold a job—or more to the point, what will she be able to do? I'm so tired of trying to figure out what and when to do things! Maybe this is partly a normal stage for kids...I wish I could believe that.

Community School Placement

Parent: Another mountain...who can teach me the ropes? Doesn't anyone understand I need the best for her? After all this work, if she falls apart, can we glue her back together again? What are my rights? How can I convince the school administrators what we need? Is ongoing therapy available in the district? Do these people know ANYTHING about head injury? Are there good teachers? Can my daughter handle this change? I'm overwhelmed thinking about it. Her old playmates are gone—it makes me so angry, but they're just kids. Will she make new friends and KEEP them? What about the relationships with her sisters? WILL THIS UNENDING FRUSTRATION EVER GO AWAY? Do we really know how to manage everything? We encourage, hope, and work for the best, but I just wish I could protect her from this pain....

Discharge from Rehabilitation

Parent: Is this it? I hope we've done our best. Have we tried hard enough? What else is there to do for her?... It seems eons ago I was pacing outside that ICU. Can I remember all the doctors and therapists? I can't believe this is the end.... Everything I've read says progress continues for several years. Hope it does.... She is so much better, but how can we ever get her ALL better? It's so scary to leave all the support we have had for so long. God, give me courage and support so we can know how to do what needs to be done—but how long can we really do it? Who is going to help us day after day now?

Discharge is not the end. For many families the complete realization of their child's deficits and changes will occur after they return home. With this awareness will often come self-doubts and grieving. Families should be forewarned of this possibility at discharge time and their continued contact with the rehabilitation staff encouraged. A follow-up plan, designed to ensure contact with the family over the following year, assures that they will receive the support, guidance, and information they might need. With time and guidance, they may be able to integrate their nightmare experiences and to resume living again.

> Parent: *Observing her has sometimes been like watching a movie on child development, but when she learned these things as a baby, everything was a lot easier for everyone, especially her. . . . It's more thrilling to watch this time. We're all cheering! She's working so hard; I just want to hug her and tell her how proud we are. . . . Her OT, PT, and CRT therapists are really helping her relearn so much. It's so nice to go out in public and not have people stare and ask stupid questions anymore — no, she's not retarded; yes, she fell. . . . Isn't she better? What is wrong with her then? If her "thinking part" will just start working as fast as her arms and legs, we'll be all set! If she could just learn to hang in there— she can do it! Each little thing is progress, so GO FOR IT!*

Responding to Common Parental Concerns

All members of the rehabilitation team should be prepared to deal responsibly with parents' questions and concerns. Because parents spend much of their time on the rehabilitation nursing unit, this is a likely setting for the expression of these concerns.

Table 3–1 lists suggested responses to concerns that are commonly expressed by family members. It can be difficult for nursing staff to remain respectful and supportive of family members who are struggling to process and integrate new information and disturbing realities. Family members may be as emotionally demanding as the patients. The key principles for nursing staff to remember when interacting with family members are the following: maintain respect; give information directly and simply; and anticipate the need for repetition.

CONCLUSION

Head injury has a devastating impact on the family as well as on the patient. Stresses on individual members and on the unit as a whole are severe and remain so over the first year and even beyond. In working with the family, professionals attempt to help them reduce stresses to a manageable level and maintain family integrity despite the crisis in their lives. To achieve these goals, the helping professional needs an awareness of characteristic family reactions in this crisis and a knowledge of the grieving process. Techniques of empathic support, clarification for families of their responses, and repetition of information about their child's injuries will enable most families, over time, to integrate their loss and to provide effective nurturing and support to their head injured loved one.

Table 3–1. Nursing Guide: Responding to Common Parental Concerns

Parent Concern	Possible Nursing Response	Comments
"What should I tell my daughter about her injury?"	"It's so difficult, but it is best to tell her what has happened. You may want me to be with you when you talk about it, or you may want to be there when we talk to her about it. It may be necessary to repeat it many times. We should keep it clear and simple so she will begin to understand where she is and why she's here."	Supportive approach to fearful and painful event and unknown response of child; offers modeling for future interaction.
"You do things very differently here. Are you sure it was a good idea for my daughter to be transferred so soon?"	"Although procedures are different here, you can rest assured that your daughter is safe. We have many fewer infections here than in a general acute care hospital. Your daughter's condition is more stable now and we want family members to understand and participate in care if they wish."	Deals with the concern respectfully; gives clear reasons why differences exist; provides reassurance regarding quality of care and safety.
"Should we bring her friends and other relatives in to visit now?"	"Although it's important for her to see familiar people, it's also very important that your daughter not be overstimulated or in situations in which others are out of control. Some people have a hard time visiting so it's probably best to have one extra visitor at a time."	States the importance of visits from important and familiar people; maintains needed control for patient, family, and staff.
"I don't feel as though my daughter is kept busy enough. If her day is filled with activity, won't it speed up her recovery?"	"Our experience has shown us that the quality of stimulation and therapy has a healthier effect than quantity. It can be frustrating and the results can sometimes seem small and slow. It's hard to see recovery taking so much	Avoids defensive posture on staff's part; acknowledges the concern; states clear rationale for approach to stimulation programming.

Table continued on following page.

Table 3-1 (continued).

	time. Talking with the therapists about their treatment programs might help you."	
"What should I be doing for my daughter?"	"On the unit you can help with those aspects of care which you feel comfortable doing safely. We will be glad to teach you procedures at your own pace and of course we will make sure it's safe. You're not expected to be an instant expert."	Assures parents that neither they nor the patient will be abandoned; extends supportive welcome to participate in care; reinforces safety.
"What should we bring from home?"	"Some children seem to be comforted by having their favorite stuffed animal, doll, blanket or other favorite things. Stories or songs on a cassette read or sung by family members can help you all to feel closer; you can make a tape as you read to your daughter right at the bedside or at home on the weekend."	Emphasizes the quality of items rather than the potential emptiness of too many things; tapes give families an opportunity to say things to their children and listen to them again themselves, thus giving them valuable feedback as well as comfort for their children.
"God will provide a miracle to cure my daughter at the proper time."	"Your faith must be a true source of hope and comfort during this difficult time. Part of the miracle that we see happening to families like yours is the unbelievable strength that you seem to have during a time when you must be exhausted and drained. It seems incredible that your daughter has survived such a devastating injury; we will surely do our best now to see that as complete as possible a recovery is achieved."	Acknowledges both the child's and parent's ordeal in a constructive way; does not offer false hope or feed into unrealistic expectations brought about by desperation; maintains honesty and respect.

REFERENCES

Beck, A. (1976). *Cognitive therapy and the emotional disorders.* New York: International Universities Press.

Bond, M. R. (1983). Effects on the family system. In M. Rosenthal, E. R. Griffith, M. R. Bond, and J. D. Miller (Eds.), *Rehabilitation of the head-injured adult* (pp. 209–217). Philadelphia: F. A. Davis.

Brooks, D. N., and McKinlay, W. (1983). Personality and behavioral change after severe blunt head injury — a relative's view. *Journal of Neurology, Neurosurgery, and Psychiatry, 46,* 336–344.

Diehl, L. N. (1983). Patient-family education. In M. Rosenthal, E. R. Griffith, M. R. Bond, and J. D. Miller (Eds.), *Rehabilitation of the head-injured adult* (pp. 395–401). Philadelphia: F. A. Davis.

Epperson, M. (1980). Families in sudden crisis: Process and intervention in a critical care center. In P. Power and A. Dell Orto (Eds.), *Role of the family in the rehabilitation of the physically disabled* (pp. 402–410). Baltimore: University Park Press.

Fleck, S. (1976). An approach to family pathology. In G. Erickson and T. Horgan (Eds.), *Family therapy: An introduction to theory and techniques* (pp. 103–119). New York: Aronson.

Herz, F. (1980). The impact of death and serious illness on the family life cycle. In E. Carter and M. McGoldrick (Eds.), *The family life cycle: A framework for family therapy* (pp. 223–240). New York: Gardner Press.

Kübler-Ross, E. (1969). *On death and dying.* New York: Macmillan.

Lezak, M. D. (1984). *Psychological implications of traumatic brain damage for the patient's family* (Unpublished manuscript).

McKinlay, W. W., Brooks, D. N., Bond, M. R., Martinage, D. P., and Marshall, M. M. (1981). The short-term outcome of severe blunt head injury as reported by relatives of the injured persons. *Journal of Neurology, Neurosurgery, and Psychiatry, 44,* 527–533.

Oddy, M., and Humphrey, M. (1980). Social recovery during the year following severe head injury. *Journal of Neurology, Neurosurgery, and Psychiatry, 43,* 798–802.

Oddy, M., Humphrey, M., and Uttley, D. (1978). Stresses upon the relatives of head-injured patients. *British Journal of Psychiatry, 133,* 507–513.

Ravenscroft, K. (1982). Psychiatric consultation to the child with acute physical trauma. *American Journal of Orthopsychiatry, 52,* 298–307.

Romano, M. (1980). Family response to traumatic head injury. In P. Power and A. Dell Orto (Eds.), *Role of the family in the rehabilitation of the physically disabled* (pp. 257–263). Baltimore: University Park Press.

Rosenthal, M., and Muir, C. A. (1983). Methods of family education. In M. Rosenthal, E. R. Griffith, M. R. Bond, and J. D. Miller (Eds.), *Rehabilitation of the head-injured adult* (pp. 407–419). Philadelphia: F. A. Davis.

Ross, B., Ben-Yishay, Y., Lakin, P., Piasetsky, E., Rattok, J., and Diller, L. (1983) The role of family therapy in the treatment of the severely brain injured. In Y. Ben-Yishay (Ed.), *Working approaches to remediation of cognitive deficits in brain damaged persons* (Rehabilitation monograph No. 66) (pp. 113–126). New York: New York University Medical Center, Institute of Rehabilitation Medicine.

Rothstein, P. (1980). Psychological stress in families of children in a pediatric intensive care unit. *Pediatric Clinics of North America, 27,* 613–620.

Weddell, R., Oddy, M., and Jenkins, D. (1980). Social adjustment after rehabilitation: A two year follow-up of patients with severe head injury. *Psychological Medicine, 10*(2), 257–263.

PART III
COMPREHENSIVE MEDICAL
MANAGEMENT

In addition to the sensory, motor, and cognitive deficits often associated with severe head injury, a variety of other problems may be present that require careful medical attention. It is not uncommon, for example, for patients to sustain internal or skeletal injuries in the accident that produced the head injury. The primary goal of medical and nursing care is to maintain the patient's overall health and to prevent complications so that rehabilitation can progress as vigorously as possible. In addition, rehabilitation nursing staff members are in a position to reinforce and potentiate all aspects of the patient's rehabilitation, including intervention with families.

In Chapter 4, Chamovitz, Chorazy, Hanchett, and Mandella discuss the physician's and dietitian's roles within a rehabilitation team in procuring all necessary diagnostic and treatment services for the patient and in overseeing the delivery of medical services. The authors discuss medical problems that occur during rehabilitation, emphasizing nutritional management and seizure control—both prominent aspects of the medical care of severely head injured children.

In Chapter 5, Yanko, Barovitch, Kozik, and O'Donnell discuss the changing focus of nursing intervention throughout a patient's rehabilitation. They emphasize the effects of essential acute care medical and nursing management on subsequent rehabilitation and the necessity of integrating nursing goals with those of other rehabilitation therapies.

Chapter 4

Rehabilitative Medical Management

Irvin Chamovitz, MD, FAAP,
Anna J. L. Chorazy, MD, FAAP,
Jeanne M. Hanchett, MD, FAAP, and
Phyllis-Ann Mandella, RD*

Severe head injury is one of the medical occurrences which catapults a healthy child into a state of chronic illness. The damage done to the brain at the moment of injury cannot be cured. Consequently, disabilities resulting from severe head injury are of great significance to the patient, to the family, and to those involved in the patient's care. The tragedy of head injury in children is incalculable because of the many years ahead of them.

The goal for rehabilitative medical management is to provide all of the necessary services that patients require to recover maximally and to compensate adequately for lost or impaired function while they continue to develop physically, cognitively, and socially to their fullest potential. To meet this goal we also attempt to prevent complications that will interfere with rehabilitative treatment and lead to further disability as well as future disease. Ideally, rehabilitation should begin in the intensive care unit and continue in the acute care setting until the child is transferred to a formal rehabilitation program (see Chapter 5).

The optimal time for transfer is the point at which children begin to show some awareness of their environment and some ability to respond to it. This is called "rehabilitation readiness." Occasionally we admit patients who are minimally responsive to the environment, particularly if it is within 3 months of the injury. Intensive therapy is provided for

*Authorship listed alphabetically at authors' request.

a 60 day trial period and the patient is discharged at that time if there is no improvement.

The capabilities of the rehabilitation setting are as important as the patient's readiness. Units that are an integral part of an acute care hospital can effectively manage patients whose conditions are less stable medically. Free-standing rehabilitation hospitals require that patients be medically stable, which includes the absence of infection and the ability to breathe independently. Hence, we generally do not accept children who are febrile or respirator-dependent. We make exceptions to this rule when the acute care hospital performs an extensive diagnostic investigation and finds that the fever is central in origin–that is, caused by hypothalamic injury. Patients with tracheostomy, gastrostomy, or nasogastric tubes are admitted, and attempts are made to remove these tubes as soon as it is medically safe. We also admit patients with orthopedic devices, such as stabilizing halos, body jackets, and braces. The physician who cares for children in a rehabilitation setting must be familiar with all aspects of child development as well as the pathologic sequelae related to head injury and their effects on a dynamically changing nervous system.

A comprehensive evaluation of head injured children includes a detailed history, parts of which, such as the "Lifeline," are obtained by other team members (see Chapter 3). The physical examination must be thorough, containing all the elements of a good evaluation, with special emphasis on the neurologic-neuromuscular systems (see Table 4–1). Outlines such as this one should be used only as a guide. Children must be considered individually in terms of their pretraumatic status, genetic background, stage of development, severity and location of head injury, associated multiple system injuries, and complications prior to admission to the rehabilitation program.

The rehabilitative medical care of children and adolescents properly belongs to the primary care physician, who shares responsibility and works closely with appropriate medical-surgical specialists and health-related professionals. Customary initial orders are outlined in Table 4–2. Computed tomographic CT scan, electroencephalograms (EEGs), or evoked potentials are not ordered routinely; typically, these have been performed during the acute care period. Such diagnostic procedures are undertaken only as indicated by such events as deterioration in neuroglogic status, significant change in seizure pattern, or evidence of increased intracranial pressure. Initial orders for all patients include consultation with medical subspecialists, including a pediatric physiatrist, neurologist, ophthalmologist, and dentist. We maintain frequent communication with the referring neurosurgeon whenever possible. On admission all patients are evaluated by a dietitian, physical therapist, occupational therapist,

Table 4-1. Admission History and Physical Examination

Name:	Physical examination
Date of Birth:	Vital signs
Date of Admission:	Weight
Reason for admission:	Height (length)
History of present illness:	Head circumference
Past medical history:	General appearance
Prenatal and neonatal	Head
Growth and development	Eyes
Behavior and personality	Ears
Diseases of childhood	Nose
Immunizations	Mouth, teeth, and pharynx
Previous hospitalizations	Neck
Surgery	Lymph nodes
Allergies	Chest
Drug allergies	Breasts
Seizures	Heart
Medications	Lungs
Review of systems	Abdomen
General health	Genitalia
Eyes and vision	Skin
Ears and hearing	Spine and back
Dental	Extremities
Cardiovascular	Neurologic
Respiratory	Mental status and developmental level
Gastrointestinal	Cranial nerves
Genitourinary	Sensory system
Musculoskeletal	Motor system
Neurologic	Reflexes
Skin	Pathologic reflexes
Endocrine	Coordination
Educational-social history	Diagnostic impressions
Family history	Plan

speech-language pathologist, cognitive rehabilitation specialist, neuropsychologist, and social worker. When medical findings on admission indicate that additional evaluations are needed, consultation may be obtained from a pediatric orthopedist, otolaryngologist, gastroenterologist, general surgeon, pulmonologist, urologist, or endocrinologist.

MEDICAL PROBLEMS DURING REHABILITATION

A variety of medical problems can occur during the rehabilitation of head injured children. Some are life-threatening whereas others are minor. All require appropriate diagnosis and care. We list below the most common problems that we encounter.

Table 4–2. Customary Initial Orders for Head Injury Patients on Admission to Rehabilitation

1. Diet
2. Vital Signs
3. Tine test or other tuberculin skin test
4. Laboratory studies: complete blood count (CBC)
   Chemscreen, anticonvulsant blood levels (if indicated)
   Urinalysis and urine culture with colony count
5. Medications
6. Institute seizure record
7. Physiatry consultation
8. Ophthalmology consultation
9. Neurology consultation
10. Psychiatry consultation, if indicated
11. Psychology consultation
12. Dental consultation
13. Nutrition consultation
14. Orthopedic consultation, if indicated
15. Physical therapy evaluation
16. Occupational therapy evaluation
17. Feeding evaluation
18. Speech-language evaluation
19. Cognitive rehabilitation therapy evaluation
20. Social service consultation
21. Neurosurgical follow-up with referring surgeon, when possible

---

Airway Problems

Aspiration is always a concern with head-inujred children, who may not chew or swallow effectively and who often lack the judgment necessary to eat safely. Each patient who is not independently eating a regular diet at the time of admission receives a complete feeding and swallowing evaluation by a feeding therapist (see Chapter 7). Despite this, the possibility of aspiration continues to be a concern with these patients. Our experience indicates that aspiration pneumonia is rare if the evaluation of feeding is thorough and the management of feeding disorders is done with appropriate caution. Certain food consistencies are particularly dangerous and should be avoided. Patients with neurogenic swallowing disorders often have greatest difficulty with thin liquids. Patients with oral motor dysfunction should not be given difficult-to-chew foods (e.g., tough meats, raw vegetables, fruits with tough skins). Patients with judgment disorders should be monitored and should not have free access to foods that could cause choking.

The most severe emergency is tracheostomy malfunction in a patient who is dependent on the tracheostomy tube to breathe. Mucus plugs, tracheal granulomas, and displaced tracheostomy tubes are the most common causes of sudden respiratory distress in these patients. They demand immediate intervention by the closest competent clinician, be it a physician or a skilled nurse. When a mucus plug is suspected, suctioning of the airway should be done. If that does not relieve the distress, removal of the tube, resuctioning, and replacement may be life-saving. Proper lubrication of the tube helps to avoid difficulty with reinsertion. It may be necessary to reinsert a smaller tube initially. Routine changing of tracheostomy tubes in tracheostomy tube–dependent patients can be dangerous. Appropriate measures should be taken to prepare for emergencies, such as inability to reinsert a tube, bleeding, or acute respiratory distress. This includes the availability of an emergency cart, oxygen, suctioning equipment, and extra tracheostomy tubes of various sizes, as well as rapid transport to an acute care facility, if necessary.

It is safest to assume that patients who have a tracheostomy may have a tracheal granuloma. We always request a direct bronchoscopic examination by a pediatric otolaryngologist before permanent removal of the tube. Prior to this referral we carefully assess the patient's ability to breathe without the tracheostomy by gradually reducing the size of the tube or covering it for short periods of time while closely observing the patient. In frightened children this sometimes must be done by the physician standing by the bedside observing respiratory effort with the tracheostomy tube open and closed. If necessary we occlude the tube playfully using the examiner's finger or using the child's own finger. Employing such methods, the physician can usually make a reliable judgment as to whether or not the patient is dependent on this airway (Stool and Beele, 1973). An additional problem that we rarely see is late-occurring tracheal granuloma or tracheal stenosis. These lesions usually present as changes in vocal quality, stridor, or croup-like symptoms. Studies such as lateral neck radiographs, pulmonary function tests, and bronchoscopy aid in diagnosis of these problems.

Seizures

This serious sequela of head injury is discussed later in this chapter.

Nutritional Problems

Some patients who have been unconscious for several weeks or more are malnourished at the time of admission to the rehabilitation program. Nasogastric and gastrostomy tube feedings with appropriate nutrient and fluid content are essential during this time. A well-trained dietitian who is readily available for consultation aids immeasureably in achieving an anabolic state during brain recovery. Obesity may become a problem in late stages of recovery, particularly among those who are wheelchair-bound. A frequently overlooked fact is that fewer calories are required to maintain weight when a patient is nonambulatory. This important topic is covered later in the chapter.

Hypertension

Transitory hypertension can occur after localized or diffuse brain trauma (Zülch, 1969). During the acute period of management of head trauma, hypertension is a frequent occurrence (see Chapter 1). In most cases this is transitory and has resolved before transfer for rehabilitation services. A small number of patients continue to manifest elevation in diastolic pressure after the period of increased intracranial pressure has subsided. When a patient is on antihypertensive medication at the time of admission to the rehabilitation facility, the medication should be continued for the first few weeks, then tapered slowly if blood pressures remain normal. Most patients are not receiving antihypertensive medications at the time of admission to our facility or are safely taken off these medications soon after admission. Rarely patients may continue to have hypertension due to structural lesions in the hypothalamus for months or years after injury.

Urinary or Urologic Problems

It is common for patients with severe head injury to have urinary tract infection during the course of treatment. Many of these infections are caused by an indwelling catheter, necessary during the acute management of injuries. Indwelling catheters should be removed as early as possible to avoid infection and to prevent urethral strictures, which are a significant long-term problem in some male patients who have had Foley catheters inserted. External urinary collecting devices (condom-catheters) can replace indwelling catheters in adolescent male patients. However, there are no satisfactory urinary devices for young boys or female patients. Prolonged bed rest and incomplete emptying of the bladder, which may occur in the severely involved, slowly recovering patient, increase the risk of infection. Since these infections are often unaccompanied by fever, we routinely order periodic urine cultures. A high fluid intake is also maintained as an additional means of preventing infection and urinary stones. When fever occurs and physical examination does not reveal an obvious cause, a urine culture should be obtained. We choose appropriate antibiotics on the basis of antibiotic sensitivities. The loss of cortical control of bladder and bowel function requires that patients be toileted regularly in order to retrain these functions. A small percentage of the most severely involved patients never regain urinary or bowel continence. Many children have a prolonged period of enuresis but ultimately do achieve day and night continence.

Fever and Infection

Fever is most often due to infection, either bacterial or viral. In children viral illnesses are much more common than bacterial infections. Careful determination of site and type of infection is important. Antibiotics a.e not helpful in viral illnesses. Cultures of the throat and urine should be routine in children with a significant fever to determine the cause of the infection and the possible need for antibiotic treatment. The most common sites of viral infection are the upper respiratory tract and pharynx. Bacterial infections commonly occur in the middle ear, urinary tract, lungs, and skin. The central nervous system must be considered as a locus of infection, especially if there has been an open head injury or ventricular shunt or if the patient has persistent rhinorrhea (discharge from the nose) or otorrhea (discharge from the ear). Careful evaluation is required to rule out meningitis or brain abscess. Central nervous system symptoms of infection may include headache, vomiting, irritability, and somnolence, in addition to fever. Neurosurgical consultation should be obtained. Patients with complicated fractures or orthopedic devices are prone to have bone and skin infections. Occasionally more sophisticated diagnostic studies are necessary to rule out infection. Thrombophlebitis and pulmonary emboli are less common in children than in adults. In a few severely head injured children, recurrent fever associated with no physical findings of infection and with multiple negative cultures leads the physician to suspect the diagnosis of fever of central origin—that is, caused by hypothalamic injury. Since there is no way to confirm central fever, it is a diagnosis of exclusion and necessitates reevaluation each time the patient develops a temperature elevation, to rule out a treatable cause of fever.

Agitation and Irrational Behavior

As severely head injured children move through the stages of recovery, agitation and irrational behavior may be a natural part of that progression. Three basic types of management are used: behavioral intervention, medication, and physical restraints. Informed staff members are generally able to handle episodes of agitation by providing a secure environment, a lower level of stimulation, a reassuring voice, rocking or patting, and redirection. It is best to avoid the use of tranquilizers whenever possible because of their reported interference with recovery after head injury (Feeney, Gonzalez, and Law, 1982; Weingartner, 1983). When medication is absolutely necessary to prevent patients from harming themselves, small does of diazepam (Valium) may be given orally or by injection. Physical restraints are rarely indicated. More information on this topic appears in Chapter 13.

Orthopedic Problems

Most head injuries occur as a result of automobile accidents and frequently injuries are multiple. Soft tissue and visceral trauma most often heal by the time the child reaches the rehabilitation facility. Orthopedic injuries may require much longer to heal. Devices such as the Hoffman apparatus for stabilizing fractures of the lower leg and halo traction for cervical fractures require careful and frequent cleaning by the nursing staff. Both of these devices are bulky and uncomfortable, and the head injured patient may require a sympathetic explanation in order to tolerate them. Confused and agitated patients often require one-to-one nursing care.

Pathologic fractures occasionally occur secondary to osteoporosis, which results from inactivity. These fractures may occur during any activity, and at times the exact cause cannot be determined.

Elevation of serum calcium level is seen primarily in teenaged boys with large bone fractures. It usually returns to normal level when the patient begins to bear weight; if it does not resolve, heterotopic ossification or primary hyperparathyroidism should be ruled out (Cristofaro and Brink, 1979). Despite the frequency of heterotopic ossification in adults and reported cases in children, it is rare in our experience. Alkaline phosphatase values are not helpful since they are elevated over adult levels in all growing children, and patients with fractures also have elevated levels.

Headache and Pain

The reported incidence of headaches following head injury in adults ranges from approximately 25 per cent to more than 50 per cent (Jennett and Teasdale, 1981). The incidence in children is much lower. Increased irritability may be a symptom of headache in nonverbal preschool children, but this is conjecture. Mild analgesics, such as acetaminophen or aspirin, are the drugs of choice in treating headaches.

Pain may also be caused by healing fractures, nerve injuries, muscle spasms, or surgical procedures. Mild analgesics usually suffice; however, some patients may need small doses of codeine in combination with acetaminophen or aspirin. Muscle relaxants may also be needed by patients with severe muscle spasms. Diazepam (Valium) is superior to baclofen (Lioresal) or dantrolene (Dantrium) in small children (Young and Delwaide, 1981). Children in general tolerate pain and discomfort at least as well as adults—and, in our experience, better than most adults.

Skin

Decubiti are rarely seen in our patients. This undoubtedly is due to the quality of nursing care. The importance of proper positioning, frequent turning, and assiduous skin care cannot be overemphasized. Plaster casts, splints, and braces sometimes cause pressure sores. A transparent, semipermeable skin dressing, such as Op-Site, is helpful when skin breakdown occurs, as well as when the skin is irritated and breakdown appears to be imminent (Chrisp, 1977). For parts of the body where it is impractical to apply this dressing, a protective dressing, such as Stomahesive, can be used.

Acne is commonly seen in adolescent patients. Steroids used during the acute phase of treatment aggravate this condition significantly, as does the anticonvulsant phenytoin (Dilantin) used for seizure control. Topical abrasives, drying agents, topical Vitamin A, or antibiotics are adequate treatment, since the acne naturally improves as the effect of steroids wears off. Systemic antibiotics are occasionally necessary. We have not found it necessary to use systemic isotretinoin.

Vision Problems

Visual impairment is very common in children who have had a severe head injury. More than 50 per cent of our patients have had one or more opthalmologic problems. Although these problems are usually caused directly by the brain injury, it is not uncommon for visual impairment to result from the associated eye injuries. The most common problems are eye muscle palsies causing strabismus and diplopia (double vision). Diplopia may also be a symptom of fracture of the orbit itself and must therefore be distinguished. We frequently see visual field defects due to injury to the optic chiasm and optic nerves as well as decreased visual acuity due to optic nerve atrophy. Other problems include ptosis of the eyelid, exposure keratitis, ruptured ciliary muscle, and cortical blindness.

Strabismus and ptosis of the eyelid improve considerably in most patients during the first six months after injury. Surgical correction should be delayed at least that long to observe the extent of spontaneous recovery. Botulinum toxin (Oculinum) injection has been used in selected patients to weaken the normal ipsilateral antagonist muscle. This will improve double vision during the time the muscle is healing (Biglan and Walden, 1984).

Hearing Problems

Fractures of the temporal bone and injuries to the middle and inner ear are not uncommon in head injury. Occasionally displacement or loss of the middle ear ossicles occurs. Sensorineural hearing loss occurs frequently (Healy, 1982), but it is rarely functionally impairing. A complete audiologic evaluation is indicated in all patients with significant head injury, and otologic consultation is obtained when a hearing loss is suspected.

Uncommon Problems

A *growing skull fracture* is occasionally observed. This is caused by a fracture with tearing of the dura at the site of the fracture, allowing the arachnoid and the brain to protrude, which does not permit the fracture to heal. A leptomeningeal cyst may result. A skull x-ray aids in the diagnosis.

Many of our patients manifest transient periods of *autonomic instability*, such as diaphoresis, shivering, piloerection, flushing, and trachycardia, which usually subside over time. In our experience permanent impairment of hypothalamic and pituitary function is rare, as is traumatic diabetes insipidus. *Anemia* may occur if there has been significant blood loss or prolonged nutritional problems. Occasionally anemia may be associated with gastrointestinal bleeding caused by stress ulcers or reflux esophagitis.

NUTRITION

Assessment

The assessment of the patients' nutritional status is a necessary component of the total clinical evaluation. An outline of our assessment protocol is presented in Table 4-3.

Nutritional Care Plan — An Interdisciplinary Team Task

Developing a nutritional care plan is an interdisciplinary team task involving the physician, registered dietitian, feeding therapist, nurse, and family.

The dietitian, using nutritional assessment data, determines adequate calorie, protein, fluid, vitamin, and mineral requirements.

1. Estimate caloric needs beginning with standard basal caloric output (see Table 4-4) and adding or subtracting calories based on the patient's activity level and need for weight gain or loss:

- usual bed activity — maximum 30% increase over basal rate;
- fever — 10 to 12 per cent over basal rate for each degree Celsius;
- weight loss — 500 additional calories per day to gain one pound per week;
- weight gain — 500 fewer calories per day to lose one pound per week.

2. A calorie-nitrogen ratio of 120:1 to 180:1 for the stressed patient will provide adequate protein.

3. For every 100 calories in the diet, 115 ml of fluid is necessary (Nelson, Behrman, and Vaughan, 1983).

4. One hundred per cent of the Recommended Daily Allowance for vitamins and minerals is necessary. Additional vitamins and minerals may be necessary due to interaction of medications, food allergies, or strong food dislikes.

Feeding therapists determine the appropriate food consistencies, positioning requirements, and feeding techniques (see Chapter 7). The

Table 4-3. Nutritional Assessment

  I. History
     A. Age
     B. Sex
     C. Usual weight prior to injury
     D. Present mobility level
     E. Feeding in acute care hospital
        1. Type of feedings (texture)
        2. Method of delivery (oral, tube, or both)
        3. Amount consumed in 24 hours
     F. Food allergies and strong dislikes
     G. Presence or absence of decubiti
 II. Present medications
III. Anthropometric measurements
     A. Present height
     B. Present weight
     C. Triceps skinfold
     D. Midarm circumference
     E. Midarm muscle circumference
 IV. Laboratory data
     A. Hematocrit
     B. Hemoglobin
     C. Serum albumin
     D. Blood urea nitrogen (BUN)
     E. Specific gravity of urine

nursing staff monitors the patient's response to the feeding program, recording intake and output and observing the length of feeding time and the patient's fatigue level and tolerance of food consistencies (see Chapter 5). The physician coordinates and supervises these activities based on the entire clinical picture of the patient.

Family involvement in the nutritional care plan has several benefits:

• Families are extremely interested in feeding activities.

• Families can personalize a portion of the child's treatment, such as suggesting favorite foods, meals, and snacks.

• Family cooperation is imperative for safety reasons. Choking or aspiration resulting from improper food consistencies, positioning, or feeding technique can occur when families are unaware of the child's current feeding program.

• Weight control programs are ineffective without family support.

The following hypothetical case history illustrates the steps in a nutritional assessment:

Table 4-4. Standard Basal Caloric Output

Weight (Kg)	Kilocalories/24 hours— Male and Female	
3	140	
5	270	
7	400	
9	500	
11	600	
13	650	
15	710	
17	780	
19	830	
21	880	
	Male	*Female*
25	1020	960
29	1120	1040
33	1210	1120
37	1300	1190
41	1350	1260
45	1410	1320
49	1470	1380
53	1530	1440
57	1590	1500
61	1640	1560

Increments or decrements:

1. Add or subtract 12 per cent of above for each degree Celsius (8 per cent for each degree Fahrenheit) above or below rectal temperature of 37.8° C (100° F).
2. Add 0 to 30 percent increments for activity.

From Nelson, W. E., Behrman, R. E., and Vaughan, V. C. (1983). *Nelson textbook of pediatrics* (12th ed.). Philadelphia: W. B. Saunders Company, p. 229. Reprinted with permission.

Case Study

I. History (obtained from the family and hospital records): 9 year old male; nonambulatory but able to move all extremities; not agitated; no decubiti and no fever for 2 weeks; 29 to 30 Kg pretraumatically; receiving gastrostomy feedings (1500 calories every 24 hours with no diarrhea or vomiting); allergic to chocolate, oranges, and soybeans; dislikes strawberries, liver, and mashed potatoes.

II. Present medication: phenytoin (Dilantin).

III. Anthropometric measurements: Height, 133 cm; weight, 22 Kg; triceps skinfold, 0.8 cm; midarm circumference, 20 cm; midarm muscle circumference, 18 cm.

IV. Laboratory data: Hematocrit, low normal; hemoglobin, low normal; serum albumin, low; blood urea nitrogen (BUN), low normal; specific gravity of urine, elevated.

We calculate the patient's caloric needs in the following way: The ideal body weight for a patient's height is determined using the NCHS* growth charts — in this case, 28 Kg (Hamill et al., 1979). Using Nelson's Standard Basal Metabolic Caloric Output in Table 4-4, we calculate the basal metabolic caloric output to be approximately 1100 calories. Because the patient is confined to bed and not physically active, a 20 per cent increase over the basal metabolic caloric output is used to calculate activity expenditure, 220 calories/24 hours. The patient has lost 6 Kg, or 21 per cent of his ideal body weight, during his hospitalization. To reach ideal weight an additional 1000 calories daily are needed for approximately 7 to 8 weeks. Therefore, this patient needs 2320 calories every 24 hours.

We calculate the protein needs in the following way: The laboratory data reveal low levels of serum albumin, indicating inadequate protein consumption levels within the past 17 to 21 days. (Tube feeding formulation in the acute care hospital had a calorie-nitrogen ratio of 200:1.) A calorie-nitrogen range of approximately 150:1 is selected because the patient is not overly stressed by fractures, decubiti, or fever. For this patient, who needs 2300 calories daily, 15.3 grams of nitrogen are needed. Daily protein needs are 95 to 96 g (1 g nitrogen = 6.25 g protein).

We calculate fluid needs in the following way: 115 ml of fluid is necessary for every 100 calories— in this patient, 2650 ml of fluid per 24 hours.

We calculate vitamin and mineral needs in the following way: 100 per cent of recommended daily allowances (RDAs) is necessary, with increased amounts of vitamins D and K because of phenytoin (Dilantin) medication.

As a result of these calculations, we find that this patient needs approximately 2300 calories, 95 g of protein, 2650 ml fluid, and a tube-feeding formulation containing no soy protein.

In our experience the following considerations are important in improving the patient's tolerance and acceptance of tube feeding:

• Isotonic formulations cause less gastrointestinal disturbances.

• Gradual increases in the size of bolus feedings or the total volume of intake in 24 hours improves tolerance.

• If the gastrointestinal tract has received no insult or if the insult

---

*National Center for Health Statistics.

is well healed, nonelemental formulations are useful in improving gastrointestinal tract function.

• Antidiarrheal medications may eliminate the need to change feeding formulations or the strength of formulation in the presence of loose stools.

• Bolus feedings that run 30 minutes to 1 hour followed by 30 minute periods of bed rest decrease the incidence of vomiting and diarrhea.

• If diarrhea persists, tube feedings prepared from foods (such as Compleat B or "homemade" foods) decrease the occurrence in some patients.

• Two to three bolus feedings at night (if patient receives six per day) will decrease the amount of time involved in daytime feedings, allowing adequate time for therapies.

Ongoing Management

Optimal nutritional status is necessary for maximizing the patient's rehabilitation potential. Monitoring tools for determining nutritional status include weekly weights, monthly measurements of triceps, skinfold, and midarm circumferences (if extremity is not paralyzed), creatinine height index (when desired intake level is achieved), monthly serum albumin levels, hematocrit, and hemoglobin levels, and analyzed food intake records (Letson, Ma, Stollar, and Hain, 1981). Monthly measurements of triceps, skinfold, and midarm circumferences are used to determine growth of lean muscle mass and to ensure that weight gain is not all adipose tissue.

Nutritional requirements change during the rehabilitation process. Adjustments in calorie and protein levels are necessary once an anabolic state is achieved. Maintaining nonambulatory patients slightly below ideal body weight is beneficial in preventing impaired blood circulation, which may lead to pressure sores (Hargrave, 1979).

When the patient can tolerate a transition from tube to oral feedings, the rehabilitation team works closely to maintain nutritional status. The dietitian provides information on total fluid and caloric needs for a 24 hour period and analyzes oral intakes to determine reductions in tube feedings. The responsibilities of the feeding therapist and nursing staff are described in Chapters 7 and 5, respectively.

Parents receive information on optimal nutrition for their child during their inpatient stay and prior to their first home visit. This includes instructions regarding food textures, weight maintenance and growth, and information regarding specific food and drug interactions.

Discharge

Nutritional status is also a component of discharge planning and follow-up. The prevention of long-term complications cannot be neglected.

Obesity is the most common nutritional complication that we see. Families require specific guidelines for feeding to maintain an acceptable body weight for the child. These guidelines include caloric levels adequate for growth, but low enough for weight maintenance, suggested meal and snack patterns, and encouragement to maintain and increase energy-expending activities.

POSTTRAUMATIC SEIZURES

Incidence

The presence of seizures (also referred to as convulsions, fits, or epilepsy) following head trauma is relatively common, but the majority of patients with a head injury do not have seizures, either in the early phase or as a late complication. Statistics vary based on the age of the patient, the severity of injury, and the length of time following the injury. The highest incidence of seizures is in patients with a missile injury, whereas the most common type of head injury is closed head injury of nonmissile origin.

In general, children have a lower incidence of seizures than do adults with similar brain injuries. Children over 2 years of age at the time of injury are less likely to develop late seizures than are younger children (Levin, Benton, and Grossman, 1982). Based on a study of over 1000 consecutive hospital admissions of head injured children and adults, Jennett (1975) demonstrated a 5 per cent incidence of late-occurring seizures. In his review of posttraumatic epilepsy in children, Hauser (1983) reported divergent incidence statistics in published studies, but concluded generally that late-occurring seizures are not common in head injured children. Mahoney and co-workers (1983) also suggest that late-occurring seizures are not a common sequela of severe head injury in children. Within the group of 5 per cent described by Jennett, the risk varies between 1 per cent and 60 per cent. Listed below are factors that alone or in combination influence the incidence of seizures in patients with closed head injury and can be helpful in predicting late-appearing seizures (Jennett, 1975). These factors should be taken into consideration before prescribing prophylactic treatment:

- appearance of seizures in the early posttraumatic period
- skull fracture
- intracranial hemorrhage
- prolonged posttraumatic amnesia
- amount of diffuse brain damage
- genetic disposition toward seizure disorder
- site and degree of focal brain damage

Seizures occurring during the first week following the injury (i.e., early-onset seizures) are correlated with a 25 per cent probability of late seizures. However, the presence of a single seizure in the early posttraumatic period does not necessarily indicate the need for prophylactic treatment. Fifty per cent of late seizures occur within the first year following the injury; 20 per cent of patients develop their first seizure 4 years or longer after the injury (Jennett, 1975). Although the presence of a linear skull fracture does not increase the risk of late seizures, a depressed skull fracture significantly increases the risk. Intradural bleeding, seen commonly with depressed skull fractures, increases the risk to about 30 per cent; diffuse brain damage increases the risk to about 25 per cent. A child's genetic susceptibility also plays a role in the occurrence of seizures, which may explain why individual patients react differently to what appear to be comparable injuries— for example, one may be convulsion-prone and the other not.

The presence of focal brain damage increases the probability of late-occurring epilepsy, as does tearing of the dura mater in combination with prolonged posttraumatic amnesia or skull fracture, or both. However, posttraumatic amnesia by itself does not alter the incidence of seizures. When all of these factors are present, the probability of seizures rises to about 60 per cent. Focal and nonfocal seizures have the same rate of recurrence, whereas temporal lobe seizures have a higher rate. Focal convulsive features occur in approximately 40 per cent of the population with posttraumatic convulsions, with temporal lobe seizures occurring most commonly (20 per cent). Jennett (1975) concluded that one third of patients with late appearing seizures continue to have frequent seizures. The variation of intracranial complications did not affect the type of seizures in Jennett's studies.

The types and character of seizures of head injured patients are no different from those occurring in the general population. Some patients have a mixed convulsive disorder. Furthermore, seizures can begin with focal features and become generalized.

Prophylactic anticonvulsant medication is usually given to patients who have two or three of the above-mentioned risk factors. The patient's social situation can also influence the prescribing of medication. The physician may hesitate to give medication to a young child in a potentially noncompliant environment in which there might be sudden withdrawal of the medication; this sudden withdrawal may cause recurrence of convulsions and possibly status epilepticus.

Identification

The International League Against Epilepsy (1981) outlines the International Classification of Seizures. We will comment on the clinical symptoms indicative of seizure activity. Rarely is there difficulty identifying seizures that have a motor component or that are associated with a definitive period of unconsciousness. Recognition of the variations of seizures with or without loss of consciousness or of motor activity can be difficult. Momentary lapses, incontinence of bowel or bladder, disturbances of visual or auditory sensations, and autonomic reactions, such as pallor, flushing, and unprovoked pupillary reactions, can be additional indications of convulsive activity. The psychic reactions of deja vu, fear, macropsia (things appearing larger than normal), and micropsia (things appearing smaller than normal) also should be considered as possibly convulsive in origin. Features that help delineate convulsive activity include an abrupt onset and duration of the episode, stereotyped activity, impaired consciousness, and postconvulsive responses (Wright, 1984). In actuality, it is the unrecognized "little seizures" which can have the most dramatic influence on the patient. These episodes can cloud the sensorium, confuse the patient, and make him or her less responsive. An EEG can be diagnostic only if epileptogenic patterns are seen concomitantly with the clinical symptoms. An abnormal EEG does not necessarily indicate a convulsive disorder, nor does a normal EEG necessarily rule out the presence of convulsive activity. When the diagnosis is still in question, prolonged video EEG monitoring can be helpful. Even with these techniques, it may be difficult to prove that these are symptoms of seizure activity. Therapeutic trials with anticonvulsant medications can be undertaken to determine whether or not beneficial responses can be achieved.

Treatment

The goal of anticonvulsive drug therapy is to achieve the greatest control of seizures without producing undesirable side effects. Wright (1984) presents an excellent review of anticonvulsant medications, appropriate treatment regimens for each, and possible side effects. We will limit our review to the most commonly used drugs and the potential side effects that are significant in a pediatric population. Whenever possible a monotherapy approach is desirable, since it simplifies the evaluation of side effects. Therapy should always be initiated with the single most effective drug for the type of seizure in question, even though it may be necessary in some instances to use a combination of medications to achieve better seizure control.

Barbiturates remain the simplest, most effective, and least expensive medications with the broadest anticonvulsive influence. However, phenobarbital can produce excitability and irritability, particularly in preschool children. These reactions are generally reduced with the use of mephobarbital (Mebaral). There is some evidence that barbiturate therapy may impair a child's learning ability (Smith and Wallace, 1982). Lethargy and skin reactions may result from barbiturates but hematopoietic dysfunction and hepatic complications are generally not a problem.

Hydantoins (Dilantin, Mesantoin) are the most popularly recommended medications in the treatment of posttraumatic seizures. As with barbiturates, there is a broad spectrum of anticonvulsive effectiveness and, as with phenobarbital, hydantoins are generally consistently absorbed and excreted, thus producing relatively stable serum levels. Although hydantoin is considered relatively safe, skin reactions can be severe. In addition, hematopoietic and hepatic dysfunction can occur. Signs of hydantoin intoxication include nausea, vomiting, double vision, dizziness, ataxia, lethargy, and speech disturbances. Hirsutism and gingival and lymph node hyperplasia also are frequently seen with hydantoin therapy.

Carbamazepine (Tegretol) has been increasingly used in the treatment of convulsive disorders. This medication has fewer clinical side effects than barbiturates or hydantoin, but it has an increased potential for producing hematopoietic dysfunction (leukopenia) and hepatic dysfunction. The half life of carbamazepine is significantly less than barbiturates or hydantoin and therefore must be prescribed in more frequent doses (three to four times per day). Barbiturates and hydantoin can be given once daily and sustain consistent therapeutic serum levels.

Primidone (Mysoline) may also be useful in seizure control. Because phenobarbital is a metabolite of primidone, prescribing these medications together may produce a toxic barbiturate serum level. Primidone, too, is a reasonably safe drug, although side effects such as lethargy, slurred speech, and skin reactions may occur. Barbiturates, hydantoin, carbamezapine, and primidone are basically useful in the control of generalized seizures with or without motor activity and variations thereof.

The following medications are helpful in absence seizures (petit mal) and simple and complex partialis episodes: (1) ethosuximide (Zarontin), (2) valproic acid (Depakene, Depakote), and (3) clonazepam (Clonopin). All of these medications have potential side effects, including lethargy, skin rash, unsteadiness, hematopoietic dysfunction, and hepatic dysfunction. Valproic acid particularly presents concern for possible production of hepatic dysfunction. It is important that frequent blood monitoring for hematologic abnormalities and liver enzymes be carried out with the use of most anticonvulsants, but particularly with valproic acid and carbamazepine. These studies should be done prior to initiating therapy and frequently thereafter.

Serum drug levels are of value in the determination of patient compliance and also in determining whether or not effective therapeutic levels have been obtained with standard dosages. Excessive blood levels should be suspected by clinical evaluation and confirmed by laboratory studies. Fortunately, most untoward side effects, such as liver toxicity, blood disturbances, and skin rashes, are reversible. Recognition of the problem and termination of the offending medication generally resolve the problem. It is important to point out that the popular anticonvulsant medications are relatively safe, but an awareness of potential side effects is mandatory. It is necessary to balance convulsion control against side effects. It may be better to permit an occasional seizure to occur than to overmedicate and produce intolerable side effects, which further interfere with a child's lifestyle and efficient learning.

The conservative approach is to continue anticonvulsive treatment for a minimum of a convulsion-free period of 3 to 4 years. It is reasonable to maintain treatment for only a 1 year convulsion-free period in low risk patients, recognizing that medication can be resumed if seizures recur. It is difficult to assess the efficacy of treatment when seizures occur infrequently. When treatment is to be terminated, it should be done gradually over a period of several months to prevent seizures from occurring on the basis of rebound activity and to decrease the possibility of status epilepticus.

REFERENCES

Biglan, A., and Walden, P. (1984). *Use of botulinim toxin in treatment of strabismus.* Paper presented at the meeting of the Pennsylvania Academy of Ophthalmology and Otolaryngology, Bedford, PA, May 24, 1984.
Chrisp, M. (1977). New treatment of pressure sores. *Nursing Times, 73,* 1202–1205.

Cristofaro, R. L., and Brink, J. D. (1979). Hypercalcemia of immobilization in neurologically injured children: A prospective study. *Orthopedics, 2,* 485–491.

Feeney, D. M., Gonzalez, A., and Law, W. A. (1982). Amphetamine, haloperidol and experience interact to affect rate of recovery after motor cortex injury. *Science, 217,* 855–857.

Hamill, P. V., Drizd, T., Johnson, C., Reed, R., Roche, A., and Moore, W. (1979). Physical growth: National center for health statistics percentiles. *American Journal of Clinical Nutrition, 32,* 607–629.

Hargrave, M., (1979). *Nutritional care of the physically disabled.* Minneapolis, MN: Sister Kenny Institute.

Hauser, W. A. (1983). Post-traumatic epilepsy in children. In K. Shapiro (Ed.), *Pediatric head injury* (pp. 271–287). Mt. Kisco, NY: Futura Publishing Company.

Healy, G. B. (1982, April). Hearing loss and vertigo secondary to head injury. *New England Journal of Medicine, 306,* 1029–1031.

International League Against Epilepsy (1981). Proposal for revised clinical and electroencephalographic classification of epileptic seizures. *Epilepsia, 22,* 489–501.

Jennett, B. (1975) *Epilepsy after non-missile head injuries* (2nd ed.). Chicago: William Heinemann.

Jennett, B., and Teasdale, C. (1981). *Management of head injuries.* Philadelphia: F.A. Davis Company.

Letson, A. P., Ma, K. M., Stollar, C. A., and Hain, W. F. (1981). *A Guide to Nutritional Care.* Chicago: Mead Johnson.

Levin, H. S., Benton, A. L., and Grossman, R. G. (1982). *Neurobehavioral consequences of closed head injury.* New York: Oxford.

Mahoney, W. J., D'Souza, B. J., Haller, J. A., Rogers, M. C., Epstein, M. H., and Freeman, J. M. (1983). Long-term outcome of children with severe head trauma and prolonged coma. *Pediatrics, 71,* 756–762.

Nelson, W. E., Behrman, R. E., and Vaughan, V. C. (1983). *Nelson textbook of pediatrics* (12th ed., p. 229). Philadelphia: W. B. Saunders Company.

Smith, J. A., and Wallace, S. J. (1982). Febrile convulsions: Intellectual progress in relation to anticonvulsant therapy and to recurrence of fits. *Archives of Diseases of Childhood, 57,* 104–107.

Stool, S. E., and Beele, J. K. (1973). Tracheostomy in infants and children: Current problems. *Pediatrics 3*(5), 1–35.

Weingartner, H. (1983, March). *Psychopharmacologic treatment in brain dysfunction.* Paper presented at Models and Techniques of Cognitive Rehabilitation, Third International Symposium, Indianapolis.

Wright, F. S. (1984). Epilepsy in children. *Pediatric Clinics North America, 31*(1), 177–188.

Young, R. R., and Delwaide, P. J. (1981). Drug therapy: Spasticity. *New England Journal of Medicine, 304*(1), 96–99.

Zülch, K. (1969). Medical causation. In E. A. Walker, W. F. Caveness, and M. Critchley (Eds.), *The late effects of head injury* (pp. 453–472). Springfield: Charles C Thomas.

Chapter 5

Nursing and
the Continuum of Recovery

The Acute Phase
Janette Yanko, RN, MN
The Rehabilitation Phase
Eleanore Barovitch, RN, BSN,
Jean L. Kozik, RN, BSN, and
Lynn O'Donnell, RN, BSN*

Patients with severe head injury present a challenge to all staff involved in their care. Throughout the phases of recovery, in acute care and rehabilitation settings, nursing services play a vital role. This service begins with a thorough assessment and individualized care plan that is appropriately revised with changes in the patient's medical status and levels of cognitive and physical functioning. Emphasis shifts from sustaining life in the acute phase to reintegrating the patient into the community after discharge from rehabilitation.

THE ACUTE PHASE

In an acute care setting, the focus of treatment is on controlling potentially life-threatening sequelae and preventing complications from the treatments employed. This section of the chapter will address these treatments and their potential complications and the manner in which crucial medical and nursing treatment may in fact hinder rehabilitation efforts in the very early stages of recovery.

*Authorship listed alphabetically at authors' request.

Management of Intracranial Pressure

Much of the management in the acute phase is aimed at preventing increases in intracranial pressure (ICP) or at reducing an already elevated ICP (see Chapter 1). Initially, critically head injured patients are in an environment filled with unfamiliar sights, sounds, and smells. They are host to an array of tubes and catheters: an endotracheal tube for pulmonary ventilation; intravenous catheters for the administration of fluids, drugs, and nutrients; venous and arterial catheters for monitoring hemodynamic status; an intracranial probe, bolt, or catheter for monitoring intracranial pressure; a urinary drainage catheter for monitoring fluid output; and a nasogastric tube initially for draining gastric contents and later for providing nutritional supplements. If the patient has additional injuries, there may be chest tubes, casts, and traction. All of these devices ultimately cause pain and stress and limit activity. They also interfere with the normal functions of communication, eating, elimination, mobility, and sleep. In the earliest stages following severe head injury, the patient is comatose and not actively performing most of these activities. Figure 5–1 depicts the unfamiliar and frightening world of the intensive care unit in which severely head injured children gradually reawaken.

Following is a brief review of the treatments used to control intracranial pressure and their consequences for early sensory, motor, and cognitive rehabilitation.

Body Position. The patient generally is placed in a supine position with the head elevated 30 degrees and with minimal hip flexion. Maintaining the patient's head in a neutral position facilitates cerebral venous drainage, which in turn prevents increases in ICP. Any flexion of the neck or turning of the head from side to side reduces the diameter of the airway, changes the position of the endotracheal tube, and compresses the jugular veins, which are responsible for the cerebral venous drainage (Lipe and Mitchell, 1980). Side-lying may cause dramatic increases in ICP. Hence, we keep the patient supine with the head elevated. Static positioning may be necessary for days to prevent dangerous elevations in ICP. This contributes to subsequent motor impairments.

The patient may also have abnormal responses to sensory stimulation, with stimuli ranging from a breeze blowing across the patient to a painful pinch. The abnormal responses range from flaccidity to decorticate or decerebrate rigidity. The degree of decorticate and decerebrate activity can vary from a barely perceptible movement to posturing so extreme that the arms cannot be straightened (decorticate) or the patient arches off the bed (decerebrate). This abnormal posturing may continue for days and makes any attempt at full range of motion or functional positioning impossible.

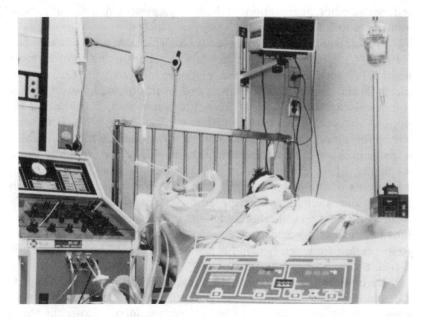

Figure 5-1. Child in an intensive care unit.

Hyperventilation. Hyperventilation by means of a mechanical ventilator reduces arterial carbon dioxide content, which in turns leads to cerebral vasoconstriction and a decrease in the cerebral blood flow (CBF). The decreased CBF creates more space for cerebral tissue expansion (see Chapter 1). If the carbon dioxide level becomes too low, cerebral ischemia may result, producing neuronal damage and seizures. The use of mechanical ventilation can cause gastric stress ulcers (Vincent, 1983), whereas artificial airways (endotracheal, nasotracheal, or tracheostomy tubes) can produce tracheal stenosis or vocal cord pathology.

Dehydration. Body fluids are closely controlled to inhibit cerebral edema formation. This is achieved by limiting fluid intake and by using osmotic (e.g., mannitol and glycerol) and loop (e.g., furosemide and ethacrynic acid) diuretics (see Chapter 1). Both mechanisms produce a dehydration effect, which could lead to electrolyte imbalances (which in turn cause weakness, among other symptoms) and the formation of emboli, which could cause cerebral, cardiac, pulmonary, or renal damage (Plumer, 1975). If the dehydration progresses to severe hypovolemia, shock and renal shutdown could occur.

Steroids. Steroids are also used to inhibit cerebral edema formation (see Chapter 1). They may, however, produce gastric stress ulcers, a steroid-induced diabetes, or alterations in the immune system, making the patient vulnerable to infection (Govoni and Hayes, 1978).

Hypothermia. Hypothermia (body temperature at approximately 86° F or 30° C) is induced to lower cerebral metabolism and to offer some neuronal protection from ischemia. Hypothermia can cause gastritis and ulcer formation, cardiac irritability, dehydration, electrolyte shifts, thrombosis formation, and, if great care is not used, frostbite and fat necrosis (hypothermia "burns") (Stevens, 1972; Zinn, 1973). Peripheral edema formation, due to sodium and water shifting into the cells, is also a major problem. The edema formation may be severe enough to cause a splinting of the extremities, limiting range of motion. We avoid rapid movements of the patient's extremities and exercise extreme caution in elevating the extremities above the level of the heart during hypothermia treatment. Elevation will cause cold blood from the extremity to be drained into an already chilled heart, which could lead to ventricular fibrillation. Resuscitation from ventricular fibrillation at a low body temperature is difficult.

Barbiturates. If it is impossible to maintain ICP with these therapies, a barbiturate coma may be induced. The patient will be given pentobarbital, phenobarbital, or pentothal to induce and maintain a specific blood barbiturate level. The barbiturates cause a chemically induced hypothermia, act as free radical scavengers to help prevent further cerebral injury, and decrease the response to noxious stimuli. In the case of the head injured patient, a simple touch may pose as a noxious stimulus. With an adequate barbiturate level, the ICP should remain basically unchanged in response to stimulation. Because of this ICP stability, it is easier to perform nursing care and rehabilitation functions. For example, range of motion exercises and suctioning of the endotracheal tube can be done without producing excessive elevation in ICP. Because of complications, such as decreased blood pressure and withdrawal seizures, barbiturate therapy is used only when other methods of reducing or maintaining ICP have failed. Barbiturates, in doses large enough to induce coma, will minimize or prevent REM (rapid eye movement) sleep. REM sleep is the dreaming stage of sleep and is associated with an increase in cortical activity. Increased cortical activity means a greater demand for oxygen and glucose, which leads to an increase in the CBF. In turn, the increase in CBF could cause an increase in ICP. Increases in ICP during REM sleep are not readily responsive to conventional treatments (i.e., diuretics, hyperventilation), so a decrease in REM sleep may be beneficial to the severely head injured patient (Marshall, Smith, and Shapiro, 1978). However, a complication of minimizing REM sleep is REM rebound. Lost REM sleep must be regained during future sleep cycles in order to prevent psychosis (Wotring, 1982).

When barbiturates are withdrawn, REM sleep resumes and will last for longer than usual periods of time. At this point, CBF will increase and cause an elevation in the ICP if compensatory mechanisms are not functioning.

Sensory Deprivation. For the severely head injured patient, simple everyday events, such as the telephone ringing or the touch of a hand, can cause significant elevations in ICP, which can ultimately lead to brain death. To prevent this disaster, we may deprive the patient of sensory stimulation and, as mentioned, even of dreams. We perform only those functions necessary to prevent life-threatening complications (such as suctioning via the endotracheal tube to prevent pneumonia). We limit activities, such as turning and range of motion exercises; the patient's eyes may also be covered to prevent light detection and the ears muffed to eliminate sound. We instruct family members and health care personnel to touch and speak to the patient only when absolutely necessary. Medically necessary procedures are scheduled at specific time intervals (Mitchell and Mauss, 1978). Each activity will raise the ICP. If the ICP is not allowed to return to baseline between activities, the increases will build on each other, raising the pressure to dangerously high levels. Rest periods are necessary and are individualized for each patient, but generally range between 20 and 30 minutes.

As the pressure begins to stabilize in response to stimulation and activity, ICP treatments are gradually withdrawn. Those therapies that have the greatest potential for complications are withdrawn first (such as barbiturate-induced coma and hypothermia). When barbiturates are withdrawn, the patient may experience tremors, agitation, delirium, hallucinations, and difficulty in controlling speech and motor movements for up to a week (Raphaely, Swedlow, Downes, and Bruce, 1980). When hypothermia is no longer necessary, we allow the patient to warm up naturally at a rate of no greater than 0.5 to 1° C per hour; otherwise "rewarming shock" may occur (Raphaely et al., 1980; Zinn, 1973). The length of time the ICP controlling treatments are necessary can vary from a few days to several weeks.

Increasing Activity and Stimulation

Each patient will have a different level of tolerance for activities. We measure the tolerance level by the amount of ICP increase in response to the activity. As the patient's condition stabilizes we initiate stimulation and activity on a trial basis. If there is only a slight or no increase in ICP, the stimulation is considered tolerable and it becomes a part of routine care.

The activities most critical in preventing complications, such as turning and range of motion exercises, are resumed first.

At this point, we encourage the family to participate actively in the care of the patient. Patients respond to their families much more readily than to hospital personnel. Family members are asked to make at least two cassette tapes for the patient — one of their voices in conversation and the other of the patient's favorite music. The tapes are played for no more than 20 minutes, with one half to one hour's rest between tapes.

For visual stimulation, we place favorite objects and photographs of the family in the patient's line of vision. This may mean placing the objects at the foot of the bed, making a special book of pictures, or hanging objects from the IV poles. A picture of the patient is placed at the head of the bed to help the hospital personnel associate the patient with a personality and specific features. Many times patients are swollen, bruised, shaved, and bandaged, which makes them barely recognizable to their families. In the midst of all the tubes and equipment, it is easy to forget that a person is there with likes and dislikes, hopes and fears.

We use touching and textured objects for tactile stimulation, and also encourage parents of small children to hold, touch, and rock them even though the child may still be attached to a variety of tubes and monitoring devices.

Other stimulation is introduced as the patient's condition permits. For example, once the endotracheal tube is removed and feeding safety is demonstrated by videofluroscopic study (see Chapter 7) or by eliciting normal swallow, gag, and cough reflexes, we begin oral feeding, preferably with favorite foods. Since the patient will be receiving either nasogastric tube feedings or intravenous hyperalimentation, the nutritional value of foods taken orally is not extremely important in the early stages of oral feeding. The patient may need to relearn taste, chewing, and swallowing, and, particularly with children, this is accomplished more readily with foods that are pleasant. Popsicles are often the number one preference, but they should be avoided if the patient has a swallowing disorder and cannot adequately handle thin liquids. As tube feedings and IV hyperalimentation are withdrawn, a balanced diet is an absolute necessity because of the higher caloric and protein requirements of the healing process (see Chapter 4).

The very early stage of recovery is not the time to introduce new objects and sensations. Because of patients' processing impairments, they respond much better to familiar sights, sounds, tastes, and textures. They also need extra time to process what they perceive and to formulate a response. What may take only a few seconds for a healthy person may take many minutes for a head injured patient. The environment should be simple and slow-paced to help prevent sensory overload. This is an extremely difficult, if not impossible, goal for an acute care setting because of the machines, procedures, and sensations that are unfamiliar and often frightening.

Summary

For severely head injured patients in an acute care setting, two medically necessary processes occur that affect rehabilitation: An abundance of "abnormal" experiences (including sounds from machinery and pain-producing procedures) and a deprivation of normal sensation and activity (including mobility and communication). As a result, when patients enter a rehabilitation program, they may first have to deal with deficits caused in part by their treatment and the deprivation necessary in the very early stages of recovery.

THE REHABILITATION PHASE

Early Stages of Recovery

When their medical condition has stabilized, patients may be ready for transfer to a rehabilitation setting. This frequently occurs while patients are still in an early stage of cognitive recovery. Characteristics of patients at this stage are given in Chapter 8, Table 8-1. Cognitive functioning ranges from inconsistent and nonpurposeful responses to stimulation at the lower end to stimulus-specific and purposeful responses, including simple communicative acts, at the upper end.

The main theme of cognitive rehabilitation in the early stage is *stimulation*. Patients need controlled sensory and sensorimotor stimulation to increase their alertness and awareness of their surroundings, leading to eventual resumption of activities of daily living. The stimulation program is discussed in Chapter 10. During this phase of recovery, the key nursing goals are in the areas of nutrition, activities of daily living, bowel and bladder care, communication, and family support.

Nutrition

Owing to the enormous nutritional needs for recovery from a serious injury, patients are frequently underweight when admitted to the rehabilitation setting. A properly balanced diet with sufficient calories and adequate hydration is essential. This requires careful weight monitoring and, until the patient is able to eat orally, nasogastric or gastrostomy tube feeding. Oral feedings are preferable since the patient is then free of extraneous equipment and tubes during active treatments and since tubes are often a source of discomfort and agitation. Tube feeding schedules may vary from several times to four times a day, depending on the patient's tolerance and needs. A schedule of four feedings a day is desirable, since it provides a more "normalized" eating pattern with fewer interruptions, especially at night, to allow for better sleep (Mauss-Clum, 1982).

By the end of the early stage of recovery, the patient may be able to begin trial oral feedings. Chapter 7 includes a discussion of criteria for resuming oral feedings as well as of radiographic procedures for determining if swallowing functions are adequate for oral feeding. Because thin liquids, such as water, are often difficult for head injured patients to swallow, a combination of tube feedings and oral feedings may be required to maintain hydration. Careful recording of intake and output is necessary if the patient is diaphoretic or has a fever.

Once oral feeding is well established, tubes, if present, may be removed. Patients may still require maximal assistance from the nursing staff to eat. Whether feeding is by mouth or by tube, nurses can use this time to provide sensory and cognitive stimulation. Oral stimulation procedures (see Chapter 7) are often best used just before or during tube feedings, unless the stimulation interferes with feeding. When oral feedings are reintroduced, we try to use previously favorite foods and encourage patients to attend to the odor and taste of the food. We also call the patient's attention to body parts (mouth, chin, lips) and movements (open, close, chew, swallow) as part of the reorientation process. Verbal and physical assistance is decreased as the patient's ability to feed independently increases. This typically does not occur until at least the middle stages of recovery.

Activities of Daily Living

While bathing, grooming, and dressing patients, nurses should incorporate relevant objectives of physical and cognitive rehabilitation. Even those patients at an early stage of recovery generally receive tub baths. This provides a more natural environment than a bed bath. It also provides proprioceptive stimulation to patients while they are in the water and feeling the soap, washcloth, and towel. This is also an ideal place to show children favorite toys and, if possible, let them play with them. The water can also lower muscle tone, making this a good time for range of motion exercises (see Chapter 6). During and after the bath, a thorough skin inspection should be done. Throughout the bathing and dressing process, the nurse talks simply and reassuringly to the child, describing the activity and naming body parts and articles of clothing.

As the patient's level of alertness increases, nurses should try to elicit the cooperation of the patient by means of simple verbal commands and physical prompts. This can be as basic as asking the patient to roll from side to side or physically moving the patient's hand through the motions of a familiar activity. Later in recovery, the nurse's verbal commands will become more complex and the patient's participation more active. The daily care also incorporates proper positioning, which will minimize impairments and maximize physical restoration.

Oral care should also be more than a daily task for the staff. This nursing activity can be part of the treatment program for patients with oral pathology (see Chapter 7), can help to orient patients to their body parts, and, for some, can make their care a pleasant experience. We use soft toothettes and soft toothbrushes rather than the commonly used lemon-glycerine swabs, which can be too "tangy" and ultimately drying to the oral mucosa. Patients receiving phenytoin (Dilantin) require especially good oral care owing to Dilantin's potential side effect of gingival hyperplasia.

Bowel and Bladder Care

An important nursing goal during the early stages of recovery is to establish a consistent means of bowel evacuation and maintenance of bladder function without the use of indwelling Foley catheters. Bowel care includes the control of diarrhea, which may result from the change in feeding regimen or other changes that occur when patients are transferred to the rehabilitation unit. Once the patient recovers from diarrhea, a regular regimen can be established by monitoring bowel patterns and by using suppositories, if necessary, to prevent constipation. Medication, such as stool softeners, may also be necessary.

When the Foley catheter is removed, the nursing staff should be aware of the possibility of urinary retention. If this is not a problem we use diapers or external catheters, or both. Intermittent catheterization is also used for some patients who are reestablishing bladder function and control.

As alertness improves, patients may begin a regimen of normal toileting. This will involve offering the toilet or urinal every 2 hours to patients who are unable to communicate their toileting needs.

Sleep and Rest

Establishing a regular sleep-rest pattern, including scheduled naps, is important for general healing as well as for reorientation to the patient's environment and routine. Sleep, feeding, therapies, and nursing care should take place at the same times every day. This consistent structuring of the day will also be helpful in the patient's reorientation as he or she moves to the middle stages of recovery.

Communication

Although easy to neglect, meaningful communication with minimally responsive patients is a fundamental nursing responsibility. Successful communication, even at a developmentally early level, is an essential part of the patient's reorientation to social reality. The communication suggestions listed in Chapter 10, Table 10-1, should be integrated into all nursing care activities with head injured patients at this stage of recovery.

Helping to reorient severely confused patients does not mean reciting in a rote manner canned "orienting information" (e.g., day, date, place, and so forth). Appropriate topics include simple descriptions, spoken slowly but with natural inflection, of objects and activities in the patient's here and now. In addition, it is useful to mention people and events that are particularly meaningful to the patient. Commands should be short and simple, with time allowed for delayed processing and with physical cues and prompts if they are needed. Tape recorded familiar voices can be played for short periods and at specific intervals to comfort and orient the patient.

Nursing staff may need to advise family members to talk to patients even if they appear unresponsive. Patients, especially young children, respond best to loved ones. Nurses should model appropriate communication for family members and also avoid "professional chatter" in the presence of both patients and their families.

Team decision making with speech-language pathologists is valuable in establishing a consistent mode of expression for the patient. Initially, this will involve responding to the patient's natural communicative acts (e.g., reaching, facial expression). Because of its importance in communication, the treatment team then attempts to create a consistent "yes-no" response. We first try to use a natural response system, such as head nods. If this is unsuccessful we explore systems such as eye blinks or hand squeezes. It is essential that all staff and family members use the same system. It is extremely confusing for patients when nurses use head nodding, physical therapists use eye blinking, and speech therapists use hand squeezing. It is helpful to post a note above the patient's bed or on the wheelchair that tells everyone which system is being used. Nursing staff should also be sensitive to subtle communicative acts (e.g., eye gaze, facial expression, tugging at pants) and respond to the implied meaning.

When patients begin to understand language, the logbook (described in Chapter 11) becomes a useful tool in communicating with patients and aiding their reorientation process. This is simply a notebook in which the patient's daily events are listed, often in the first person as if the patient were writing it. Several times a day family members or nursing staff review with the patient the events recorded in the logbook. This serves as a memory "jogger" for the patient and can also enhance communication among therapists, family members, and other caregivers. The logbook may also contain labeled photographs of the patient's treatment staff members as an additional orientation cue. Finally, we place appropriately labeled family pictures in a photograph album or on a bulletin board by the patient's bed. This plays a role in the patient's reorientation and also helps the staff to know and respond to the patient as a person.

Family Support

Since family members often interact more with nursing staff than with other rehabilitation professionals, family support and education are essential components of nursing care. This should begin in the acute care setting and be continued throughout the patient's recovery. Once the patient is in a rehabilitation setting, family support moves gradually away from critical medical issues to helping the family deal with what they may not yet understand about the long road to recovery and their role in this process. The role of the nursing staff in working with families is discussed in Chapter 4.

Middle Stages of Recovery

Cognitive characteristics of patients at this broad phase of recovery are outlined in Chapter 8, Table 8-1. These include the following:
- heightened alertness and activity
- disorientation to person, place, time, and schedule
- weak attention and concentration

- severe deficits in processing information, including memory for recent events
- inappropriate or incoherent verbalization
- noncompliant and at times agitated and combative behavior

Over the course of the middle stages of recovery, these cognitive and psychosocial deficits gradually decrease in severity. Motor impairments range from severe to minimal. Despite cognitive deficits, middle-stage patients are capable of adaptive behavior in a highly structured and simplified environment and with adequate cueing and assistance. Group and individual therapy sessions increase in frequency, with a growing focus on cognitive rehabilitation in the areas of deficit listed above.

Family members may renew their hope as they observe the patient's increase in alertness and activity, but they also express concern and often shock at the uninhibited behavior that they may have thought the child incapable of. Relatives and friends often misinterpret such behavior as signifying a step backward or a psychiatric disorder.

Nursing goals are discussed at this stage under the headings of feeding, activities of daily living, bowel and bladder control, safety, rest and sleep, socialization and play, communication, and patient-family teaching. Since consistency and structure are keys to treatment at this stage, nursing staff must work closely with all other treatment staff in helping patients to achieve their goals (Mastrain, 1981).

Feeding

The patient with no oral pathology may begin self-feeding. With occupational and physical therapists, optimal positioning and adaptive equipment are determined for those patients with motor deficits. Since patients have significant attentional and processing deficits, feeding time must be highly structured. A staff member is always available for monitoring, assisting, and supervising. Feeding should occur in an environment free of distractions. We use simple, reassuring instructions and feedback as a means of orienting patients to the task and encouraging improvement: for example, "This is your spoon," "Those are nice, small bites." Preparation of the food should take place before putting it in front of the patient. Agitated patients may push food off the table, whereas patients with impaired judgment may place large quantities of food in their mouths and choke. With these patients we present only one item of food at a time and carefully monitor their eating.

Since patients often show an uncontrolled appetite, we take care to prevent overeating and excessive weight gain. This problem is compounded by severe memory deficits: The patient might not recall having eaten only 30 minutes ago. Together with feeding therapists, the nursing staff trains parents in feeding principles and techniques so that they can actively participate in feeding (see Chapter 7). Often parents have a strong need to provide this nurturing activity for their child, and this may alleviate some of their feelings of helplessness.

We continue to record intake of food and liquids and monitor the patient's weight until a well-established pattern of feeding is present. As patients improve in motor and cognitive functioning and especially in judgment, we gradually decrease verbal and physical assistance and allow the patient to eat in a more natural environment. Owing to the patient's impaired judgment, monitoring of eating may be necessary despite otherwise normal functioning.

Activities of Daily Living

While providing basic nursing care, staff members should focus on the same physical and cognitive objectives as other team members. The maintenance of a highly structured and predictable environment on the nursing unit is a high priority. In addition we make use of self-care activities (e.g., dressing, bathing) to reinforce cognitive goals such as sequencing and direction following. As patients improve, they are required to sequence and organize increasingly large tasks and to follow increasingly long instructions. We also encourage increasing independence in the patients' initiation and completion of tasks. Treatment planning meetings with therapists are necessary to integrate efficiently nursing goals with the goals of the other therapies.

With confused and highly distractible children, self-care activities should occur in an environment with few distractions. We start with simple tasks that were overlearned prior to the injury. Using one-step directions, patients may be asked simply to brush their hair or wipe their faces with a washcloth. A knowledge of the patient's pretraumatic developmental level and interests is necessary for selecting the best tasks to begin training in self-care. For instance, children who were not expected to dress themselves before the injury should be given developmentally simpler self-care tasks. Chapter 11 includes an extensive discussion of task analysis and the systematic progression from simple to complex tasks for patients in the middle stages of recovery.

Given the demands of a busy nursing unit, it is easy to neglect details in grooming, such as jewelry and matching clothing, which contribute to the patient's sense of dignity and self-worth. Attention to such details also helps families see the concern of staff for their patient.

Bowel and Bladder Control

Patients may be unaware of body signals, such as bladder distention, or may not remember how to respond to these signals. Having patients use the toilet regularly and frequently helps to promote continence, and giving them clear and simple instructions and feedback is also useful in helping them to relearn these functions.

Safety

As patients become more active, safety becomes one of the highest priorities of nursing care. Careful monitoring of the patient and adequate staffing are essential to ensure safety. Basic safety precautions include the following:
- Keep the bed in the lowest position when not administering care
- Use padded side rails
- Have the suction machine equipped and ready to use
- Use weighted IV poles for suspending feedings to prevent tipping

For patients who attempt to remove tracheostomy or feeding tubes, mitts are used, but only during the feeding or when staff or family members are not present. One-to-one attention is preferable, but if mitts must be worn extensively, they should be removed at least once per shift for range of motion exercises and washing of the hands.

Proper positioning and safety are concerns for patients in wheelchairs. Safety belts must be secured in such a way that the patient cannot fall. We make the safety buckle inaccessible to patients with impairments of judgment or behavior by placing it behind the chair. Wheelchair positioning is discussed in Chapter 6. Among the options are inserts and head straps for alignment and head control, and reclining wheelchairs or lap trays for general positioning. We use footstraps to keep the feet in place and prevent them from dragging and being injured.

The middle recovery stage may include a period of agitation and combativeness, which compounds the normal safety hazards. This period may last a few hours or persist indefinitely. Control of the environment is important both to reduce the agitation and to enhance safety. Staff members should restrict traffic through the patient's room, limit visitors, and keep the room quiet (Brigman, Dickey, and Zegeer, 1983). It may be helpful to pull the curtains around the patient's bed. Only one person at a time should talk to the patient, speaking slowly in a soft, soothing voice. We do not argue with patients or escalate a verbal confrontation, but rather attempt to redirect them or ignore agitated behavior. If this period lasts more than a few days, the behavioral consultant will recommend an intervention strategy to be followed by all staff members (see Chapter 13).

We plan physical nursing care so that it can be completed as quickly and smoothly as possible while allowing necessary rest periods for the patients. With heightened activity there is a risk of abrasions and excoriations, which requires frequent examinations of the skin. Restraints may increase agitation and cause injury to patients as they attempt to free themselves. In selected cases, however, the restraints may be necessary. The use of pharmacologic agents for severe behavioral disturbances is discussed in Chapter 14.

Confused patients who are ambulatory often wander aimlessly. One-to-one supervision may be necessary, with special attention to building security since patients may decide to walk home, however unrealistic that intention may be.

A number of rehabilitation centers have created useful procedures to ensure safety for high risk patients. At the Thoms Rehabilitation Hospital in Ashville, North Carolina, "[a] green dot is used to identify and communicate to hospital staff and volunteers those patients who need assistance or those who need to be monitored closely or observed. . . . This system is intended to make everyone more aware of high risk patients" (Seymour, 1984, p. 32). At the Santa Clara Valley Medical Center, San Jose, California, the stairway doors have alarms to prevent patients from leaving unnoticed (Berrol and Cervelli, 1982).

Rest and Sleep

Because of the increase in activity and the demands of therapies, patients need rest periods in their daily schedules. Disturbances in sleep patterns may also develop during this stage of recovery, requiring 24 hour monitoring and intervention to ensure adequate sleep (Kroner, 1979).

Socialization and Play

We use play and leisure activities on the nursing unit to meet cognitive rehabilitation objectives without turning play into work. Consultation with occupational therapists or cognitive rehabilitation therapists assists in individualizing a specific program. With preschool children we use representational play while gradually increasing demands on their attentional and organizational abilities. With older children we begin with simple board and card games, gradually increasing their complexity so that children can begin to plan and use strategies. Video games, which are highly motivating and can be used to enhance cognitive recovery, can also be used. Including family members in these games teaches them the therapeutic value of selected recreational activities.

Although it can be therapeutic, play should continue to be fun. We try not to place excessive demands on the patient's cognitive or social abilities or cause frustration. Initially the activities are highly structured and individualized; later the patient progresses to small peer group activities.

Communication

Strategies for communicating with confused patients are outlined in Chapter 11. Talking to patients, encouraging their communication, and helping them to communicate more effectively are important areas for all nursing staff. Since nurses spend much time with patients and their families, they are in an excellent position to model appropriate communicative behaviors.

Family Teaching

In preparation for the patient's first home visit, we teach the parents the skills they will need to care for their child, including the use of special equipment. We also give them written care guides for reference at home and advise them to call nursing staff members if problems develop. We invite parents to bring the patient back early if they become overwhelmed. Because patients at this stage are severely impaired in their ability to learn new information, no attempt is made to teach them new procedures until the later stages of recovery.

Late Stages of Recovery

Table 8-1 in Chapter 8 outlines a set of cognitive and behavioral deficits frequently observed in patients in the late stages of recovery from severe head injury. Many children and adolescents who are severely injured reach a plateau in recovery at earlier levels. Among those who continue to recover cognitively, some have moderate to severe motor deficits, which may prolong their inpatient stay in a rehabilitation facility. Children with few physical sequelae but with significant behavioral, psychosocial, and cognitive problems may also continue inpatient programming in order to receive intensive cognitive rehabilitation services and behavioral and psychosocial intervention.

Patients at this stage are generally alert and oriented to the environment and, consistent with their developmental level, capable of independent and appropriate goal-directed behavior within a familiar and structured environment. The range of such behavior may, however, be restricted to routine tasks performed in a mechanical way. With disruptions in their schedules or changes in their environment, these patients may easily become disoriented and again behave unpredictably and inappropriately.

Although memory problems may persist, patients are now better able to learn new information and skills. Older children and adolescents may begin to engage in independent problem solving. Most patients, however, have difficulty thinking abstractly and organizing large amounts of information. Rarely do patients understand the extent and implications of their residual impairments. This lack of self-awareness combined with impaired judgment places them at risk for additional injuries and places a responsibility on rehabilitation professionals to address the issues of patient safety and effective social reintegration. Because these deficits are not readily apparent, family and friends often question the need for further rehabilitation services.

The two primary themes of rehabilitation at this stage are independent functioning in increasingly normalized settings and compensation for residual deficits. Within this context, the nursing team has four main goals: (1) to promote independent physical functioning with a focus on self-care; (2) to promote cognitive recovery with a focus on independent planning and execution of daily living activities; (3) to promote self-awareness, self-acceptance, and social recovery; and (4) to educate the patient and the family in necessary nursing care procedures. Within these areas, nursing intervention is coordinated with that of relevant therapists and specific plans are created for each patient.

Physical Independence

Nursing staff members work closely with occupational and physical therapists in encouraging patients to practice and habituate those new skills that they are learning in their therapies. This may include using adaptive feeding equipment correctly, walking with a walker, or using compensatory methods for dressing and grooming. The process of generalizing therapy achievements to the nursing unit is often time-consuming for nursing staff. Helping a child to practice new bathing, grooming, or dressing techniques that are necessary for independent functioning may take twice the time that it would take for the nurse to complete the task for the patient. However, the value of independence for patients is well worth it.

Treatment integration between nursing staff and therapists is also valuable in that nurses can describe to therapists the successes and failures experienced by patients on the nursing unit and in this way help therapists to fine-tune their treatment.

Cognitive Functioning

Together with occupational therapists, speech-language pathologists, and cognitive rehabilitation therapists, nursing staff select activities that encourage cognitive growth. On the nursing unit, cognitive recovery and independence can be promoted by creatively using self-care and recreational activities. During the middle stages of recovery confused patients can be helped to function adaptively by creating a highly consistent, simplified, and structured environment and by giving cues and physical assistance as needed to the patients. Children in the late stages of recovery may have grown comfortable with this degree of dependence, and nurses and parents may have difficulty relinquishing their nurturing roles.

We gradually encourage patients to take increasing responsibility for their own care. The degree of independence expected depends on both the child's pretraumatic developmental level and his or her residual cognitive and physical impairments. For example, nurses may request that children plan and appropriately sequence their prebreakfast activities, including selecting clothes, dressing, and attending to bathroom needs. Working with cognitive therapists, nurses may create a reminder card with words or pictures to help patients complete these and related tasks independently despite deficits in planning and organizing skills.

Recreational activities, including games and TV watching, can be used to meet therapeutic objectives while remaining fun to do. Earlier in this chapter the use of representational play and card, board, and video games in cognitive rehabilitation for middle-stage patients was described. These activities are continued with late-stage patients by placing increasing demands on their ability to attend, to remember, to organize larger amounts of information, and to use strategies and problem-solving procedures in order to play effectively. Games that are played in groups are most useful in that they also encourage socially appropriate behavior and help children to win or lose gracefully. (Chapter 11 contains more detailed information on gradually increasing the cognitive, perceptual, and social demands on children during structured recreational activities.) Television watching, although not encouraged for extensive periods of time, can be therapeutic if family or staff members engage patients in discussion of main ideas of the plot versus incidental details, or of problems that occurred in the show and in what alternative ways they could have been resolved.

Self-Awareness and Self-Acceptance

Since patients and their families spend much of their time on the nursing unit, nursing staff members cannot avoid the issues of self-awareness of deficits, denial, self-acceptance, and hope. Chapter 14 outlines counseling procedures for head injured patients and Chapter 3 includes a discussion of intervention procedures for family members who may share with their head injured loved one problems in the areas of awareness of deficits, denial, hope, and acceptance. Chapter 3 also discusses the nurse's role in responding to family members' hopes, fears, and needs.

Nursing staff members can help patients whose focus is solely on deficits and who see no progress, by reminding them of their earlier, more severe problems and by demonstrating the progress that has occurred. We use patients' logbooks to remind them in a concrete and objective way of the skills that they previously lacked and have now mastered. On the unit we set goals for patients that are easily reached and which generate a high rate of success. We encourage patients and offer hope, acceptance, and respect, at the same time attempting to avoid communicating unrealistic optimism. Since these issues are of such complexity and intensity for patients and their families, integration between nursing and other treatment staff members is essential.

Patient and Family Education

Prior to discharge nurses teach all necessary nursing procedures, including the use of special equipment, to family members and also—in the case of older children and adolescents—to the patients. This teaching process includes the nurse's demonstration of a skill or procedure, a thorough explanation, a demonstration by the parent or patient, and reteaching as often as necessary. It is essential to send written instructions home to serve as a reference and invite parents to call the nurse's station if they have any questions. Figure 5–2 illustrates these home instructions.

Figure 5–2. Illustration of home instructions for nursing care: misting a tracheostomy.

Misting a Tracheostomy

In normal respiration, the nose and mouth moisten and filter the air that is breathed into the lungs. When a person has a tracheostomy, this natural system is bypassed and the air reaching the lungs is very dry. The lungs respond to dry air by producing abnormal amounts of mucus. The drier the air in the lungs, the thicker the secretions from the lungs. Misting is one way to moisten the air, and thereby to keep the secretions fluid, and easily discharged.

Mist is humidified air — air with water added to it. It is cool and damp and some people find it uncomfortable.

When to Mist

• As ordered by M.D.

• If secretions become thick and viscous.

• If there is a persistent dry cough or hack.

Generally, mist is used continuously during sleep, and for an hour in the morning, afternoon, and evening.

[A small child tends to chew the mask or pull on it on going to sleep. If your child does this, try putting the mist mask in place after your child is asleep.]

Equipment Needed

Mist machine
2 mist masks
2 sets of corrugated tubing
2 water bottles
Sterile water (1 pint bottle per 8 hours of misting)
Mild liquid detergent
Solution of 1 part vinegar to 3 parts water

How to Use the Mist Mask

1. Make sure the water bottle is filled to the *full* line with sterile water (see diagram *A*).

2. Attach the water bottle to the machine tubing (see diagram *A*).

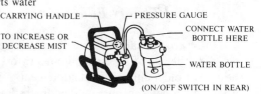

A. Mist Machine

Figure 5–2. (Continued)

3 . Make sure the valve on the water bottle is opened to 100 per cent oxygen (see diagram *B*).

4 . Attach corrugated tubing to the water bottle (see diagram *C*).

5 . Attach the other end of the corrugated tube to the mist mask (see diagram *C*).

6 . Turn on the mist machine and check to see that a stream of mist is coming from the mask.

7 . Place mask over tracheostomy. Attach elastic around the back of the neck and snap it in place on the other side. You should be able to slide two fingers comfortably under the elastic.

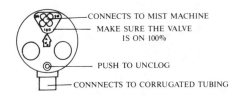

B. Top of Water Bottle

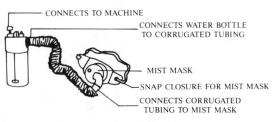

C. Mist Mask and Water Bottle

NOTE: If the water bottle becomes clogged, push the unclog button (see diagram *B*).

Care and Cleaning of Mist Equipment

Clean equipment twice a day so that you always have one drying and ready for use when the other is in use.

1. Take tubing, mask, and bottle apart.

2. Soak for 15 minutes in warm (not hot) soapy water.

3. Rinse thoroughly in clear water.

4. Soak for another 15 minutes in vinegar and water.

5. Rinse in clear water.

6. Place all pieces on a clean towel to air dry. Hang corrugated tubing over a shower bar or hook so that it will drain and dry.

Table 5–1. Rehabilitation Nursing Goals

Area	Early Stages of Recovery	Middle Stages of Recovery	Late Stages of Recovery
Special Care	Provide life-sustaining measures	Prevent complications Prevent infection	Maintain wellness
Bathing-Dressing-Grooming	Provide basic hygene	Reestablish self-care skills	Promote independence in self-care skills
Maintaining Posture	Maintain proper position Enhance function Minimize impairments Promote skin integrity	Maximize functional ability Prevent-decrease impairments	Promote independent mobility
Bowel-Bladder	Establish regular bowel regimen	Promote continence	Facilitate independent eating
Feeding-Nutrition	Provide optimal nutrition-hydration	Establish self-feeding program	
Cognitive	Provide sensorimotor stimulation Control sensory input	Use consistent approach Use structured activities	Facilitate compensation for residual deficits Promote independent planning Prepare for community reentry
Safety	Prevent injuries	Begin safety teaching	Practice safety and judgment
Communication	Talk meaningfully to patient	Provide adequate time for communication	Provide adequate time for communication
Emotional-Developmental	Control daily routine	Structure play-social activities Normalize appearance	Promote independent play-socialization Enhance self-image Provide emotional support
Family	Develop trust Involve family in care	Provide family teaching Prepare for home visits Assist family in expression of grief	Prepare for discharge

CONCLUSION

Recovery from a severe head injury is a long, hard, and emotionally intense process for patients, for their families, and for the rehabilitation team members. The staff on the nursing unit play an important role in this process at each stage of recovery. Table 5-1 presents an outline of the primary rehabilitation nursing goals and their place within the total process of recovery.

REFERENCES

Berrol, S., and Cervelli, L. (1982). Description of a model care system. *Head Injury Rehabilitation Program Final Report.* San Jose, CA: Santa Clara Valley Medical Center.

Brigman, C., Dickey, C., and Zegeer, L. J. (1983). Agitated aggressive patient. *American Journal of Nursing, 83,* 1408–1412.

Govoni, L. E., and Hayes, J. E. (1978). *Drugs and nursing implications* (3rd ed.). New York: Appleton-Century-Crofts.

Kroner, K. (1979). Dealing with the confused patient. *Nursing 79, 9*(11), 71–78.

Lipe, H. P., and Mitchell, P. M. (1980). Positioning the patient with intracranial hypertension: How turning and head rotation affect the internal jugular vein. *Heart and Lung, 9,* 1031–1037.

Marshall, L. F., Smith, R. W., and Shapiro, H. M. (1978). The influence of diurnal rhythms in patients with intracranial hypertension: Implications for management. *Neurosurgery, 2*(2), 100–101.

Mastrain, K. G. (1981). Of course you can manage head injury patients. *RN, 44,* 45–51.

Mauss-Clum, N. (1982). Bringing the unconscious patient back safely: Nursing makes the critical difference. *Nursing 82, 12*(8), 34–42.

Mitchell, P. H., and Mauss, N. K. (1978). Relationship of patient-nurse activity to intracranial pressure variations: A pilot study. *Nursing Research, 27*(1), 4–10.

Plumer, A. L. (1975). *Principles and practice of intravenous therapy* (2nd ed.). Boston: Little, Brown, and Company.

Raphaely, R. D., Swedlow, P. B., Downes, J. J., and Bruce, D. A. (1980). Management of severe pediatric head trauma. *Pediatric Clinics of North America, 27*(3), 715–727.

Seymour, N. (1984). Green dot program. *Hospital Topics, 62*(1), 32.

Stevens, V. C. (1972). Clinical hypothermia: Some nursing concepts. *Journal of Neurosurgical Nursing, 4*(1), 33–42.

Vincent, J. E. (1983). Medical problems in the patient on a ventilator. *Critical Care Quarterly, 6*(2), 33–41.

Wotring, K. E. (1982). Using research in practice: What effect do drugs given in critical care areas have on patients' sleep? *Focus, 9*(5), 34–36.

Zinn, W. J. (1973). Hypothermia in the critical care unit. *Heart and Lungs, 8*(1), 58–61.

PART IV
PHYSICAL REHABILITATION

In discussions of *groups* of head injured patients, physical sequelae are often characterized as less pervasive and less significant than cognitive and behavioral sequelae in the long-term management of patients as well as in the effects on patients and their families. We must, however, not underestimate the impact of a severe or even a mild motor impairment on *individual* patients, whose activities are thereby curtailed and whose goals may be dramatically altered. This is especially true of children and adolescents, whose self-concepts and social acceptance depend heavily on physical appearance and motor integrity.

Taken individually, motor impairments following severe head injury are similar to those caused by prenatal and perinatal insults (cerebral palsy) and by acquired brain lesions that are not diffuse (e.g., strokes). Furthermore, treatment techniques that have been developed for use with other groups of neurologically impaired individuals are also useful in the physical rehabilitation of head injured patients.

Following severe head injury, however, motor deficits often exist in complex combinations, and treatment is additionally complicated by accompanying cognitive, behavioral, and social deficits. These unique complexes of motor, cognitive, behavioral, and social impairments pose a great challenge to professionals attempting to help patients to restore lost function or compensate for residual deficits.

In Chapter 6, a unique collection of rehabilitation professionals— physiatrist, physical therapist, occupational therapist, and speech-language pathologist—addresses issues of common concern among these four professions as well as issues specific to each. The authors discuss impairments and treatment options under the headings of severe, moderate, and mild physical involvement, and they highlight the important relationships between physical rehabilitation on the one hand and developmental issues and cognitive-behavioral impairments on the other. The joining of members of these four professions in the writing of this chapter underscores the importance of an integrated approach to head injury treatment.

In Chapter 7, Ylvisaker and Logemann discuss the assessment and treatment of feeding and swallowing disorders, emphasizing disorders of the reflexive pharyngeal stage of swallowing. Swallowing disorders are given special treatment in this textbook in part because of their medical significance (with respect to nutritional status as well as the danger of choking and aspirating) and frequency of occurrence following severe head injury, and in part because professional training in the assessment and treatment of swallowing disorders is far less common than training in other areas of physical restoration. Although most of the techniques of intervention have been developed for feeding and swallowing disorders caused by conditions other than head injury, Ylvisaker and Logemann, like the authors of Chapter 6, give special attention to the influence of cognitive impairments on this type of treatment.

Chapter 6

Intervention for Motor Disorders

Mata B. Jaffe, PhD, CCC/Sp,
Joyce P. Mastrilli, OTR/L,
Cindy Black Molitor, LPT, MS, and
Anne S. Valko, MD*

A severe head injury produces damage of varying degrees in many separate parts of the brain and can result in a wide variety of sensory, motor, cognitive, and behavioral changes. The extent of damage is not always readily apparent; conversely, motor deficits may be temporary and resolve partially or completely. Motor deficits may appear as cranial nerve signs, weakness, abnormal muscle tone, and extraneous movements.

The patient and family often focus on the more obvious physical results of head injury, equating physical recovery with overall recovery. Unfortunately, this equation is not accurate. Furthermore, since the prognosis for full motor recovery is better than for full cognitive recovery (see Chapter 2), patients and their families often develop unrealistic expectations for overall recovery based on the return of motor function.

Physical rehabilitation is based on the principle of plasticity of the brain. The child is at an advantage because the immature brain is thought to have greater potential for relearning. The professional team attempts to help children relearn normal movement patterns and inhibit abnormal patterns. Kottke's engram theory (Kottke, 1982) states that movement patterns a patient actively practices will be imprinted on the brain and ultimately will be performed spontaneously. If a patient practices abnormal patterns, these engrams must be "erased" before the more normal, functional patterns can evolve.

Rehabilitation ideally begins in the intensive care unit. At this point, life-sustaining measures are more important than concern about frequent

*Authorship listed alphabetically at the authors' request.

positional changes to prevent skin breakdown, contractures, or secondary nerve injuries (see Chapter 5). It is thus understandable that some patients develop contractures that must be treated before therapeutic intervention toward functional activity can be effective.

The remainder of this chapter addresses typical motor sequelae of head injury, general principles of therapy, and specific treatment for gross and fine motor disorders and motor speech disorders. The treatment section is organized according to the degree of motoric involvement: severe, moderate, and mild.

MOTOR SEQUELAE AND FUNCTIONAL IMPLICATIONS

The literature is limited regarding the physical outcome of children and adolescents who have suffered a head injury. In both adult and pediatric populations physical outcome has been investigated in terms of age, duration of coma, type of injury, and site of injury. Table 6-1 summarizes outcome results of three pediatric head injury studies.

Brink, Imbus, and Woo-Sam (1980) investigated the occurrence of types of motor deficits in 344 patients under the age of 18 years who were 1 year post trauma. Ten per cent of those tested had normal results. Residual motor deficits included spasticity (38 per cent), ataxia (8 per cent), spasticity and ataxia (39 per cent), "soft" signs (3 per cent), spinal cord injury (1 per cent), and peripheral nerve injury (1 per cent).

Following traumatic head injury, patients may show one or more of the neuromotor signs of dysfunction outlined in Table 6-2. For further neurophysiologic background, refer to Chusid and McDonald's book (1962).

In addition, any sensory modality may be impaired, which significantly affects treatment for the motor deficits. Hypersensitivity or hyposensitivity may exist in visual, auditory, olfactory, gustatory, tactile, proprioceptive, and kinesthetic senses. (Aphasia may also be present in some children and adolescents, further interfering with physical rehabilitation. Aphasia is a communication disorder characterized by complete or partial impairment of language comprehension, formulation, and use.)

GENERAL CONSIDERATIONS

Before presenting specific treatment guidelines, general considerations of the nature of head injury and of the recovery of head injured children and adolescents are discussed.

Table 6-1. Physical Outcome for Head Injured Children

	Number of Subjects	Age Range	Duration of Coma	Time Post Injury	Outcome
Brink, Imbus, and Woo-Sam, (1980)	344	4 months to 18 years	≥ 24 hours	1 year	73% Independent (including 10% motorically normal) 10% Partially dependent 17% Totally dependent
Bruce, Schut, Bruno, Wood, and Sutton (1978)	53	4 months to 17 years	≥ 6 hours	≥ 6 months	83% Good recovery 7% Moderately disabled 2% Severely Disabled 2% Vegetative survival 4% Death
Ylvisaker (1981)	27	5–16 years	≥ 3 days	≥ 1 year	31% Normal 23% Mild, nonhandicapping 35% Moderate motoric involvement 11% Severe motoric involvement

Table 6–2. Motor Sequelae and Functional Implications

Dysfunction	Probable Site of Damage	Functional Implications
Rigidity: marked resistance to movement in any range, unrelated to speed or direction of movement. Often present initially, generally resolves.	Extrapyramidal lesions (decorticate): resistance primarily in extensors. Decerebrate: rigidity in antigravity muscles.	Prevents active movements and good positioning.
Spasticity (hypertonicity): velocity-dependent increased tonic stretch reflex; exaggerated deep tendon reflexes, clonus, Babinski's or Hoffman's sign seen. Primarily in upper extremities in flexion, or in lower extremities in extension, but also seen in neck, trunk and face.	Upper motor neuron syndrome: release of cortical inhibition, extrapyramidal tract, cerebral cortex internal capsule, brain stem or spinal cord.	Major problem in head injury. Limits full range. Can lead to contractures. Interferes with purposeful movements. Clonus interferes with weight bearing over extremities.
Hypotonicity: low muscle tone, which occurs primarily in the trunk but is also seen in extremities.	Impaired muscle proprioceptive or motor innervation. Cerebellum or muscle.	Prevents initiation of balanced muscle contraction for stability.
Ataxia • limb ataxia or dysmetria: loss of ability to coordinate smooth movements ("past pointing"). • truncal ataxia: wide-based gait, unsteady, staggering on turning.	Cerebellum	Lack of equilibrium control to regain balance during movement; lack of graded control of trunk and extremities.
Tremors: involuntary movements resulting from alternating or rhythmic contractions of opposing muscles. Often combined with spasticity or ataxia. • resting tremors: usually diminish with action. May occur later in recovery. • cerebellar tremors: with volitional movement, usually are intensified at termination of act. Rhythmic and large in amplitude.	Resting: basal ganglia Intentional: cerebellum	Hinder smooth graded control of movements. May limit patient's gross motor ability or may limit only accuracy in fine motor tasks.

Table 6-2. (Continued)

Dysfunction	Probable Site of Damage	Functional Implications
Apraxia: difficulty in planning, organizing, and carrying out sequential movements. Patient cannot execute motion on command, but may be able to automatically.	Precentral gyrus or supramarginal gyrus of dominant cerebral hemisphere	May affect gross, fine, or oral motor tasks. Limits spontaneous movements.
• Apraxia of speech (non-linguistic disorder): impaired ability to motor plan articulatory postions and to sequence movements (respiratory, laryngeal, and oral) for volitional speech.		Apraxia of speech affects verbal communication. Most severe impairment can cause speechlessness. Mild disorder (sometimes termed "dyspraxia") causes difficulty mostly with multisyllabic words.
Dysarthria: collection of motor speech disorders. Lack of control of volitional and automatic oral motor actions, such as chewing, swallowing, and tongue and jaw movements.	Central or peripheral nervous system	May affect phonation, respiration, articulation, resonance, prosody, feeding, and swallowing. Most severely dysarthric patients are nonverbal. Mildly dysarthric speech may be intelligible although disordered.

Cognitive Considerations

Although they are related, cognitive recovery and physical recovery do not necessarily correspond. At any level of cognitive functioning, physical deficits can range from mild to severe. Likewise, a patient who is severely involved physically may be at an early, middle, or late stage of cognitive recovery and functioning (see Chapter 8). A patient who attains full physical recovery may remain limited in function because of residual cognitive deficits, such as impaired safety judgment and impulsiveness.

Cognitive deficits significantly affect the planning, methods, and strategies of physical rehabilitation. The characteristic cognitive impairments of head injured patients distinguish their therapy from that of other motorically involved patients. Treatment changes as the patient responds more appropriately to the environment and to the demands of therapy.

Patients in the earliest stage of cognitive recovery are generally passive recipients of sensorimotor treatment, regardless of motoric level. Treatment for these patients focuses on increasing purposeful and functional motor skills. Because agitated and confused patients typically resist therapy, however, behavior management often takes precedence over therapy goals. Techniques that have an inhibitory effect on the central nervous system, such as using dim lights, soft music, or slow rocking motions, help reduce agitation. Therapists should also include energy-expending activities in the patients' schedules to fatigue and calm them, as well as familiar tasks, which often improve attention.

Late in the middle stage of cognitive recovery, patients actively assist in therapy if distractions are minimal and directions are simple. Because patients may be inattentive or may perseverate on one activity, frequent changes of activity may be necessary. In the late stage of cognitive recovery, they usually can learn new or compensatory behaviors; however, self-monitoring of these compensatory behaviors may be limited to therapy sessions or nonstressful situations.

Specific cognitive deficits affect the treatment of patients' motor deficits. Those with deficits in orientation often resist treatment because of poor awareness and understanding of motor problems and their ramifications. The therapist can work through resistance by structuring treatment around favorite activities. Patients with poor judgment or impulsivity require close supervision to prevent subsequent accidents or another head injury. Patients with an attentional deficit who may fixate on irrelevant details or perseverate on motor activities may respond to environmental restructuring, redirection, or novel stimuli. It is important that patients with a memory deficit have a program that is consistent with regard to schedule, therapist, location, and sequence within the session. Patients who are confused or who have receptive language difficulties perform better when the therapist simplifies verbal directions, uses gestures and environmental contexts, or gives visual and tactile cues. Patients with frontal lobe damage, a typical result of closed head injury, may present with adynamia, which is a state of apathy and lethargy in which the patient does not initiate motor activity or communication. Physical or verbal prompting, highly motivating situations, and overlearned activities may encourage initiation.

Developmental Considerations

It is important to consider the patient's pretraumatic and present levels of development and try to attain and surpass the pretraumatic level. Thus, infants and young children must not only regain former developmental and motor functions but also gain additional motor components to set a foundation for further development. Older children, on the other hand, who had developed all physical components of motor skills, must relearn previously integrated movements. Patients' motivation in treatment varies with chronological and developmental age. A 7 year old child, for instance, may be interested only in getting back on a bike, whereas an adolescent may be concerned primarily with physical appearance.

Behavioral Considerations

Behavior significantly affects treatment and is related to cognitive and developmental levels. Because young children who are injured need familiar people and settings, their adjustment to the rehabilitation team is generally more difficult than an adult's. Also, it is often difficult for parents to share or relinquish their role in their child's physical care.

Maladaptive behaviors may be a continuation or an exacerbation of pretraumatic behaviors or may be a result of the head injury. In either case, they reduce the effectiveness of treatment. Children who are easily frustrated and have poor emotional control resist the continual treatment that is necessary for maximal physical recovery. Most patients go through a stage of depression, which often intensifies this problem. Consultation with the family and a psychologist is important so that behaviors that interfere with treatment are managed consistently (see Chapter 13).

Orthopedic Considerations

Head injured patients often sustain fractures or internal injuries that prevent or postpone their full participation in therapy activities. For example, a clavicular fracture postpones upper extremity weight bearing; recent abdominal surgery precludes aggressive therapy for trunk mobility. A fractured jaw with mandibular wiring prevents oral feeding and oral motor treatment.

Physical Recovery

The physical recovery of head injured patients is not always a continuous or predictable process. Periods of slow and fast recovery may alternate, and periods of progress may follow periods of plateau. The cessation of physical recovery, which may occur at any point, may leave patients with residual physical disabilities.

Recovery of gross, fine, and oral motor function reflects a close relationship among these skills. Fine motor skills, such as pointing to a communication board, depend on the development of gross motor control, particularly trunk stability and balance. Although brain damage from head trauma is most often diffuse, localized damage may occur as a result of penetrating head injury, surgery, skull fracture, coup and contrecoup contusions, or hematoma. Depending on the area and severity of damage to the central nervous system, isolated oral, fine, or gross motor deficits may persist in greater severity or in isolation. Thus, for example, a patient occasionally regains much of his or her pretraumatic cognitive and gross motor abilities but retains a severe speech disability because of verbal apraxia or dysarthria.

In the treatment section that follows, intervention with patients who have severe, moderate, and mild involvement in gross, fine, and oral motor (or motor-speech) areas is discussed.

TREATMENT

Severe Physical Involvement

Patients with severe involvement are either in the initial posttrauma phase of decorticate or decerebrate rigidity or, following the resolution of rigidity, remain dependent in all areas because of the severity of motor disability. Patients often have abnormal muscle tone in the form of spasticity. Primitive reflexes, such as tonic labyrinthine, symmetrical or asymmetrical tonic neck reflexes, positive supporting reflex, and palmar or plantar grasp, may be dominant or interfering. Severely affected patients are essentially nonverbal. Eating problems and drooling are common because of abnormal muscle tone and movement patterns and associated paralysis, weakness, or incoordination. Dysarthria and apraxia of speech (with or without aphasia) may be temporary and may improve spontaneously or may persist as a residual impairment.

Gross Motor Treatment

The goal of postcoma treatment is to elicit increasingly adaptive responses to the environment by means of structured stimulation (see Chapter 10). One method of stimulation is movement, which elicits tactile, proprioceptive, vestibular, visual, and auditory sensations. Functional and meaningful patterns of movement are incorporated into treatment to give patients the sensations of normal movement. The active components may initially be missing when therapists are treating severely involved patients, but they are introduced as patients begin to respond actively to treatment.

Movement from the supine to an upright sitting or standing position helps to reorient the patient to the environment and to regain a healthy physiologic status. To avoid overstressing the patient, blood pressure, pulse, and other physiologic signs should be monitored during these transitions. Total body movements are preferable to basic range-of-motion exercises of the extremities because they help patients to regain mobility in the trunk and extremities. They prepare the trunk for the development of active control for balancing and for maintaining stability, which in turn allow free arm and leg use. Total body movements are also used to decrease hypertonicity by incorporating tone-reduction techniques, such as slow, rhythmic rocking, vibration, and proprioceptive stimulation. These movements can help calm patients and reduce their extraneous activity when they are agitated. Table 6–3 gives some examples of total body movements that are used to develop mobility.

It is often during these types of movement that patients first initiate active movements and sounds. It is important to document these responses and the stimuli that elicit them (see Chapter 10).

Therapy is not limited to exercise mats and mat tables but includes the use of other equipment such as therapy balls, bolsters, and a pool. Therapy in a pool with lukewarm water decreases spasticity, a reduction that allows freer motions of the trunk and of the extremities to develop. The water lessens the effect of gravity so that patients can move actively with less effort, and this greater ease can decrease overflow to spastic muscles. Although warm water can have a calming effect, we are cautious about taking agitated patients into the pool if their behavior is difficult to manage.

The mobility that is gained during treatment sessions is maintained throughout the day and night by proper bed positioning as suggested by Bobath and Bobath (1974), by proper wheelchair and standing positioning, and by the use of splinting and casting shown in Tables 6–4 and 6–5.

Splints and casts are used to regain and maintain mobility and are an important adjunct to treatment; uses are listed in Table 6–5.

Patients who remain severely physically impaired but who regain the necessary cognitive processing ability may be able to exercise control over the environment. There are many switch options that require only a minimum of physical ability to operate environmental control systems and electric wheelchairs (Williams, Csongradi, and LeBlanc, 1982).

Table 6–3. Examples of Total Body Movements to Gain Range of Motion

Movement	Motion Achieved
Supine	
Flex legs to chest, head and neck flexed by pillow; rock side to side	Hip flexion; trunk flexion with elongation of back and neck extensors (body-on-body movement)
Rock hips over small ball or roll, knees extended (hip extension)	Internal-external rotation of hips; hip extension; mobility between pelvis and hips and between trunk and pelvis; lateral elongation of trunk; can achieve hip abduction
Rolling to side-lying	Trunk rotation; neck rotation, rotation of shoulders and hips
Side-lying	
Counter rotation of shoulders and hips	Mobility between shoulders and trunk and between hips and pelvis; scapula moves on thorax; elongation of lateral trunk muscles; internal-external rotation of bottom hip and shoulder joints
Prone Over Wedge	
Rocking hips from side to side	Hip extension; knee extension; mobility between pelvis and hips; back extension
Sitting Against Large Firm Ball	
Side-to-side movements of trunk	Mobility between pelvis and hips (internal-external rotation); trunk rotation and elongation
• Controlling from the head	Mobility between neck and shoulders and between shoulders
• With arms abducted	Increased elongation of trunk
• With arms above head	Increased elongation of trunk; thoracic extension and expansion; shoulder elevation-abduction (be careful that the humerus does not sublux or pull the scapula too far laterally)
Leaning and rocking back on elbows or straight arms	Internal-external rotation of shoulders; thoracic extension; elongation of pectoral muscles; lateral trunk mobility; neck elongation if head is supported; mobility between neck and shoulders and between pelvis and trunk; possible elbow flexion
Rocking forward over legs with flat feet	Trunk flexion; hip flexion; mobility between pelvis and trunk; elongation of heel cords (preparation for standing)

Table 6–4. Guidelines for Positioning to Maintain Range of Motion

Objective	Procedure
Bed Positioning (Supine)	
Reduce retraction of shoulders.	Gently move outstretched arm forward, guiding scapula along back. Place small pillow or towel roll under scapula and arm.
Reduce retraction of hips.	Place towel roll or pillow under pelvis and buttocks (affected side).
Reduce tightness of neck capital extensors.	Build up pillow behind head so neck flexes forward.
Bed Positioning (Side-lying)	
Reduce influence of abnormal reflexes which increase hypertonicity.	Use alternating side-lying positions instead of supine
Decrease severe extensor tone.	Side-lying, flex top leg toward chest and block with pillows or sandbags.
Reduce retraction of more affected side and avoid painful weight bearing on head of humerus in hemiplegic patient.	Always place more affected shoulder and hip forward of less affected side. Support position with pillows behind back, between legs, and supporting forward arm. If both sides are affected, underside is placed forward.
Reduce tightness between neck and shoulder on one side.	Build up pillows under head when side-lying to affected side. Flatten pillows or remove when side-lying to unaffected side.
Wheelchair Positioning	
Give adequate support to body.	Use solid seat inserts in chair (can adapt for pressure relief). Can recline back *slightly* for severely involved patient.
Reduce extensor spasticity; give adequate support to body.	Hips are flexed, placed back in chair, and secured snugly by seat belt across hips. Can use wedged seat. Body is symmetrical, with pelvis even. Knees are flexed to be same height as hips. Feet are flat on foot pedals.
Support arms, encourage elbow weight bearing; prevent disregard of hemiplegic side.	Use wheelchair lap tray attached to chair at elbow height.
Maintain head in midline with neck slightly flexed; reduce neck extensor tightness; improve orientation to environment.	Use supporting head rest attached to chair insert. May need to recline chair back *slightly* so head stays in head rest. Most useful in conjunction with lap tray of adequate height.
Prevent overstretching of neck extensors.	Foam neck collars are useful until patient gains some head control.
Reduce shoulder retraction.	Towel rolls behind scapula bringing shoulders forward.

Table continued on following page.

Table 6–4. (Continued)

Objective	Procedure
Maintain hips and pelvis even.	Place towel rolls between hips and side of chair.
Keep knees slightly apart.	Place towel roll or foam square between knees (not thighs).

Supported Standing	
(Tilt Table, Supine Stander, Prone Stander)	
Reduce hip and knee flexion and heel cord tightness while supporting trunk.	Stand patient on tilt table or supine stander with three straps (across lower chest, making sure underarms are cleared; across hips; just above knees). Body is symmetrical; feet are flat and directly under hips.
Support for weight bearing on elbows; encourage flexion; increase orientation to environment; increase feeling of security.	Use tilt tables and supine standers with trays attached at elbow height or place high table (elbow height) in front of stander.
Encourage extension; support for weight bearing on elbows.	Use prone standers for children. Secure straps across buttocks and at feet. Lean against table at elbow height.

Motor-Speech Treatment

When the nonverbal patient is in the early postcoma stage, a differential diagnosis among dysarthria, apraxia of speech, and aphasia is difficult. Furthermore, these disorders often coexist. Single-process impairments due to twelfth cranial nerve damage, isolated neurogenic velopharyngeal incompetence, and unilateral vocal fold injury or paralysis (from extended endotracheal intubation) are not common but may be present. Patients with impaired phonation should be evaluated by an otolaryngologist.

Dysarthrias are more common than apraxia of speech in patients with severe physical involvement. In our clinical work, we have seen that there is a higher incidence of persistent dysarthria among adolescents than among young children, whereas apraxic-like disorders appear more frequently among youngsters. When children begin to speak, they often have symptoms of both dysarthria and apraxia. If abnormal muscle tone and movement patterns improve, usually only motor planning problems remain.

Head injured patients may recover to any degree of cognitive functioning and still remain severely dysarthric or apraxic. Speech therapy

Table 6-5. General Guidelines for Using Splints and Casts

Type	Area of Application	Objective and Procedure
Resting splints: Prefabricated or individually constructed. Metal, plastic, plaster, or foam for fingers and toes.	Fingers, wrists, elbows, knees, ankles, between toes.	Maintain range of motion and proper alignment of joint; reduce influence of spasticity. Worn on schedule (usually 2 hours on, 2 hours off or to tolerance) to prevent skin breakdown. Plaster can be too heavy for infants and may interfere with developing movements.
Serial casting: Series of cylindrical plaster casts.	Wrists, fingers, elbows, knees, ankles, feet.	Regain motion through prolonged stretch and progressive casting. Worn continuously for 1 to 2 weeks. Must be well padded. Can be paired with weight bearing.
Drop-out casts: Plaster.	Fingers, wrists, elbows, knees, ankles.	Maintain prolonged stretch and permit free range into desired movement. Worn continuously 1 to 2 weeks. Can be paired with Functional Electric Stimulation (Baker et al., 1983).
Bivalved positional casts: Plaster (sometimes with Fiberglas for extra strength). Lower extremity casts can incorporate molded foot plates (Cusick and Sussman, 1981).	Elbows, wrists, knees, ankles.	Maintain range of motion, ensure proper alignment. Casts at ankles are used for weight bearing and weight shifting. Worn to tolerance or scheduled 2 hours on, 2 hours off.

requiring active relearning or compensation is seldom effective until the period of significant confusion has passed. In the early stage of physical and cognitive recovery, treatment for severe oral motor deficits consists of graded facial and oral stimulation and of feeding therapy in a structured environment, such as described in Chapter 7. Patients usually begin to eat before they begin to talk. Gross and fine motor treatment methods (presented in this chapter) to normalize muscle tone, coordination, posture, and strength can influence speech production and improve dysarthric speech. As trunk and head control and mobility improve, vocalizations may occur spontaneously during yawning, sighing, and other physical movements. By reinforcing and shaping any vocalizations that may be used communicatively, the therapist can help patients acquire a core vocabulary of easily articulated words for functional communication. As the patient's skills progress, we stimulate sound combinations that require more breath support and coarticulation. A mirror provides visual feedback for the patient who has poor internal feedback.

Hypernasality can result from incomplete (weak) or inappropriate and uncoordinated action of the velopharyngeal mechanism, hyper- or hypotonicity in the muscles of the articulators, and abnormal tongue positioning. Videofluoroscopic evaluation is indicated for patients who have resonance problems. A palatal lift prosthesis or surgery should be considered in cases of severe hypernasality. A palatal lift produces a mechanical obstruction between the oral and nasal cavities by elevating the soft palate to the posterior pharyngeal wall. The lift can give more normal resonance and may have some impact on articulation as well. Extremely spastic, nonmoving palates do not respond well to this kind of management. A prosthesis should not be considered until the patient is sufficiently recovered cognitively and behaviorally to cope with evaluation, fitting, and daily usage. The patient should have concurrent speech therapy for the best results. An advantage of a prosthesis is that it can be removed or modified. Surgical procedures include Teflon injection and pharyngeal flap surgery. Palatal surgery is contraindicated for patients with respiratory problems. The decision for prosthetic or surgical intervention is highly individualized and is generally not made until at least a year post trauma. Although neither intervention produces normal speech, our experience supports the general premise that prosthetic management is superior to surgical management.

Patients with severe involvement or who are in an early recovery phase often manifest apraxia of phonation: they may mouth words and later whisper without phonation. This condition may either resolve spontaneously or require intervention. As with dysarthria, vocalizations may occur spontaneously with yawning, laughing, or sighing. Movements during physical or occupational therapy sessions and in the therapy pool sometimes elicit phonation. All therapists can make the patient aware of the sounds produced, alternate in making the sounds with the patient, and encourage their repetition. Oral movements that may facilitate phonation are chewing (Froeschels, 1952), grunting, coughing, humming, and making sounds like an animal or inanimate object (e.g., a clock). Gesturing may also facilitate phonation. The speech-language pathologist may vibrate the larynx or apply rapid pressure below the ribs as a more direct way of stimulating sound. Some head injured children with whom we have worked have regained speech as late as 18 months post trauma.

One method for teaching the severely apraxic patient to position the speech musculature for speech sounds is a phonetic placement technique (Vaughn and Clark, 1979; Young and Hawk, 1955). Since this method depends on verbal description and oral manipulation, it cannot be used with either apraxic or dysarthric patients who have significant processing problems or disturbed oral sensitivity. Phonetic derivation (Van Riper and Irwin, 1958) teaches new sounds and movements by modifying those that are in the patient's repertoire by means of progressive approximation. Employing the key-word approach, the therapist uses a word over which the patient has gained control to help transfer the target sound to other words. Often patients can produce sounds only in automatic activities, such as counting, singing, and rhyming. Also, words and phrases sometimes can be cued by the cloze technique (e.g., "glass of _____").

Assessment and experimentation with a variety of switches begin early with severely involved patients. Nonvocal patients may require some kind of call signal to gain the attention of others, particularly in an emergency. Many commercial devices require only a light touch and may be attached to the bed, sheet, or wheelchair. Usually the therapist then attempts to teach reliable signals for "yes" and "no" to facilitate early communication. All staff and family members should work together to teach and reinforce the selected symbols and systems. It is helpful to attach a sign to the bed and wheelchair describing the patient's particular yes-no signals. Some options are eye blinking, head turning, pointing thumb up and down, and writing or pointing to yes and no signs. The most natural responses, such as shaking and nodding the head, are best. They are easiest for the patient because of pretraumatic use and are most easily understood by others. In general, responses must be readily distinguishable from random movements to be communicatively effective.

Other staff and family members are then urged to assume most of the responsibility for communication, a task that includes presenting single yes-no questions and accepting the patient's mode of response. Because apraxic patients are less likely than dysarthric patients to have severe physical involvement, they are usually better able to supplement speech with one or more expressive modalities, such as gesturing, pantomiming, signing, drawing, writing, or using a communication board. However, all expressive modalities may be impaired in the early recovery stage. Concomitant aphasia in many apraxic patients also limits the effectiveness of language-dependent communication modes. The presence of generalized or limb apraxia limits acquisition of manual sign language, such as Ameslan, or a gesture code system, such as Amer-Ind (Skelly, 1979).

Factors that are important for the selection, use, and effectiveness of nonspeech communication systems are cognitive status, motor ability, receptive language functioning, inner language status, desire to communicate, and the specific communication mode or combination used (Silverman, 1980). In selecting an augmentative system, the therapist should observe the patient's spontaneous communication, which is generally the most successful modality.

Much has been written about augmentative communication systems (Capozzi and Mineo, 1983; Cohen and Shane, 1982; Musselwhite and St. Louis, 1982; Shane and Bashir, 1980; Vanderheiden, 1978), but not about their use with head injured patients. It is often tempting to introduce an augmentative communication system before these patients are ready. Patients require sufficient cognitive recovery to integrate new learning and to appreciate an alternative system as a means of communication. Patients who are not ready for an alternative or augmentative system may reject it; they sometimes become angry when staff members encourage them to take the communication aid to their scheduled program and to use it. Initially, a lapboard or book with pictures, words, or other symbols is probably best for orientation, visual scanning or matching, auditory processing, facilitation of negation or affirmation, and highly cued and prompted responses. During the early and middle stages of cognitive recovery, the amount of visual information must be reduced. Four to six pictures are often appropriate. Head injured patients often require a long period of time to initiate the use of a system, although they may use it in therapy sessions when modeled or prompted. Staff and family members should consistently give cues for the use of the system. Patients with severe frontal lobe damage and generalized cognitive deficits may seldom or never initiate communication, regardless of the system.

Changing of levels of cognitive and motor functioning necessitates continual reassessment of communication needs and subsequent changes in communication systems. The therapist who spends a great deal of time fabricating a language board may have to abandon it if the patient regains speech or to design others as the patient progresses. A patient may use a variety of selection modes and output systems, progressing from simple clinician-made communication boards to sophisticated computerized systems. Sometimes families need to be convinced of the potential usefulness of an alternative communication system. In general, we find that head injured patients do not readily accept voice output systems, probably because they have lost speech and do not consider artificial speech their own.

Table 6-6. Drugs Used in Treatment of Spasticity

Name	Site of Action	Dose	Complications
Dantrolene (Dantrium)	Periphery— extrafusal muscle fibers	25 mg bid (maximum, 100 mg qid depending on size)	Drug hepatitis rare, most common in women over age 35; weakness
Diazepam (Valium)	Spinal cord and supraspinal limbic system	1 mg bid (5 qid depending on size)	Drowsiness, weakness; potentiate other drugs; paradoxical reactions
Baclofen (Lioresal)	Spinal cord and supraspinal	5 mg bid or tid (maximum, 20 mg qid)	Lethargy; rare hallucinations; need to raise or lower gradually

Pharmacologic Treatment

Various pharmacologic approaches have been used in the treatment of spasticity. Table 6-6 summarizes the most commonly used oral medications. For further information, refer to Young and Delwaide (1981a,b).

Surgical Intervention

Late in the course of rehabilitation, orthopedic procedures are sometimes indicated. Lengthening of the Achilles tendon may lessen the effect of lower extremity spasticity and may improve the patient's ability to transfer, stand, and walk. Tendon transfers or releases in upper and lower extremities have had varying degrees of success. Surgery should be coupled with an intensive physical or occupational therapy program.

Interdisciplinary and Family Team

Teamwork is essential to the rehabilitation process. Team members, including therapists, doctors, nursing staff, dietitians, and family members, constantly exchange information to coordinate intervention that is directed toward a commonly accepted goal. Physical, occupational, and speech-language therapists also often treat together. From the beginning, family members play an active part by joining therapy sessions whenever possible, providing significant background information (such as the patient's favorite activities or foods), and participating in team decisions. Because family members are more familiar to the patient, they may elicit different responses; they themselves might also find their involvement therapeutic. Excluding family members from the rehabilitation process can compound their loss (see Chapter 3).

Family members also need information on how to move the patient, both for their own safety and to facilitate the patient's recovery. Since patients often go home for weekends, therapists train the family in bed and wheelchair positioning, transfers, the use of casts or splints, feeding techniques, oral exercises, and communication. As family members show interest and ability, they are instructed in movement activities. Even if the family cannot participate in treatment, therapists maintain regular contact with family members regarding the patient's progress and needs, and they discuss realistic expectations for further recovery. The development of a good family and treatment staff relationship is essential to the rehabilitation of head injured patients.

Moderate Physical Involvement

At this stage of motor recovery, patients have emerging active control of movements but still exhibit abnormal muscle tone and movement patterns. They may still have cognitive deficits that limit their full participation in therapy, or they may be too young to cooperate fully.

Gross Motor Treatment

Therapy at this stage is a very active process for the patient. Therapists incorporate active movements that provide normal sensory feedback on a subcortical level to facilitate the patient's motor learning or relearning. According to Bly (1980), we learn the sensations of movements. To promote normal sensorimotor development, therapists inhibit abnormal motor patterns because those patterns interfere with regaining functional, energy-efficient movements (Ayres, 1973; Bobath, 1969, 1971). Direct physical handling provides sensory input to facilitate and modify automatic balanced use of the neck and trunk muscles during weight shifting, balancing reactions, and equilibrium responses. Physical cues are preferable to verbal cues, which may actually inhibit the desired response (Moore, 1980) and may confuse the disorganized patient. At this stage active weight shifting and balancing are the primary goals for the improvement of gross motor skills. As head and trunk control develop, the resulting stability frees the arms for use and allows pelvic and hip control to develop for weight bearing and weight shifting. Within a session, treatment progresses from gaining proximal control to gaining distal control and follows the normal developmental sequence.

Familiar activities, such as playing with a favorite toy or swinging a tennis racket, are used to facilitate normal movements on a subcortical level. We incorporate movements such as transfers and activities of daily living into functional activities to encourage independence. These activities must be practiced to habituation.

Bed and wheelchair positioning, casting, and splinting continue to augment direct therapy. We use positional bivalved casts in therapy to aid the development of standing balance and weight shift control, both of which prepare patients for walking.

Functional electrical stimulation (FES) can be used to gain range of motion or to activate either weakened muscles or antagonists to spastic muscles (Baker, Parker, and Sanderson, 1983; Benton, Baker, Bowman, and Waters, 1981). This effect is then incorporated into functional movement patterns to facilitate normal motor learning. For example, FES can help improve ankle dorsiflexion so that components of gait can be facilitated.

The use of electromyography (EMG) biofeedback can help patients learn to decrease spasticity in muscle groups and to move functionally while maintaining the reduction in spasticity. EMG biofeedback also augments the feedback loop for improved movement control for the patient with inadequate proprioception or other sensations. Biofeedback is not effective unless the patient eventually can be weaned from it and can develop an internal feedback mechanism. For more information, see the reports by Basmajian (1981) and Brudny and co-workers (1976).

EMG biofeedback and FES are used only when cognitive recovery and developmental levels are adequate. Patients who are unable to attend for long periods or who have short-term or immediate-recall memory deficits are not appropriate candidates.

Working in front of a mirror also provides external feedback and gives the therapist a better view of the patient's movement responses. Because the change in physical appearance can be upsetting we prepare patients before asking them to look at themselves in the mirror. Videotaping also provides useful feedback and can show patients or family members the changes over time that are too subtle to notice on a daily basis. Because older children at this stage of recovery become aware of their physical limitations and become frustrated with seemingly slow progress, recognizable success is a strong motivator.

Reducing physical restrictions is also motivating. The therapist arranges some form of independent or semi-independent mobility that still incorporates normal postural tone and movements. An infant may be positioned to allow active supine play, such as reaching for knees or a mobile. A tricycle may be an alternative to walking for the young child who has poor balance or uses abnormal patterns in gait. Some adolescents can move a wheelchair with their hands or feet. A motorized cart or electric wheelchair is useful if other transportation is too difficult or if it increases overflow to spastic muscles. Wheeled or regular walkers provide stability for balance during walking.

Fine Motor Treatment

Fine motor functioning in patients at this level is limited by spasticity or movement disorders. Active control may be only unilateral or may be limited to gross grasp. Fine motor control is closely related to proximal stability, which provides a base for reaching. Treatment focuses on developing graded control in the upper extremities by means of dynamic weight bearing and weight shifting with normal postural alignment. Therapy also develops a patient's isolated and controlled reach and grasp. Therapists often improve the patient's distal control by providing proximal stability and guidance that inhibit abnormal movements.

Visual-Perceptual-Motor Treatment

Visual-perceptual-motor function is generally related to cognitive level. Oculomotor skills should be evaluated, since deficits will affect functioning in all therapies and in school. Perceptual evaluation should distinguish between sensory discrimination abilities (especially visual and tactile), visual-motor abilities, and perceptual-motor integration. Therapy may utilize a sensorimotor approach (Ayres, 1973), a direct transfer-of-training approach (Frostig and Horn, 1964), or a functional activities approach (Siev and Freishtat, 1976). Therapy should avoid developing splinter skills but rather should provide a foundation for further development and generalization to daily activities.

Activities of Daily Living

Evaluation of activities of daily living can begin if the patient is able to attend briefly and follow directions and if he or she is at an appropriate developmental level. In a structured setting the child or adolescent is familiar and successful with these activities, which often involve automatic and habitual motor patterns. Repetition and the technique of backward or reverse chaining (Banus, 1979) work well with head injured patients. (In reverse chaining patients are trained to accomplish an activity by beginning with the final step and progressing backward until all steps are learned.)

While adaptive equipment may be necessary because of motor limitations, the patient's cognitive level must be adequate for tool usage, new learning, and memory. Environmental structuring may be needed for optimal independence, and adaptive aids may be necessary as a result of cognitive limitations. For example, checklists can help sequencing; drawer labels can aid memory.

If a child or adolescent has the potential to return to the community, therapists must evaluate community skills. Community mobility is related to motor function, praxis, and cognitive level. Therapists should not, however, draw broad inferences about patients' ability to function independently in the community on the basis of their performance in therapy. In an overstimulating or stressful environment, patients may not retain the level of physical functioning observed in therapy sessions.

Motor-Speech Treatment

The speech of a patient with moderate oral motor or motor planning involvement is fairly intelligible. At this stage of recovery from head injury, the most typical dysarthric symptoms are a soft and breathy voice, inaccurate articulation, hypernasality (sometimes with nasal emission), monopitch, and slow rate; in each case, muscle groups rather than single muscles are involved. The soft palate, lips, and tongue move slowly and within a limited range. Alternating tongue movements are markedly slow and effortful. In addition to the motor component, communication may be disordered because of the patient's cognitive deficits, confabulation, confused language, lapses in attention and responsiveness, word-finding problems, and aphasia.

Therapy for the aforementioned motor-speech symptoms is similar to that described by other authors (Rosenbek and LaPointe, 1978), although certain aspects of therapy, such as the level and type of stimuli that will correspond to the patient's cognitive and development level, concomitant sensory deficits, and gross and fine motor limitations, are taken into account. Systematic drill and practice are used only with patients who can cooperate and actively participate in treatment. Team treatment in a therapy pool can improve voice volume and quality and can also be a pleasurable activity that does not require much conscious effort. Improved physiologic support typically produces better speech.

Apraxic patients usually become more intelligible by reducing the rate of speech and by pausing between words to allow motor planning time and careful articulatory executions. Techniques such as contrastive stress drills, melodic intonation therapy, gestural reorganization, motokinesthetic training, emphasis on the visual modality, and use of a pacing board (Jaffe, 1984; Wertz, La Pointe, and Rosenbek, 1984) can be used with an apraxic child or adolescent to the extent that cognitive functioning allows.

Some types of augmentative or backup communication systems may be appropriate to enhance communication for patients who are verbal but whose speech is not always intelligible. If gross and fine motor and motor planning abilities are adequate, the patient may be able to augment speech by writing, typing, drawing, gesturing, pantomiming, or signing. A more physically involved patient may be able to point to a phrase, word or letter card, board, or booklet. These items can be carried in a pocket or purse. Generally there is no need for the most sophisticated and expensive augmentative communication systems. One relatively inexpensive option is an electronic aid that was designed for the nonhandicapped population as a desk note writer and calculator with a crystal display and hard-copy output. Specifically designed keyguards and hardware for mounting the aids to desks or wheelchairs can make them more accessible to physically handicapped patients.

Family Involvement

The family is still an important part of the team. Family members now learn ways to help the patient to move actively and to use functional, more normal movements. They should be encouraged to support their child's independence in self-help areas.

Mild Physical Involvement

The patient at this stage generally is motorically functional but has some residual physical limitations. Independence is closely tied to the patient's cognitive and developmental level. It is the cognitive level that determines how patients use their available motor control for functional tasks. Therapy focuses on the refinement of skills and compensation for residual deficits.

Gross Motor Treatment

Some deficits in balance reactions and fine weight-shift control may remain. Treatment focuses on fine tuning the components of gross motor skills to develop efficiency and ease of movements. In some settings patients are discharged from therapy prior to their refinement because they are "functional." It is important, however, to consider the patient's long-term goals. Refinement means setting the stage for further development so that more normal, functional, and energy-efficient movement develops later. Among the aims of refinement are the improvement of quick balance and protective reactions that increase the patient's safety in movement and decrease the risk of another injury as the patient reenters the community and school.

Refinement also achieves more "normal-looking" movements, which are important to the development of a positive self-image, especially during the self-conscious adolescent years. In adult life, appearance may effect employability as the patient enters the job market. Treatment prepares patients to be physically safe and enables them to conserve energy for future job tasks.

In refining motor skills the patient's developmental level must be considered. For instance, the therapist must be aware of the differences between the gait of a toddler and that of a seven year old. Also, equilibrium reactions of the infant are different from those of the adolescent.

The subtle weight-shift control of equilibrium responses may be improved by the use of many age-appropriate and developmentally appropriate activities, such as sitting or standing on a balance board, balancing on a therapy ball, shifting weight with roller skates, climbing and descending stairs with reciprocal steps, or playing ball.

Another focus of treatment is development of compensatory strategies. Working in front of a mirror can be especially helpful with older children, who can monitor their own behavior and incorporate the reinforcing feedback. EMG biofeedback is useful for refining movement control, especially in the extremities. Other strategies are introduced to allow patients to use more refined movements without bringing these movements under conscious control. For example, if the tone of a patient's arm has increased as a result of motor overflow while walking, he or she may be taught to walk with the hand in a pocket. This cue may be sufficient to keep the arm relaxed without requiring the patient to concentrate on the arm.

At this stage bracing and other assistive devices compensate for residual motor deficits. They are used to assist in functional activities, to maintain range of motion and normal muscle tone, and to decrease energy consumption.

Fine Motor Treatment

Fine motor dysfunction affects coordination, manipulation of objects, visual motor control, and bilateral motor coordination. Deficits in speed and dexterity, writing speed and accuracy, and visual motor reaction time are common even in those patients with little to no obvious neurologic involvement (Ylvisaker, 1981). Visual or visual-perceptual deficits may remain and interfere with daily living and academic activities.

Neurodevelopmental activities are used at this stage to decrease the effects of residual neuromuscular involvement. Self-monitoring and compensatory strategies are utilized to optimize functioning. For example, hemiplegic adolescents may be taught to bear their weight forward on the involved elbow (adding proximal stability and decreasing associated reactions) to improve control of the involved hand.

Deficits in coordination, manipulation, speed, and dexterity can be improved through the therapeutic use of developmentally appropriate games, such as marbles, jacks, or quick-reaction card or video games. Sometimes it is necessary to emphasize specific and functional skills, such as shoelace tying or cutting. Games and activities that can improve bilateral coordination include scooter board, balloon volleyball, Tinkertoys, or ball games. Therapy for specific visual or visual-perceptual-motor deficits may continue. When the physical considerations of therapy become less important, it is possible to involve patients in appropriate perceptual activities, such as computer games.

Compensation may be necessary if the child or adolescent is involved in a school program in which fine motor demands are great. A typewriter or small communication system with hard-copy printout is often a good substitute for handwriting. If a student is required to take notes, a tape recorder can compensate for decreased speed or accuracy in writing. The teacher may need to reduce time constraints to optimize the student's performance.

Motor-Speech Treatment

Patients often have imprecise articulation, mild hypernasality, soft volume, slightly monotonal and breathy voice quality, reduced rate of speech, and reduced length of utterance per breath unit. Some patients with breathy or weak vocal production may be in the early stage of general physical recovery. In this case, mildly dysarthric speech sometimes reflects physical weakness or decreased responsiveness to and interaction with the environment. More commonly, it is a residual, rather than transitory, deficit. Therapy focuses on refining these speech parameters and on teaching compensatory strategies. The therapist may focus on phrasing, specific phonemic productions, modifications of the oral resonating cavity, motor planning, exaggerated oral posturing, and intonation patterns.

If the cognitive, behavioral, and developmental aspects discussed earlier indicate that a patient is an appropriate candidate, we may use EMG biofeedback for deeper breathing, relaxation of the shoulder girdle and facial muscles, and other, similar objectives. The patient may use a voice amplifier, especially in noisy or group communication situations, such as the classroom. These aids were developed to amplify the voices of speakers who use an artificial larynx.

Family Involvement

We explain to parents and other family members that even though patients look functional and independent, they may need supervision owing to poor safety judgment or inattention, lack of impulse control, or other cognitive deficits. Parents are cautioned to allow their child to resume full participation in gym class, bike riding, or other activities only gradually.

HOME AND COMMUNITY REENTRY

Long before discharge the team must complete a home assessment for those severely and moderately involved children and adolescents who will be discharged to home. This is also important for patients who go home for weekend visits. On the one hand, the team may suggest simple modifications that would make the home more accessible, such as removing throw rugs, rearranging furniture, adding a bath seat, or stabilizing the patient's bed against a wall. On the other hand, major structural changes may be needed, such as wider doorways, relocated bathroom and shower facilities, lowered light switches, entrance ramps, or an additional room. Several authors have provided information on home modifications for the disabled (Chasin, 1978; Chasin and Saltman, 1978; Wittmeyer and Barrett, 1980).

If the patient goes to a long-term care facility, therapists visit the facility and demonstrate program recommendations to the staff. Written instructions with photographs depicting activities, proper positioning, and the use of equipment have proved useful.

Since many patients return to their school and community, we prepare the student to be safe in school settings where halls, stairs, and playgrounds are crowded. The therapist, patient, and family visit the school to review class locations, to determine accessibility to the building, classroom, and lavatories, and to train teachers to use adaptive equipment. Demands on the student's physical energy should be minimized to allow the student to perform as well as possible in the classroom. These predischarge efforts all help to ensure an easy and successful reentry.

REFERENCES

Ayres, A. J. (1973). *Sensory integration and learning disorders*. Los Angeles: Western Psychological Services.

Baker, L. L., Parker, K., and Sanderson, D. (1983). Neuromuscular electrical stimulation for the head injured patient. *Physical Therapy, 63*, 1967–1974.

Banus, B. S. (1979). Treatment/management. In B. S. Banus, C. A. Kent, Y. Norton, D. R. Sukiennicki, and M. L. Becker (Eds.), *The developmental therapist* (pp. 203–233). Thorofare, NJ: Charles B. Slack.

Basmajian, J. V. (1981). Biofeedback in rehabilitation: A review of principles and practices. *Archives of Physical Medicine and Rehabilitation, 62*, 469–475.

Benton, L. A., Baker, L. L., Bowman, B. R., and Waters, R. L. (1981). *Functional electrical stimulation: A practical clinical guide* (2nd ed.). Downey, CA: Rancho Los Amigos Rehabilitation Engineering Center.

Bly, L. (1980). The components of normal movement during the first year of life. In D. S. Slaton (Ed.), *Development of movement in infancy* (pp. 85–123). Chapel Hill, NC: University of North Carolina at Chapel Hill, Division of Physical Therapy.

Bobath, B. (1969). The treatment of neuromuscular disorders by improving patterns of coordination. *Physiotherapy, 55*, 18–22.

Bobath, B. (1971). *Abnormal postural reflex activity caused by brain lesion* (2nd ed). London: William Heinemann Medical Books Limited.

Bobath, B., and Bobath, K. (1974). *Positioning and moving of hemiplegic patients for nurses and therapists*. London: The Western Cerebral Palsy Centre.

Brink, J. D., Imbus, C., and Woo-Sam, J. (1980). Physical reovery after severe closed head trauma in children and adolescents. *Journal of Pediatrics, 97*, 721–727.

Bruce, D. A., Schut, L., Bruno, L. A., Wood, J. H., and Sutton, L. N. (1978). Outcome following severe head injuries in children. *Journal of Neurosurgery, 48*, 679–688.

Brudny, J., Korein, J., Grynbaum, B. B., Friedman, L. W., Weinstein, S., Sach-Frankel, G., and Belandres, P. V. (1976). EMG feedback therapy: Review of treatment of 114 patients. *Archives of Physical Medicine and Rehabilitation, 57*(2), 55–61.

Capozzi, M., and Mineo, B. (1983). Nonspeech language and communication systems. In A. H. Holland (Ed.), *Language disorders in children* (pp. 173–209). San Diego, CA: College-Hill Press.

Chasin, J. (1978). *Home in a wheelchair*. Washington, DC: Paralyzed Veterans of America.

Chasin, J., and Saltman, J. (1978). *The wheelchair in the kitchen*. Washington, DC: Paralyzed Veterans of America.

Chusid, J. G., and McDonald, J. J. (1962). *Correlative neuroanatomy and functional neurology*. Los Altos, CA: Lange Medical Publications.

Cohen, C. G., and Shane, H. C. (1982). *An overview of augmentative communication*. In N. J. Lass, L. McReynolds, J. L. Northern, and D. E. Yoder (Eds.), *Speech, language and hearing*. Vol, II pp. 875–890. Philadelphia: W. B. Saunders.

Cusick, B. D., and Sussman, M. D. (1981). *Short leg casts: Their role in management of cerebral palsy* (unpublished manuscript). Charlottesville, VA: Children's Rehabilitation Center.

Froeschels, E. (1952). Chewing method as therapy. *Archives of Otolaryngology, 56*, 427–434.

Frostig, M., and Horn, D. (1964). *The Frostig Program for the Development of Visual Perception*. Chicago: Follett Publishing Company.

Jaffe, M. B. (1984). Neurological impairment of speech production: Assessment and treatment. In J. M. Costello (Ed.), *Speech disorders in children* (pp. 157–186). San Diego, CA: College-Hill Press.

Kottke, F. J. (1982). Therapeutic exercise to develop neuromuscular coordination. In F. J. Kottke, G. K. Stillwell, and J. F. Lehmann (Eds.), *Krusen's handbook of physical medicine and rehabilitation* (pp. 403–426). Philadelphia: W. B. Saunders.

Moore, J. C., (1980). Neuroanatomical considerations relating to recovery of function following brain lesions. In P. Bach-y-Rita (Ed.), *Recovery of function: Theoretical considerations for brain injury rehabilitation* (pp. 9–90). Baltimore: University Park Press.

Musselwhite, C. R., and St. Louis, K. W. (1982). *Communication programming for the severely handicapped: Vocal and non-vocal strategies*. San Diego: College-Hill Press.

Rosenbek, J. C., and La Pointe, L. L. (1978). The dysarthrias: Description, diagnosis and treatment. In D. F. Johns (Ed.), *Clinical management of neurogenic communication disorders* (pp. 251–310). Boston: Little, Brown and Co.

Shane, H. C., and Bashir, A. S. (1980). Election criteria for the adoption of an augmentative communication system: Preliminary considerations. *Journal of Speech and Hearing Disorders, 45*, 408–414.

Siev, E., and Freishtat, B. (1976). *Perceptual dysfunction in the adult stroke patient*. Thorofare, NJ: Charles B. Slack.

Silverman, F. H. (1980). *Communication for the speechless*. Englewood Cliffs, NJ: Prentice-Hall.

Skelly, M. (1979). *Amer-Ind gestural code*. New York: Elsevier–North Holland.

Swaan, D., VanWieringen, P. C. W., and Fokkemn, S. D. (1974). Auditory EMG feedback therapy to inhibit underused motor activity. *Archives of Physical Medicine and Rehabilitation, 55*(6), 251–254.

Vanderheiden, G. C. (Ed.) (1978). *Non-vocal communication resource book*. Baltimore: University Park Press.

Van Riper, C., and Irwin, J. V. (1958). *Voice and articulation*. Englewood Cliffs, NJ: Prentice-Hall.

Vaughn, G. R., and Clark, R. M. (1979). *Speech facilitation: Extraoral and intraoral stimulation technique for improvement of articulation skills*. Springfield, IL: Charles C Thomas.

Wertz, R. T., La Pointe, L. L., and Rosenbek, J. C. (1984). *Apraxia of speech in adults*. Orlando, FL: Grune & Stratton.

Williams, J. R., Csongradi, J. J., and Le Blanc, M. A. (1982). *A guide to controls: Selection, mounting, application*. Palo Alto, CA: Children's Hospital at Stanford.

Wittmeyer, M., and Barrett, J. E. (1980). *Housing Accessibility Checklist*. Seattle: University of Washington, Health Resource Center.

Ylvisaker, M. (1981, October). Cognitive and behavioral outcomes in head injured children. Paper presented at the International Symposium on the Traumatic Brain Injured Adult and Child, Boston.

Young, E. H., and Hawk, S. S. (1955). *Moto-kinesthetic speech training*. Stanford, CA: Stanford University Press.

Young, R. R., and Delwaide, P. J. (1981a). Drug therapy: Spasticity (1st of 2 parts). *New England Journal of Medicine, 304*(1), 28-33.

Young, R. R., and Delwaide, P. J. (1981b). Drug therapy: Spasticity (2nd of 2 parts). *New England Journal of Medicine, 304*(2), 96-99.

Chapter 7

Therapy for Feeding and Swallowing Disorders Following Head Injury

Mark Ylvisaker, MA, and
Jerilyn Logemann, PhD

Although there are no reported data on the incidence of feeding and swallowing problems following severe head injury in children, it is safe to say that transient impairments at an early stage of recovery are pervasive and significant residual problems requiring long-term therapeutic management are not uncommon. Swallowing disorders are singled out for special treatment in this book for two reasons. First, because none of the rehabilitation professions routinely trains its members in dysphagia treatment, most agencies have less expertise in this area than in other areas of motor restoration. Second, swallowing disorders can have serious medical implications and must be managed accordingly.

There is currently no agreement in the use of the terms "feeding" and "swallowing." Following Logemann's usage (1983), in this chapter the term "feeding" includes (1) placement of food in the mouth; (2) manipulation in the mouth (e.g., chewing and bolus formation); and (3) posterior movement of the bolus by the tongue into the pharynx. The term "swallowing" generally encompasses these three feeding processes as well as triggering of the swallowing reflex and the movement of the bolus through the pharynx and esophagus into the stomach. Occasionally, the term "swallowing" is used in a narrower sense to refer to the aspects of deglutition that commence with the triggering of the swallowing reflex.

Although treatment techniques for oral motor feeding disorders are listed here (Appendix 7-1), this chapter focuses primarily on diagnosis and treatment of disorders of swallowing that occur after the oral phase of deglutition. These disorders are less well understood and are more serious medically than oral motor feeding problems. Furthermore, oral motor dysfunction by itself, regardless of the severity, need not interfere with oral intake of food, since special placement techniques (e.g., syringe) or diet changes (liquid only) can bypass the oral phase of swallowing entirely. The reflexive or pharyngeal phase of the swallow cannot be bypassed.

The ultimate goal of treatment for dysphagic patients is complete recovery of normal eating patterns while, at the same time, maintaining the patient's health and nutritional status. Unfortunately, some head injured patients cannot achieve this goal because of apparently permanent impairments of deglutition. For these latter patients, more restricted goals may be identified:

- Oral feeding using compensatory techniques or some degree of primitive or abnormal oral patterns, or a restricted range of food consistencies
- Combined oral and tube feedings, with tubes used primarily to maintain hydration
- Minimal "recreational" oral feeding (for long-term, severely involved patients)

Secondarily, the dysphagia (swallowing disorders) program for head injured patients in the early stages of cognitive recovery is part of the sensory stimulation program described in Chapter 10, which is designed to increase the patient's alertness and adaptive responses. Improvement in oral feeding also serves to heighten a patient's motivation and sense of normalcy while at the same time providing a naturally pleasurable experience.

The objectives of this chapter are the following:

- to describe neurogenic swallowing disorders, emphasizing those that are particularly common following head injury
- to introduce anatomic and physiologic concepts relevant to an explanation of these disorders and their treatment
- to describe evaluation, including radiographic procedures, and the purposes and limitations of these procedures
- to emphasize special considerations for cognitively impaired patients who have feeding or swallowing disorders
- to present treatment options

Therapists responsible for the assessment and treatment of swallowing disorders should consult Logemann (1983) for a more thorough and highly informative discussion of the issues addressed in this chapter.

DISORDERS OF SWALLOWING FOLLOWING HEAD INJURY

Disorders of feeding and swallowing can result from anterior cortical (motor strip) lesions or from damage to the brain stem. With very severe head injury, there is a strong possiblility of combined focal, multifocal, and diffuse cortical, subcortical, and brain stem damage, which makes it difficult to localize the lesion responsible for a feeding or swallowing problem. However, lower brain stem — especially medulla — damage usually results in significant problems in the reflexive swallow.

Specific swallowing disorders will be described under the four stages of swallowing: oral preparatory, oral, pharyngeal, and esophageal. These stages — and corresponding disorders — are discussed in greater detail in Logemann (1983).

The Oral Preparatory Phase

The oral preparatory phase of swallowing includes placement of food in the mouth and oral manipulation for bolus preparation as well as for the pleasure of eating. This involves the jaw, lips, tongue, cheeks, teeth, and palate. Graded and refined jaw movements are required to open the mouth to allow food to enter and to reduce food to a consistency ready for bolus formation by the tongue. Lateral tongue movements move the food particles to and from the molars for chewing. Refined lip movements are needed to form a seal on the cup, straw, spoon, or fork and to keep food in the mouth during the preparatory stage. Cheek (buccal) tension keeps food out of the lateral sulci (spaced between teeth and the cheeks) during chewing and assists in posterior propulsion of the food for swallowing. Active pressure of the soft palate against the back of the tongue creates a posterior seal and prevents food from trickling into the pharynx prematurely. Posterior elevation of the tongue against the soft palate helps to create the posterior seal. When oral preparation is completed, a variety of refined tongue movements collect the food particles from any location in the oral cavity to form a cohesive bolus prior to the beginning of the oral stage of the swallow. The duration of the oral preparatory stage varies with food consistency as well as with individual style. The processes are voluntary in neurologically normal individuals beyond infancy. Normal breathing continues during this phase, and the airway is open.

Disorders. Common disorders in the oral preparatory phase resulting from central nervous system dysfunction following head injury include the following.

Primitive or pathologic reflexes. Developmentally primitive or pathologic reflexes including the rooting reflex, tonic or clonic bite, and food ejection are often present after head trauma and interfere with normal patterns.

Abnormal muscle tone. Hypo- or hypertonicity of the lips, cheeks, jaw, and tongue interferes with the normal preparatory stage functions of these structures described earlier.

Abnormal sensation. Hypersensitivity to touch may elicit pathologic reflexes or tonal changes, such as lip pursing or retraction, jaw clenching or hyperextension, tongue protrusion or retraction, or total head hyperextension or deviation. Hyposensitivity may result in food particles being lost in the mouth, falling out of the mouth, or prematurely falling into the pharynx. The direction in which the food falls will depend on head position, the consistency of the food, and the amount of food.

Movement disorders. A combination of abnormal reflexes, sensation, and muscle tone creates characteristic movement disorders following head injury: difficulty in opening the mouth to receive the food, difficulty in closing the lips around a cup or utensil, loss of food from the mouth or into the pharynx before the swallow, and a suckle-swallow pattern that excludes tongue lateralization and bolus formation and often requires several suckle movements before a swallow can be initiated. Disorders of sensation, muscle tone, and movement patterns can easily result in food entering the pharynx *before* the swallow is initiated, with the possibility of aspiration before the swallow despite an otherwise adequate swallowing mechanism.

Oral Phase

The oral phase of swallowing begins when the tongue initiates an anterior-posterior squeezing or stripping movement against the palate (Blonsky, Logemann, Boshes, and Fisher, 1975; Miller, 1982; Shedd, Kirchner, and Scatliff, 1961). The oral phase ends when the bolus passes the anterior faucial arches and the swallowing reflex is triggered. The oral phase is voluntary and normally takes approximately one second to complete (Blonsky et al., 1975; Mandelstam and Lieber, 1970).

Disorders. The tone, sensation, and movement disorders of the tongue already described dramatically interfere with this phase. Suckle-swallow or munch patterns (Morris, 1982), not uncommon following head injury, result in bolus dispersion as well as inefficient and slow anterior

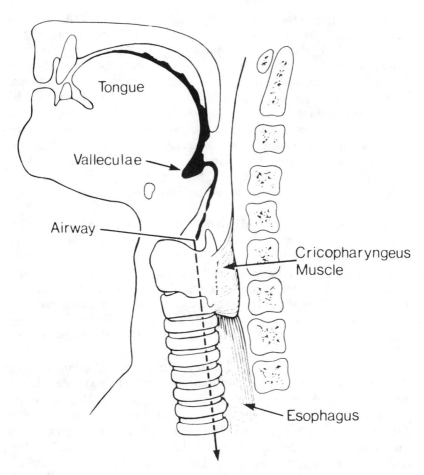

Figure 7-1. Lateral view of the head and neck with food trickling over the tongue and into the airway during the oral phase of the swallow before the swallowing reflex triggered.

to posterior movement of the tongue. Food can trickle over the back of the tongue *before the swallow* and either collect in the vallecular space or fall into the airway or pyriform sinuses, as shown in Figure 7-1. Inadequate labial and buccal tension will also decrease the efficiency of this phase.

Pharyngeal Phase

This phase begins with the triggering of the swallowing reflex as the bolus passes into the oropharynx and ends when the bolus passes through the cricopharyngeal sphincter (or pharyngoesophageal segment) and into the esophagus. The four physiologic processes that define the pharyngeal phase are all triggered or programmed by reflex: (1) the nasopharynx is closed by active movements of the velum and pharyngeal wall; (2) food is propelled toward the esophagus by coordinated pharyngeal wall peristaltic action; (3) the airway is protected by the elevation of the larynx and by three valving actions: the epiglottis and aryepiglottic folds are pulled down over the larynx, and the false and the true vocal folds adduct; (4) the cricopharyngeus, normally closed to keep esophageal contents out of the pharynx, relaxes momentarily to allow passage into the esophagus (Bosma, 1957; Curtis, Cruess, and Berg, 1984; Miller, 1982). During this phase, the bolus divides evenly as it passes over the epiglottis and passes through the two pyriform sinuses.

The swallowing reflex is in part voluntary and in part reflexive (Miller, 1982). The tongue propulsion in the oral phase represents the cortical or voluntary input into the triggering of the reflex. The four neuromuscular functions described in the last paragraph occur reflexively and in sequence to actualize the reflex in the pharyngeal phase of the swallow. The pharyngeal phase of the swallow normally takes no more than one second, and respiration is temporarily halted for the portion of the pharyngeal stage when the airway is closed (Blonsky et al., 1975; Mandelstam and Lieber, 1970).

Disorders. Our experience as well as that of other clinicians suggests that the most common posterior swallowing disorder following head injury is a delayed or absent swallowing reflex (Logemann, 1983). If the reflex is not delayed more than 3 or 4 seconds, and if very small quantities of food are given and the patient is well positioned, a delayed reflex simply means that food will collect in the vallecular space before the swallow (Fig. 7-1). If larger quantities are given or if the patient's head is hyperextended, the food will enter the pharynx and collect in the pyriform sinuses or enter the airway, which is unprotected until the swallowing reflex is triggered. Inadequate velopharyngeal closure, if severe or if accompanied by uncoordinated pharyngeal peristalsis, will result in nasal regurgitation. Failure of the three airway protection valves to close can result in aspiration *during* the swallow. Not all of the valves need be efficient, however, and alert patients can facilitate protection by holding their breath during the swallow and immediately coughing and spitting, then swallowing again (supraglottic swallow, described below). Failure of the airway protection mechanisms *during* the swallow is not, in our experience, a common disorder following head injury. Failure of the larynx to be elevated can result in residue left on top of the larynx *after* the swallow and in aspiration *after* the swallow when the patient opens the larynx to inhale.

Uncoordinated or weak pharyngeal peristalsis results in residue in the pharynx and possible aspiration *after* the swallow. This is not uncommon following head injury, and the weakness may be unilateral or bilateral. Poorly timed cricopharyngeal relaxation or complete spacticity of this sphincter results in minimal or no penetration of the bolus into the esophagus, with the likelihood of significant aspiration *after* the swallow. Since the pharyngeal recesses are large enough to hold several cubic centimeters of food, this disorder is often misdiagnosed as fatigue, since the patient may not cough or sputter until after trying to swallow four to five spoonfuls. Cricopharyngeal disorders have also been observed following head trauma (Logemann, 1983) but are not common.

If combined oral and pharyngeal transit time with the best food consistency is greater than 10 seconds, supplementary tube feedings will probably be required to maintain nutrition even if airway protection is not a problem (Logemann, 1983).

Esophageal Phase

The esophageal phase begins with the entrance of the bolus into the esophagus and ends with passage of food through the gastroesophageal sphincter into the stomach. It is completely involuntary and normally takes 8 to 20 seconds (Mandelstam and Lieber, 1970). This phase will not be discussed, since esophageal disorders are not assessed or treated by feeding-swallowing therapists, although they occasionally masquerade as swallowing disorders if they result in reflux and aspiration.

ASSESSMENT OF SWALLOWING

Assessment and treatment of swallowing disorders should be a team process. The attending physician, together with a nutritionist and, if indicated, ENT, pulmonary, and gastroenterological medical specialists, evaluates the patient's medical history and current nutritional, physiologic, and general health status relevant to feeding decisions. The swallowing therapist, who may be a speech-language pathologist, an occupational or physical therapist, or a nurse specifically trained in dysphagia management, should complete a bedside examination of oral structures and function and, indirectly, of laryngeal function and swallowing effectiveness. (In our facilities speech-language pathologists play this role.) If posterior swallowing disorders or aspiration is suspected, a videofluorographic swallowing study should be performed by a radiologist working together with the swallowing therapist. Since the majority of serious swallowing disorders in this population are pharyngeal in origin, a radiographic study is often necessary.

With all of the relevant information assembled, the team makes a decision regarding the initial treatment regimen. The most common possibilities are the following:

- Nasogastric tube (NG) or gastrostomy feeding only, with a program of oral motor and swallowing therapy with no food
- NG or gastrostomy feeding for nutrition and hydration, with oral treatment to include trial oral feeding with small quantities of food and close monitoring of responses
- Combined oral and tube feeding, systematically decreasing the latter as oral intake increases
- Exclusive oral feeding, with a systematic normalization of methods of intake (e.g., from syringe to tongue blade to spoon to self-feeding) and of food consistencies. Pudding or apple sauce *may* have consistencies easiest for head injured patients, followed by thick nectars and blenderized solid foods. Dry or multitextured solid foods are often difficult for dysphagic patients to handle. Thin liquids may be the most difficult for head injured patients because of bolus formation problems, a delayed swallowing reflex (if present), and the rapid movement of thin liquids through a slowly responding system. It is important to note, however, that the choice of food consistency for a particular patient will depend on knowledge of that patient's disorder(s).

In making initial decisions regarding a treatment regimen, it is extremely important to remember that feeding and swallowing disorders can be treated as effectively or more effectively with *no* food or *very small quantities* of food as with large quantities of food. There is no treatment advantage to a potentially dangerous and premature resumption of oral feedings. On the other hand, there is reason to proceed aggressively with exercises directed to improving those neuromotor functions necessary for normal swallowing and early trial oral feeding treatment, since normalization of eating patterns may be foremost in the minds of patients and their families, and this normalization may be importantly related to behavior management and cognitive reorientation.

Bedside Assessment

The feeding therapist's bedside examination should include careful observation of the patient's overall positions, muscle tone, and reflex patterns, as well as the anatomy, reflexive and nonreflexive functioning, and sensation of oral structures (Logemann, 1983; Morris, 1978).

Assessment of pharyngeal intactness and airway protection can be done only indirectly at bedside, and inferences from gross observation of swallowing symptoms are known to be unreliable (Logemann, Lazarus, and Jenkins, 1982; Linden and Siebens, 1983).

Four reflexes are triggered in the posterior oral cavity and larynx. These reflexes should be triggered, if possible, and their responses assessed for intactness of muscle contraction.

Palatal Reflex. *Stimulus:* Touch the soft palate in the midline just posterior to the hard palate juncture. *Response:* Upward and backward movement of the velum, without pharyngeal wall movement; may require several stimulations.

Gag Reflex. *Stimulus:* Touch the back of the tongue or posterior pharyngeal wall. *Response:* Strong contraction of the pharyngeal wall and soft palate; forward propulsion to clear the pharynx.

Protective Cough Reflex. *Stimulus:* material in airway. *Response:* cough (diaphragm contracts, larynx elevates, pharynx constricts). Note: The voluntary cough and the cough reflex are neurologically independent of one another. Many head injured patients have no reflexive cough in response to food entering the airway.

Swallow Reflex. *Stimulus:* Material in contact with the base of the anterior faucial arches, posterior pharyngeal wall, and possibly posterior tongue, epiglottis, larynx, and lower pharynx. The presence of material to be swallowed and beginning tongue movements are also part of the eliciting mechanism. *Response:* Reflexive swallow characterized by the neuromotor movements noted earlier.

Two points must be stressed. Of these four reflexes, only the swallowing reflex is required for adequate oral intake of food. Second, these reflexes are neurologically independent in that the presence or absence of one does not necessarily indicate the presence or absence of any of the others. Hence, it is unacceptable to draw strong conclusions regarding the status of the swallowing mechanism, as is often done, from the presence or absence of a gag reflex (Logemann, 1983).

Swallowing Efficiency and Aspiration

Currently, all bedside assessments of aspiration and the pharyngeal aspect of swallowing have a high error rate (approximately 40 per cent). Four tests are described.

Four Finger Test (Logemann, 1983). At bedside, secretions can be stimulated with oral stimulation and spontaneous swallowing observed.

Alert patients can also be instructed to swallow. Following stimulation, place the index finger lightly under the patient's chin anteriorly, the second finger on the hyoid bone, the third and fourth fingers above and below the thyroid cartilage. From this placement the following information can be collected: initiation of tongue movements, number of tongue movements prior to a swallow, initiation of hyoid movement with the swallow reflex, and timing and strength of laryngeal elevation. This provides a rough indication of the presence or absence of the swallowing reflex as well as oral transit time. It is *not* an indication of pharyngeal efficiency. A cough following the swallow indicates a cough reflex, but it also is strongly suggestive of aspiration.

Blue Dye Test (Manly, 1983). For patients with tracheostomy tubes, four drops of methylene blue dye can be placed on the tongue so that the colored saliva will not escape as drool. After several minutes, the patient should be suctioned. The presence of dye in the suctioned material is positive evidence of aspiration. The absence of dye does not guarantee the absence of aspiration. The test should be repeated several times if the results are negative. The presence of a tracheostomy tube is very useful during the initial stages of oral feeding, both for diagnostic purposes and for suctioning.

Phonation Test. Alert patients are asked to vocalize following a swallow. A wet, hoarse quality to the voice suggests aspiration (Linden and Siebens, 1983). If patients are unable to follow instructions, the therapist should listen for spontaneous breathing, vocalizing, and coughing. If breathing is noisy or if the voice or cough following trial oral feeding is hoarse or wet sounding, then again aspiration should be suspected.

A Positive History of Pneumonia. Pneumonia or suspicious lung sounds are further indications of possible aspiration.

Radiographic Assessment

Those patients whose bedside examination or pathophysiologic and medical history indicate the possibility of aspiration or pharyngeal dysfunction during the swallow without aspiration are referred for a videofluorographic swallowing study. The purpose of the study is to provide the swallowing therapist with diagnostic information relevant to the following questions:

- Should oral feedings be reintroduced?
- How efficiently do the oral, pharyngeal, laryngeal, and upper esophageal structures function during swallowing?

- How adequate is the patient's airway protection under varying conditions?
- In what ways do position, food consistency and amount, method of presentation, physical prompts, and instructions affect swallowing?

In summary, this radiographic procedure provides information that is otherwise unavailable, but which is essential to effective dysphagia therapy. From a medical point of view, the key issue is to determine the amount of aspiration relative to food consistency, position, and method of intake. For swallowing therapists it may be equally important to identify pharyngeal dysfunction in patients who may or may not aspirate, and to document the best food consistency and feeding technique radiographically. Ideally, the feeding therapist will have a working relationship with the radiologist so that experimentation with positioning, food consistency, and method of intake can occur during the radiographic study.

Because the questions to be answered in the videofluorographic study of oral and pharyngeal aspects of swallowing differ dramatically from those at issue in standard barium swallows studies (i.e., esophageal anatomy and motility), procedures also differ dramatically. Most importantly, the patient should be upright (possibly seated or strapped onto a tilt table) and very small quantities of food given. Positioning for neurologically impaired patients often requires advance preparation, time, and ingenuity. The patient is given one third to one half teaspoon of barium-injected pudding or apple sauce, followed by one third to one half teaspoon of thin liquid barium (often more difficult for head injured patients to swallow), and a small piece (one quarter) of barium paste–coated cookie, if indicated.

The study begins with a lateral view to measure oral and pharyngeal transit times and to observe location of stasis in the oral cavity and pharynx, swallowing reflex, general pharyngeal efficiency, and, finally, amount of and reason for aspiration. One or two swallows are repeated in an anteroposterior view to detect possible unilateral pharyngeal disorders, as well as to examine vocal fold functioning. To assess vocal fold movement, the patient's neck is hyperextended and the patient is asked to say, "ah, ah, ah."

Radiographic swallowing studies are particularly important for cognitively impaired patients and young children suspected of having pharyngeal disorders, since these patients are rarely able to recognize or describe their swallowing problems. With young children, taste experimentation prior to the study may be necessary to avoid contamination of the results because of taste aversions. Logemann (1983) gives additional details on the procedures and purposes of this videofluorographic swallowing study, known as the modified barium swallow, or "cookie-swallow test."

TREATMENT

Appendix 7-1 includes a large number of intervention procedures, organized according to the anatomic or physiologic dysfunction they address. These procedures, which should be selected following a complete team assessment and careful identification of the disorder, have been compiled from a variety of sources, including Morris (1982, 1978) and Logemann (1983). The treatment suggestions fall under five major categories.

Neuromuscular Treatment. Neuromuscular treatment involves inhibitory and desensitizing stimulation for hypersensitivity, hypertonicity, and hyperreflexia, and excitory stimulation and strengthening exercises for hyposensitivity, hypotonicity, and hyporeflexia.

Position. The best position of the total body and the head in relation to the body is used to normalize tone and reflexes, to create the most efficient movement of food, and to maximize patient safety.

Food. The best consistency, taste, and temperature are used to control movement of the food, to effect efficiency of swallowing and airway protection, and to avoid taste aversions. Of these, consistency is most important.

Swallowing Technique. Alert patients can learn compensatory food placement or compensatory swallowing techniques to enhance food movement and airway protection.

Medical-Nutritional Issues. Issues to be considered include adequate nutrition and hydration, adequate airway protection and pulmonary function, prosthetic devices, and surgical intervention.

It is generally preferable to have several short (10 to 15 minute) oral stimulation-swallowing therapy sessions per day than one or two extended sessions. We give written instructions to alert patients who can exercise independently and tell them to exercise at least five times per day. Exercises should be done in front of a mirror and followed by a functional task (facial expression, speech, eating).

With cognitively and motorically involved patients, sometimes family members, nursing staff, and stimulation team members are included in the dysphagia program. However, because dysphagia treatment requires considerable skill, and treatment can be aversive and even frightening, treatment staff should be well trained and establish a good relationship with the patient. Following intervention sessions, it is important to leave patients upright and observe them for several minutes to monitor delayed responses.

Family members often have strong emotional feelings associated with oral feeding. Mothers of young children may have an intense, but unspoken, need to feed the child as an act of nurturing. Consequently, careful and sympathetic counseling is necessary to gain parents' acceptance of what they may perceive to be a slow reintroduction of oral feeding. The therapist must explain the intervention process thoroughly at each stage of recovery. If a radiographic study has been completed, family members often benefit from seeing the videotape recording of the study to help them understand the nature of the patient's swallowing disorders and the reason(s) why the patient should not feed by mouth.

Table 7–1 outlines principles of positioning and communication useful in preparing patients for feeding or swallowing treatment sessions.

Treatment of Patients with Severe Cognitive Deficits

Some decrease in cognitive functioning almost always accompanies disorders of feeding and swallowing following head injury. Cognitive and behavioral deficits compound the already difficult task of helping patients to improve their feeding and swallowing patterns. It may, for instance, be impossible to treat patients at a stage of severe agitation. Furthermore, treatment techniques that require patients to follow verbal instructions are not options in the very early stages of recovery. Even cognitively well recovered patients may have difficulty acquiring compensatory swallowing techniques because of a depressed ability to learn new routines.

The following guidelines are useful in treating cognitively impaired patients:

Environment. The environment in which feeding therapy occurs should be quiet, adequately lighted, and free of distractions. Treatment personnel should be familiar to the patient and should choose times for treatment when the patient is known to be most alert.

Behavior and Judgment. Since feeding treatment can be unpleasant and even frightening for patients, the therapist must be skilled in preparing, reassuring, calming, and redirecting them. Techniques of behavior management are discussed in Chapter 13. These techniques should be used to complement the positive effects of a good relationship with the patient.

Confused patients with minimal neuromotor involvement continue to require attention. Because of impaired judgment, these patients often put far too much food into their mouths, placing them at increased risk

Table 7-1. Preparation for Treatment Sessions

Muscle Tone
   Consult occupational or physical therapist regarding procedures to normalize total body tone before proceeding with feeding or oral treatment.
Positioning
   Frequent position: Upright sitting; hips flexed 90 degrees; knees flexed 90 degrees; feet supported; shoulders relaxed; arms forward; head in midline and slightly flexed.
   Exceptions: Severely involved patients may be treated semi-upright in bed, head and knees propped with pillows. A chin tuck position (head flexed forward) is often important for head injured patients since it widens the vallecular space, adding a dimension of safety for patients with a delayed swallow reflex. Tilting or turning the head may be indicated for specific pharyngeal disorders (see Appendix 7-1), as may having the patient lie down. Other positions may be necessary, depending on the nature of the patient's swallowing problem.
Communication
   Prepare all patients with simple descriptions of what is to be done (see Chapter 10). Give specific instructions (e.g., "Lift your tongue now") only if the patterns cannot be reestablished on an automatic basis. Similarly, feedback should remain general (e.g., "Nice job") rather than specific (e.g., "You swallowed too quickly that time") unless a decision has been made to bring the process under voluntary control. Make the session pleasant and encouraging; discontinue temporarily in the face of agitation.

for aspiration. It is essential to keep food out of reach and to slow the rate of eating for these patients. After a meal, we check the oral cavity for residue that could be aspirated.

New Learning. Patients who are no longer significantly confused may continue to have difficulty learning and generalizing new procedures, such as compensatory feeding techniques. Because of this depressed learning rate, repeated instruction and ongoing cuing will be necessary.

REFERENCES

Blonsky, E., Logemann, J., Boshes, B., and Fisher, H. (1975). Comparison of speech and swallowing function in patients with tremor disorders and in normal geriatric patients: A cinefluorographic study. *Journal of Gerontology, 30,* 299–303.

Bosma, J. (1957). Deglutition: Pharyngeal stage. *Physiological Reviews, 37,* 275–300.

Curtis, D., Cruess, D., and Berg, T. (1984). The cricopharyngeal muscle: A video recording review. *American Journal of Radiology, 142,* 497–500.

Linden, P., and Siebens, A. (1983). A dysphagia: Predicting laryngeal penetration. *Archives of Physical Medicine and Rehabilitation, 64,* 281–284.

Logemann, J. (1983). *Evaluation and treatment of swallowing disorders.* San Diego: College-Hill Press.

Logemann, J., Lazarus C., and Jenkins, P. (1982, November). The relationship between clinical judgment and radiographic assessment of aspiration. Paper presented at the American Speech Language Hearing Association Annual Meeting, Toronto.

Mandelstam, P., and Lieber, A. (1970). Cineradiographic evaluation of the esophagus in normal adults. *Gastroenterology, 58,* 32–38.

Manly, C. A. (1983, October). *Dysphagia assessment.* Workshop presented at the conference Technology in the 80's: Impact on Speech and Language Services, New York.

Miller, A. (1982). Deglutition. *Physiological Reviews, 62,* 129–184.

Morris, S. (1982). *The normal acquisition of oral feeding skills: Implications for assessment and treatment.* New York: Therapeutic Media, Inc.

Morris, S. (1978). Oral-motor problems and guidelines for treatment. In J. M. Wilson (Ed.), *Oral-motor function and dysfunction in children.* Chapel Hill, NC: University of North Carolina.

Shedd, D., Kirchner, J., and Scatliff, J. (1961). Oral and pharyngeal components of deglutition. *Archives of Surgery, 82,* 371–380.

APPENDIX 7-1
TREATMENT OPTIONS

Key: *Can be done regardless of the patient's level of alertness, unless medically contra-indicated. In some cases, the patient must be sufficiently alert to be aware of food in the mouth.

†Requires that the patient be able to process simple instructions.

‡Requires that the patient be able to learn new procedures.

I. ORAL-FACIAL DYSFUNCTION
  A. *Hypersensitivity to stimulation: grimace, pathologic reflexes, hypertonicity of oral structures*
    *1. Gradual *desensitization:* Firm pressure with a warm wash cloth, fingers, or other implement. Begin at some distance from the face. Gradually move closer to the mouth, always stopping short of eliciting the pathologic responses.
    *2. *Oral stimulation:* Use a glycerin swab, finger, or other implement (note infection control issues with finger stimulation). Use jaw control during stimulation, if needed.
      a. Firmly rub gums, one side, then the other; first upper, then lower. Start with one rub, increase to four per quadrant. Use pureed food on the swab or the finger if the patient can swallow and production of saliva is desired.
      b. Firmly rub front to back on the palate, first one side, then the other, then the midline. Stop short of a gag.
      c. Firmly tap down on the tongue, front to back on midline. Stop short of a gag.
      d. Stimulate across the surface of the tongue for tongue flattening.
      e. Stimulate lightly along the lateral edges of the tongue for lateralization.
      f. Holding the tongue between index and middle fingers, vibrate side to side for range and tone reduction.
      g. With index finger inside and middle finger outside, vibrate cheek muscles out to reduce cheek tone.
    Note: Give the patient time to swallow after each stimulation. Always stop short of an abnormal response. Do not overstimulate. Gradually increase the amount of stimulation that the patient can tolerate. Be sensitive to the offensiveness of fingers in the mouth. Use a swab or other implement if indicated. Do not place fingers or a fragile implement in the oral cavity of a patient with a tonic bite reflex.
  B. *Hyposensitivity or hypotonicity*
    a. Orofacial musculature: Several strengthening exercises are listed below for specific structures. Most exercises are facilitated by first stimulating the belly of the muscle being exercised. Possible forms of stimulation: tapping firmly or flicking with finger; quick stretch of the muscle, rapid brushing; light application of ice, then wipe dry. Wait briefly after stimulation before beginning the exercise. These forms of sensory stimulation can be initiated before the patient is cognitively capable of deliberately exercising the structures.
    b. Intra-oral hyposensitivity: Experiment with food temperatures (especially cold) and tastes (especially spicy). Place food on the more sensitive side of the oral cavity.
II. LIPS
  A. *Hypertonic: poor closure, loss of food, drooling*
    *1. See hypertonicity suggestions above (I.A.).
    *2. Firm pressure below the nose to lower tone. Do not pull down on a hypertonic upper lip.

*3. Allow time for closure on the spoon or tongue blade or cup during feeding. Do not scrape food off the spoon using upper teeth.

*4. Use a straw to encourage lip closure. This can initially be done using the straw as a pipette, with the therapist holding one end of the straw to control the amount.

B. *Hypotonic: weak closure, loss of foods, drooling*

*1. See hypotonicity suggestions above (I.B).

†2. Place a button held by a string inside the patient's lips in front of the teeth. Pull on string, requiring the patient to hold the button by pursing his or her lips.

†3. Have the patient hold tongue blade(s) between his or her lips and resist outward pull. Decrease the number of blades as lip closure improves, to increase task difficulty.

†4. Instruct the patient to smile or pucker or raise or lower the upper or lower lip, all against finger resistance. Gradually increase resistance.

†5. Instruct the patient to suck on a straw (no food) with end held closed to offer resistance. If the patient can swallow, practice sucking heavy liquids through a straw.

†6. Have the patient hold exaggerated facial expressions.

†7. Instruct the patient to alternate between an exaggerated smile (or "ee") and exaggerated pucker (or "oo"). Increase the length of time in each posture.

†8. Gradually increase the amount of time the patient can maintain continuous, firm lip closure.

†9. Have the patient practice words with bilabial consonants (m, b, p, w) in all word positions with exaggerated ariculation.

*10. In feeding, wait for the patient to bring his or her upper lip down on the tongue blade, spoon, or cup. Do not scrape food off the spoon using upper teeth. Do not simply pour liquid into the mouth. Use a tongue blade or shallow spoon before proceeding to a deep bowl spoon.

III. CHEEKS

A. *Hypertonic: grimace, pseudosmile, poor lip closure.* See hypertonicity suggestions above (I.A).

B. *Hypotonic: loss of food in lateral sulci, weak facial expression*

*1. See hypotonicity suggestions above (I.B).

†2. Instruct the patient to exaggerate facial expressions involving cheek muscles. Hold the expressions for increasing periods or against finger resistance, or both.

†3. Instruct the patient to alternate rapidly between an exaggerated smile and an exaggerated pucker.

†4. Instruct the patient to puff out his or her cheeks by filling them with air. Gradually increase finger resistance against the puffed cheeks.

*5. During feeding:
   a. Apply external pressure on the affected cheek to keep food out of the sulcus.
   b. Place food on the unaffected side and tilt the head slightly toward that side.

IV. TONGUE

A. *Hypertonic: tongue bunched; forward thrust to initiate the swallow*

*1. See suggestions for hypertonicity stimulation above (I.A).

†2. Use textured food and molar placement as much as possible. Use jaw control unless the jaw control itself increases hypertonicity.

†3. Mild to moderate tongue thrust: Instruct the patient to position his or her tongue on the alveolar ridge and initiate a swallow with up or back tongue movement.

B. *Hypertonic: tongue retraction*

*1. Apply firm pressure on the belly of the tongue with a spoon or tongue blade; gradually bring the spoon or tongue blade farther forward on the tongue.

C. *Reduced tongue lateralization*

   *1. Stroke lightly along the lateral edges of the tongue with a toothbrush, swab, or similar instrument.

   †2. Instruct the patient to press his or her tongue laterally against a tongue blade.

   †3. Use a piece of gauze for the patient to practice chewing. First, place the end of a gauze roll on the patient's tongue at the midline. Then ask the patient to move to the end of the gauze to each side of his or her mouth and back to the midline.

   *4. Begin feeding with pureed food: gradually add texture. Place small pieces of crunchy food on the molars to encourage lateralization; facilitate a chew.

D. *Hypotonic: reduced tongue elevation*

   †1. Instruct the patient to elevate the front of the tongue, hold, and release. Elevate the back of the tongue, hold, and release.

   †2. Instruct the patient to push the tongue up against a tongue blade.

   †3. Instruct the patient to push up against a wad of gauze (juice-soaked if the patient can swallow). The therapist should hold the end of the gauze. The size of the gauze wad can be diminished as tongue elevation improves.

   †4. Have the patient practice hard contact consonant-vowel (CV) syllables beginning with /t/ and /k/.

   *5. During feeding, regularly check the patient's palate for packed food.

   *6. If there is a residual elevation impairment, consider consultation with a maxillofacial prosthodontist to discuss a prosthetic appliance to lower the roof of the mouth to meet the tongue.

E. *Reduced bolus formation and cupping of the tongue*

   †1. Use a licorice whip, a long piece of gauze soaked in juice, or a Lifesaver on a string with the therapist firmly holding one end. Place the other end in the patient's mouth. Have the patient move his or her end to all extremities of the oral cavity, retrieve it, and return to midtongue. Gradually increase range, accuracy, and speed of movement.

   †2. Give the patient a small amount of pudding. As him or her to hold the bolus with the tongue, move the bolus around in the mouth, and then spit it out. Check for residue. When the patient can manipulate the pudding bolus satisfactorily, gradually liquify the material. Ask the patient to hold each bolus with the tongue, move it around the mouth, bring it to the middle of the tongue, and hold it again. The patient should then spit the material out, and the therapist should check the oral cavity for residue.

F. *Reduced anterior-posterior movement to start the swallow*

   †1. Place a long piece of juice-soaked gauze front to back along the patient's tongue. Have the patient squeeze the juice out of the gauze by pressing the tongue against the gauze, anterior to posterior. The patient should swallow at the end of the movement.

G. *General tongue dysfunction*

   *1. If the tongue is mildly to moderately involved, tilt the patient's head toward the stronger side to keep food from being lost on the weaker side.

   *2. If the tongue is severely involved but the reflexive swallow is adequate, use a syringe or straw to place the food directly in the back of the oral cavity.

   *3. Patients with primitive suck-swallow or munch patterns should be able to eat pureed foods adequately (if the reflexive swallow is normal). However, a diet of nothing but pureed foods will not improve tongue patterns. Hence, textured and crunchy foods placed on the molars should be introduced as soon as possible, consistent with patient safety. Alternate sides of the mouth. If the patient cannot safely handle textured or crunchy foods, use gauze to practice chewing and tongue lateralization, as decribed in IV. C.3.

* 4 . *Drinking.* Thick liquids (thick nectar or milkshake consistency) are easier to handle, usually less likely to be aspirated and less likely to worsen the patient's primitive oral patterns than are thin liquids. If excessive secretions are a problem, reduce the intake of milk and milk products.

V. JAW

A. *Hypertonic: jaw thrust*
   *1. Use good positioning (see above) and jaw control during feeding and oral stimulation. Do not use jaw control if it increases the force of the thrust pattern. See suggestions for hypertonicity stimulation above (I.A).

B. *Hypertonic: bite reflex (tonic)*
   *1. See suggestions for hypertonicity stimulation above (I.A.2).
   *2. Press firmly on the belly of the patient's masseters to release. Do not try to pull the spoon out of the mouth during a tonic bite reflex, as this usually increases the reflex.

C. *Hypotonic: reduced range*
   *1. See suggestions for hypotonicity stimulation (I.B).
   † 2 . Have the patient move his or her jaw in all directions (open-lateralize), hold for 1 to 2 seconds, and release. Add resistance.

D. *Weak vertical and rotary chewing movements*
   * 1 . Place small pieces of fruit in a juice-soaked gauze sleeve; the therapist holds both open ends of the sleeve. Place the fruit between the patient's molars and facilitate chewing movements.
   * 2 . Use a combination of pureed foods and easily crunchable foods placed directly on the molars. Manually assist with chewing motions if necessary. When starting with pureed foods, gradually thicken them as the patient progresses.

VI. VELUM: *Hyporeflexive, Hypotonic*
   *A. Touch lightly with a cold metal object (e.g., size 00 laryngeal mirror) the patient's soft palate on midline slightly posterior to the hard palate/soft palate juncture. Look for reflexive lifting.
   † B . Have the patient repeat hard attack "ah" sounds. This can be preceded by thermal stimulation.

VII. SWALLOW REFLEX: *Delayed or Absent* (possible aspiration before the swallow)
   *A. With a cold size 00 laryngeal mirror, lightly touch the base of the anterior faucial arch. Repeat 5 to 10 times; look for some movement of the soft palate or larynx. Then immediately ask the patient to swallow or (if safe) present a very small amount of ice water or ginger ale, held in a straw (used as a pipette) at the base of the anterior faucial arch. Place the liquid in the same area that has been stimulated and ask the patient to swallow. Repeat this procedure several times daily until the swallow reflex occurs and the delay decreases. Gradually increase the amount of liquid to be swallowed or switch to a liquid of thicker consistency presented at the faucial arches.
   * B . If the swallow reflex continues to be mildly delayed when oral feeding is initiated, the patient's head should be tilted forward to keep food out of the airway before the swallow. If the delay is significant (more than several seconds), oral feeding should be avoided.
   † C . If the patient is alert and the swallow reflex is mildly delayed, use the supraglottic swallow technique (VIII.B).

VIII. LARYNX: *Reduced Glottic Closure* (possible aspiration during the swallow)
   †A. Adduction exercises. Instruct the patient to hold his or her breath (requires glottic closure) while pushing down or pulling up on a chair. Hold breath while pulling

or pushing and produce a clear voice. Repeat short "ah's" with hard glottal attack. Produce "ah" with hard glottal attack and hold voice. Place hand on patient's forehead. Patient pushes head against therapist's hand while holding breath or phonating.

‡ B . If airway protection continues to be weak, teach the patient to use the "supraglottic swallow":

  a. Take a deep breath and hold it at the height of the inhalation.

  b. Keep holding breath while swallowing.

  c . Cough or clear throat immediately after swallowing (do not inhale before coughing).

  d. Spit or swallow again.

This process should be practiced without food before introducing food.

‡ C . Train the patient to cough or clear his or her throat and then to spit or swallow whenever he or she notices a wet, hoarse quality to the voice. The patient should phonate frequently during eating and after every swallow at the outset to check for residue on the vocal folds.

* D . Consider a Teflon injection for residual unilateral vocal fold paralysis.

IX. PHARYNX

A. *Pharyngeal Apraxia or Dyscoordination*

  *1. Use small amounts of food; pudding-type consistency.

B . *Unilateral Pharyngeal Dysfunction: residue or pooling on one side*

  *1. *Tilt* the patient's head toward the stronger side to encourage food to proceed along the more efficient channel. If the condition is severe, have the patient eat in a side-lying position.

  * 2 . *Turn* the patient's head toward the weaker side to close the pyriform sinus on that side and prevent pooling.

  ‡ 3 . *Teach* the patient to clear his or her throat and spit or swallow again after every swallow.

  * 4 . *Alternate* solid and liquid swallows so the liquid washes the solid food through the pharynx.

C . *Reduced Peristalsis*

  *1. Alternate foods of semisolid and liquid consistencies.

  *2. Avoid solid and sticky foods.

  †3. Instruct the patient to swallow several times with each presentation of food.

  ‡ 4 . Teach the patient to clear his or her throat and either spit or swallow again if there is any suspicion of residue in the pharynx.

  * 5 . Reevaluate the patient's swallowing radiographically at 1 to 2 month intervals. Reduced peristalsis may recover within the first 6 months after the head injury.

X. CRICOPHARYNGEUS MUSCLE

A. *Dyscoordination: sphincter opens but not sufficiently or at the appropriate phase of the swallow cycle.*

  ‡1. Have the patient use small amounts of food; use repeated swallows or supraglottic swallow technique. Emphasize all airway protection techniques.

B . *Achalasia: sphincter does not open*

  * 1 . Wait for spontaneous recovery. Cricopharyngeal dysfunction in head injured patients will often recover spontaneously in 3 to 4 months. Patients with this disorder should be reevaluated radiographically every 1 to 2 months to assess recovery.

  ‡2. Voluntary control of cricopharyngeus muscle

    a. Teach a process similar to that used for esophageal voice air intake.

    b. Use biofeedback with esophageal motility manometer.

Note: These procedures are highly experimental and not of known efficacy.

† 3 . Progressive dilatation (ENT procedure): Stretch cricopharyngeus muscle by passing tubes (bougies) of increasing diameter through the sphincter (questionable long-term effectiveness).

† 4 . Cricopharyngeal myotomy (ENT procedure): Surgically open the sphincter by cutting the muscle along a vertical plane (controversy exists as to effectiveness). Should not be done within 6 months of the head injury.

PART V
COGNITIVE REHABILITATION

Over the past decade, a dramatic increase in clinical interest and research has occurred in the area of cognitive recovery and residual cognitive impairments following closed head injury. At the same time, clinicians have systematically explored the application of varied intervention techniques to these problems. Many of the intervention techniques and strategies that fall loosely under the general headings "cognitive rehabilitation" and "cognitive retraining" have a long history of use with other disability groups by occupational therapists, speech-language pathologists, special educators, psychologists, and other professionals. Some of the techniques are new, either capitalizing on recent technological developments (e.g., the microcomputer) or targeting more precisely the types of cognitive deficit characteristic of closed head injury. Although there is some research evidence that certain cognitive rehabilitation techniques are effective with head injured adults, the application to children is still in a formative stage.

In Chapter 8 Szekeres, Ylvisaker, and Holland present a framework for pediatric cognitive rehabilitation based on current theories in cognitive and developmental cognitive psychology, on models of cognitive rehabilitation that have proved their clinical value in the rehabilitation of head injured adults, on recent developments in special education intervention and research, and on characteristic constellations of cognitive deficits as they are manifested over broad stages of recovery in head injured children. The discussion of stages of cognitive recovery forms the backdrop for many of the chapters on intervention in this textbook, while the section on forms and principles of cognitive rehabilitation outlines themes that are explored further in Chapters 10 to 12.

In Chapter 9 Baxter, Cohen, and Ylvisaker discuss comprehensive cognitive assessment of head injured children from the points of view of neuropsychological, language, and educational assessment and also with a focus on issues common to all three disciplines. Since a thorough treatment of these issues would require a separate volume, the scope of this chapter is limited. The authors emphasize assessment that is directly relevant to creating rehabilitation plans and monitoring progress, stressing those cognitive deficits that occur most commonly following closed head injury. Thus, for example, in the section on language assessment, little attention is paid to specific linguistic impairments that are central in the assessment of children with congenital language disorders. Rather, the focus is on communicative deficits that are generally secondary to more general cognitive impairments. The authors stress the importance of integrating assessment data from each discipline and of integrating results of formal assessment with informal observations and diagnostic treatment.

In Chapters 10 to 12, members of the interdisciplinary cognitive rehabilitation therapy team at The Rehabilitation Institute of Pittsburgh, with backgrounds in occupational therapy, speech-language pathology, and special education, outline intervention strategies and techniques for patients in the early, middle, and late stages of recovery from severe head injury. Clinicians will find in these three chapters treatment ideas that they may have expected to find in separate chapters devoted to the traditional rehabilitation disciplines. The integration of intervention by an interdisciplinary treatment team, illustrated in these chapters, is necessary to avoid contributing to the cognitive fragmentation that plays a leading role in the tragedy of head injury.

Chapter 8

Cognitive Rehabilitation Therapy: A Framework for Intervention

Shirley F. Szekeres, MA, CCC/Sp,
Mark Ylvisaker, MA, CCC/Sp, and
Audrey L. Holland, PhD

On the surface, closed head injury seems an unusual diagnostic category around which to structure a rehabilitation program. Individual differences among head injured children are legion, encompassing pretraumatic intellectual level; cognitive style, personality, and other developmental differences; the nature and severity of the injury; and, finally, the variable interaction of individual children's brain damage with their pretraumatic characteristics and posttrauma environment.

Most head injured children and adolescents come from the broad range of normally developing children, but there are also significant numbers from the group with disorders of learning, attention, judgment, and behavior (Levin, Benton, and Grossman, 1982). Head injury can exaggerate these preexisting differences and possibly deprive the children of the learning and coping strategies on which they relied pretraumatically. Mass lesions may result in varying types and degrees of motor and sensory deficits in some of the children, whereas others show no signs of residual neurologic dysfunction.

Despite these differences, there is a thread that knits this diverse group together: generally depressed cognitive and psychosocial functioning. These deficits are presumably related to widespread shearing and commonly occurring anterior frontolimbic and temporal lobe contusions described in Chapter 1. This theme helps to unify the population of severely head injured children and serves as a focus for rehabilitation efforts.

In this chapter, we shall briefly (1) outline a conceptual framework that guides rehabilitation planning for children and adolescents; (2) describe broad stages of recovery from severe head injury; (3) distinguish forms of intervention; and (4) list basic principles that govern cognitive rehabilitation therapy (CRT) services at each stage of recovery.

A CONCEPTUAL FRAMEWORK

Clinical activity, unstructured and without the direction of a conceptual framework, is blind; models and theories, uninformed by clinical experience and therapeutic skill, are empty. As clinicians, we use theories of cognition, cognitive development, and brain-behavior relationships for three major reasons:

- To organize descriptions of patients' deficits and to define criteria for measuring progress
- To organize intervention at the level of general program development as well as to select goals, objectives, and therapeutic activities for individual patients
- To generate novel intervention procedures while measuring their value ultimately against patient progress, not academic acceptability.

A clinical program inevitably involves assumptions regarding both the nature and the interrelationships of the deficits to be treated as well as of the normally functioning system that has become impaired. If unstated and unexamined, the program easily assumes a haphazard and inefficient "workbook" approach to treatment. With underlying hypotheses explicitly stated and examined, a conceptual framework becomes an open source of principles for treatment and the framework itself is more easily evaluated and readjusted in response to patients' performance and progress.

Pediatric cognitive rehabilitation programs face a particularly severe challenge with respect to selecting a framework. There are conflicting conceptions of the nature of the cognitive system (Flavell, 1977), varied explanations of cognitive development (Kail and Bisanz, 1982), and insufficient information regarding the nature of brain-behavior relationships in children (Rutter, 1981). It is clear, however, that pediatric programs must account for the fact that patients not only are in a process of recovery from brain injury but also are undergoing normal cognitive development and biologic maturation. The interaction of these processes is not well understood. Therefore, in searching for a framework, we have relied on a variety of theoretical perspectives as well as the large body of special education research conducted with children whose learning impairment is congenital.

Our framework for cognitive rehabilitation includes concepts from behavioristic (Bandura, 1977; Miller and Dollard, 1941; Skinner, 1969), structural-organismic (Flavell, 1977; Piaget, 1983), and information processing (Dodd and White, 1980) models of cognition and cognitive development, as well as a model of brain-behavior relationships and of the effects of brain damage on established systems within the brain (Luria, 1963). To a great extent, our descriptions are stated in information processing terms because of the comprehensiveness of this approach to cognition and the clinical usefulness of the categories. From the perspective of the information processing model, cognition is viewed broadly as a complex system with which an individual processes information, for particular purposes, within certain mental structures and environmental constraints (Dodd and White, 1980). The information processing framework has been used increasingly to explain developmental phenomena (Kail and Bisanz, 1982) and to serve as a framework for intervention with learning impaired students (Hagen, Barclay, and Schwethelm, 1982.)

Aspects of Cognition

Although we make considerable use of information processing categories to describe cognitive functioning and recovery from head injury, we do not wish to imply or recommend a resolute commitment to any particular model of cognition. Clinicians should remain free to use what is useful and ignore what is not, regardless of current academic trends. Table 8-1 (pp. 230-235) outlines the descriptive cognitive categories that have proved to be of clinical usefulness and lists typical cognitive symptoms following closed head injury.

The complexity of cognition and the dynamic interrelationships involved in cognitive functioning make even more challenging the development of a comprehensive and coherent framework for cognitive rehabilitation therapy. We have elected to describe cognitive functioning and recovery from head injury with focus on three major aspects. First, *component processes* (attending, perceiving, learning or remembering, organizing, reasoning, and problem solving) are described. Second, *component systems* (working memory, permanent storage, response system, and executive system), which are organized structures composed of basic and acquired processes and knowledge, are discussed. Third, the *functional-integrative performance* of an individual, which includes the complex interaction of the entire cognitive mechanism with the environment, is described. The purposes or goals of the individual, executive functions, interrelations of cognitive processes and systems with structures of knowledge, the generation of responses, and the environment (including task variables) are all involved in the functional-integrative performance of real-world tasks.

Component Processes and Systems

The categories of this cognitive taxonomy (processes, systems, and functional-integrative performance) overlap, as the list of head injury sequelae demonstrates (see Table 8–1). There are dynamic interrelationships within the categories of processes and systems. For example, basic attentional processes may be impaired selectively or may only *appear* to be impaired as a reflection of deficits in organizing processes. Encoding may be impaired selectively, or the deficit may result from an impairment in basic perceptual processes. The same is true of cognitive systems. The permanent knowledge store may be inadequate (in amount or organization) or may only *appear* to be so because the patient lacks motivation or direction to initiate and maintain an adequate search (impaired executive system) or because the patient lacks an efficient means of expressing what has been located in storage (impaired response system).

Clinically, we have found these distinctions to be valuable. By distinguishing components (process *and* system) from global functional-integrative performance, areas of deficiency can be pinpointed better for precise planning of treatment. Furthermore, careful differential diagnosis between processes and systems can result in an increase in the efficiency of treatment. For example, if it has been determined that the capacity of the working memory system is significantly reduced, treatment may focus on strategies a patient could use to compensate for this deficit. On the other hand, if the set of symptoms is thought to result instead from impaired attentional processes, treatment that is focused directly on strengthening attention could be initiated.

Performance Variables

Because the interaction of cognitive and environmental factors is so complex, there is great potential for variation in an individual's performance. For instance, it is well established that the increase in rate amount, duration, or complexity of task stimuli results in disproportionate deterioration in performance of head injured patients (Hagen, 1981). To facilitate the identification and tracking of these variations and the subsequent planning of treatment, performance is described in the following terms:

1. *Efficiency* refers to a time-productivity consideration (how much was accomplished and in what amount of time, including reaction time).

2. *Scope* refers to the types of situations in which performance is effective. Very generally, scope may be defined in terms of structured, semistructured, quasinatural, or "real-life" situations, or it may be defined in terms of specific situations (e.g., classroom recitation) or *categories* of situations (e.g., classroom).

3. *Level* refers to the conceptual or developmental level of cognitive functioning (points of reference may be grade level for academic activities, chronological age for social appropriateness, developmental level and age for recreational activities, etc.).

4. *Manner* refers to the characteristic way in which individuals approach a task, including dependent-independent and impulsive-reflective continua.

Any targeted cognitive function can be rated and tracked along any or all of these continua, noting interactions among variables. Charts from data can be extremely useful in recording characteristics of and changes in the performance of the patient and in evaluating the effectiveness of intervention.

As indicated by this cognitive framework, the potential focus for treatment in cognitive rehabilitation is broad.

Cognitive Development

With children, the professional is dealing not only with recovery from the head injury, but also with the facilitation of cognitive development itself. Questions about which aspects of cognition develop with age and how development occurs currently are being investigated by cognitive psychologists (Flavell, 1977; Siegler, 1983; Stevenson, 1983). Attempts have been made to identify significant factors of development in order to concentrate intervention effectively in areas that are clearly related to cognitive development and to discover new and neglected areas (Brown, 1979). A better appreciation of the factors involved in normal cognitive development will yield a more complete understanding of the nature of recovery from head injury at any particular age. The clinical implications of these developmental factors are discussed in Chapters 11 and 12.

Probably the most familiar change in the cognitive system is the acquisition of *new information* and its integration into storage. This knowledge base increases with age and training and is typically measured by school achievement tests. As new information is acquired, a progressive restructing of internal knowledge and organization occurs that results in quantitative and qualitative changes in knowledge and thinking.

Changes in the *efficiency* or *capacity* with which the cognitive system operates have also been identified. The speed of processing (Gitomer, Pellegrino, and Bisanz, 1983; Kail and Bisanz, 1982), the capacity of working memory (Chi, 1978), and the flexibility of the retrieval system (Ceci and Howe, 1978) have all been found to increase with age while reaction time decreases (Kail and Siegel, 1977). It is difficult to determine if these changes are due to a general maturation of the nervous system (Hebb, 1949) or to an increase in the amount or organization of knowledge (Chi, 1978; Gitomer et al., 1983).

Recent research has concentrated on the use of strategies in normal and handicapped children as well as on the effectiveness of strategy training in improving cognitive performance. It has consistently been found that the use of strategies increases with age (Flavell, 1977; Hagen, Jongeward, and Kail, 1975; Lodico, Ghatala, Levin, Pressley, and Bell, 1983). A number of developmental variables have been identified as significant factors in the increasingly effective use of strategies.

1. *Goal directedness and acceptance of task,* which involve deliberate and persistent thinking about problems (Gordon and Flavell, 1977) and the motivation to succeed.

2. *Content and organization of the knowledge base,* which involve the knowledge and principles of organization necessary to guide strategic behavior (Chi, 1978; Hall, 1980; Nelson, 1978; Roblinsky and Cruse, 1981).

3. *Situational discrimination* (Campione, 1980), which involves awareness of appropriateness of particular strategies in a given situation.

4. *Awareness of self and limitations,* which also involves awareness of the need to use strategies and of their value in improving performance (e.g., awareness of the relation between organization and improved recall [Tenney, 1975]).

5. *Internal memory monitoring* (Lodico et al., 1983; Wellman, 1977), which involves the monitoring of one's own comprehension and either requesting that information be repeated or taking notes. This ability is closely related to that of predicting how much and what kind of information can be remembered and under what conditions.

6. *Knowledge monitoring* (Markman, 1979), which involves listening to and applying instructions and mentally confronting problems in application, both of which lead to realization that understanding or

information is incomplete (e.g., people who listen passively would not encounter problems because they would not realize that they had failed to comprehend).

Variables 4, 5, and 6 are referred to as *metacognitive* (Loper, 1983), which signifies an awareness of an individual's own cognitive functions (Flavell, 1977). These factors, which develop with age, are often used to explain a common finding that even though some young children may be trained to use a strategy effectively, they will not do so unless prompted (Flavell, 1977). Flavell calls this phenomenon a "production deficiency," which implies that if a child is to use strategies independently and effectively, metacognitive development will be a primary factor in training. Chapters 11 and 12 discuss the clinical relevance of those developmental factors.

It should be apparent by this point that virtually all aspects of the cognitive system have a developmental dimension. Furthermore, the development of each component is related to developments elsewhere in the system, as well as to the environment, in ways that are complex and have not yet been fully identified. Intervention thus cannot be directed solely to any one aspect of cognition. Rather, attempts must be made to improve processing efficiency, growth of the knowledge base (including concepts, procedures or strategies, and organizing processes), executive functions (including metacognitive factors), and an individual's ability to set goals and maintain motivation. Above all, professionals must help patients to become effective problem solvers, that is, to analyze their own needs and explore potential strategies to compensate for deficits that interfere with achieving meaningful goals.

The focus in intervention, then, will change as a function of the patient's stage of cognitive recovery, level of cognitive development, and specific cognitive deficits identified as barriers to achieving short-term and long-term goals.

Facilitating Change in Cognitive Performance

The mechanisms of cognitive change are a special concern in intervention with head injured children and adolescents. The development of cognition does not depend solely on biologic maturation but results partly from the nature and quality of experience and sociocultural demands made on the developing organism (Flavell, 1977; Fowler, 1977). Although the information processing framework has been used in the explanation of cognitive change and growth (Kail and Bisanz, 1982), our understanding of the mechanisms of change in the cognitive system has also been influenced by four additional sources:

1. Piaget's notions of assimilation and accommodation—which are two aspects of adaptation to the external environment—provide a guideline for controlling tasks and environmental factors in treatment. According to Piaget, the mind develops by means of repeated environmental interactions that involve interpretation of external objects and events in terms of what individuals already know (assimilation), at the same time taking into account unknown properties and relations (accommodation). Cognitive growth depends on a balance between assimilation and accommodation. With this balance a child both understands and has some facility with a task and also takes account of its new and unfamiliar aspects (Flavell, 1977; Piaget, 1983). Therefore, controlled presentation of a task can facilitate change or restructuring of existing knowledge. Since its goal is to challenge without overwhelming patients, cognitive rehabilitation programming strives to control their environment so that this balance can be achieved.

2. Concepts of learning theory are used that emphasize social, emotional, and cognitive feedback or reinforcement to motivate and direct change in the individual. The children's attention is focused on target objectives through instructions (including task goals), materials, and response alternatives; they are informed of the adequacy or appropriateness of a response with informative feedback; and an attempt is made to create and maintain internal motivation with significant reinforcement (Harter, 1978; see also Chapter 13 and 14).

3. Procedures of Cognitive Behavior Modification (CBM), which emphasize self-instruction (overt or covert) as a means of controlling and mediating behavior (Meichenbaum, 1977),are used. CBM has been reported to be useful in effecting behavioral changes (Keogh and Glover, 1980), including the reduction of disruptive behavior in the classroom (Kneedler, 1980; Loper, 1983), and it has been particularly effective in altering attentional strategies of impulsive (Meichenbaum and Goodman, 1971) and learning disabled children (Hallahan et al., 1983). These problems and deficits closely parallel those of head injured children.

4. Efforts to effect change in the cognitive functioning of an individual with acquired brain damage must take account of the nature and severity of the damage as well as the areas of the brain that remain relatively intact. We have borrowed heavily from Luria's functional systems model, including the dynamics of functional system disruption following brain damage and of compensatory restoration by means of alternative functional systems (Luria, 1963).

It is beyond the scope of this book to provide an in-depth account of any of these models of cognition and cognitive development. The reader is referred to the sources cited for excellent reviews and further information.

STAGES OF COGNITIVE RECOVERY

For any individual patient it is possible to identify a large number of distinguishable stages of recovery that would not necessarily be identical to those of any other head injured patient. Given different mass lesions, patterns of deficits at a given stage of recovery may vary from child to child. For instance, of two equally confused children, one may have intact surface language function while the other experiences severe transient aphasia. Furthermore, the rate of recovery can vary dramatically from patient to patient, as can the ultimate recovery level.

Why then identify broad stages of recovery? We make these relatively arbitrary divisions in the course of recovery for two reasons: (1) an understanding of the typical complexes of behaviors during the recovery process is important for helping professionals, family members, and even patients to predict and understand behavior that would be distressing under ordinary circumstances; and (2) stages provide reference points for multidisciplinary program development and planning, and help to establish an overall focus in intervention. The three stages outlines in Table 8–1 correspond to three qualitatively distinct phases of rehabilitation.

Early Phase. The focus is on sensory and sensorimotor stimulation to increase arousal and adaptive responses to the environment.

Middle Phase. The focus is on channeling recovery for confused patients by means of highly structured environmental compensations and on retraining cognitive components using tasks that increase gradually in difficulty so that a patient develops greater cognitive and behavioral adaptability.

Late Phase. The focus is on increasing independence and adaptability of the patient by withdrawing environmental supports, training functional-integrative skills in progressively more natural settings, and equipping patients with strategies to compensate for residual impairments.

In acute care settings, the Glasgow Coma Scale (Teasdale and Jennett, 1974) is useful to describe recovery quantitatively from deep coma to relatively normal functioning, but the scale is not sufficiently precise or complete to be useful to rehabilitation efforts. The Rancho Los Amigos Hospital's Levels of Cognitive Recovery (Hagen, 1981), an eight-stage recovery scale, is widely used with adolescents and adults to describe recovery along cognitive parameters similar to those described here. The usefulness of any scale, however, lies not in the precise placement of a patient in a particular category, but rather in accurate description of the patient along relevant cognitive parameters, in careful consideration of the interrelationships among deficits, and in a flexible use of those descriptions in rehabilitation planning.

Care should be taken not to confuse "early," "middle," and "late" with the length of time following an injury. Some patients reach a plateau and never move beyond the early or middle stages of recovery. Furthermore, the stages should not be identified with motor recovery. It is as much a mistake to infer significant cognitive deficits from severe motor involvement as it is to infer cognitive integrity from normal walking and talking.

Table 8–1 summarizes typical cognitive behaviors or deficits at the early, middle, and late stages of recovery. They are presented within the present descriptive framework and are based on our clinical experience with a large number of severely head injured children and adolescents over a large span of recovery time, as well as on the growing body of literature on outcome summarized in Chapter 2. The first column further defines the terminology of our conceptual framework grouped under the general headings *component processes, component systems,* and *functional-integrative performance.* In columns two through four, characteristic behavior, inferred cognitive abilities and disabilities, and recovery sequences are listed for the early, middle, and late stages of recovery.

FORMS AND PRINCIPLES OF COGNITIVE REHABILITATION

Cognitive rehabilitation therapy (CRT) is a major part of a head injured patient's program, even in agencies that lack a formally designated CRT program. Much of the territory covered by cognitive rehabilitation has a traditional home in occupational therapy, speech-language therapy, special education, behavior management, and psychosocial or psychiatric counseling. Since, however, a fragmented program can do little to remediate the cognitive and social fragmentation typically seen with head injury, there is great value in integrating and focusing cognitive rehabilitation efforts within a tightly knit interdisciplinary program.

The term "cognitive rehabilitation" is used here in a very broad sense to stand for the treatment of those deficits listed in Table 8–1, such as cognitively based communicative, behavioral, and psychosocial deficits, as well as more narrowly defined deficits in component systems and processes. Since the scope of CRT is so broad, an attempt is made to make it more manageable by distinguishing forms of intervention and by listing general therapeutic principles (see Table 8–2) that guide treatment decisions at each stage of recovery.

Forms of Intervention

Rehabilitation efforts may be directed toward facilitating spontaneous recovery, retraining pretraumatically acquired functions, developing new skills, compensating for residual deficits, or, finally, creating environmental compensations that permit effective performance despite residual deficits.

Facilitation. Spontaneous neurologic recovery occurs for several months following a severe insult to the brain. Spontaneous recovery can be effectively channeled within the context of a rehabilitation environment that provides patients with forms of stimulation and activity that are correctly chosen and modulated for that patient (see chapters 10 and 11). Cognitive development can be advanced as well, by providing the patient a progression of graded tasks to engage higher level processes.

Direct Retraining of Cognitive or Task Components. Retraining can expand and make optimally functional the residual cognitive functions that are no longer recovering spontaneously, by means of carefully targeted drill and practice. Objectives for the patient range from basic level (e.g., selective attention) to higher level (e.g., logical reasoning) components. Furthermore, tasks can be separated into increasingly smaller parts and practiced separately.

Retraining Functional-Integrative Skills. This form of intervention is distinct from component retraining in that the skills practiced are actual functional behaviors (e.g., conversing, reading a meaningful story, organizing a job task), rather than cognitive components that are part of or presupposed by functional goal behaviors. For purposes of enhancing generalization, training takes place in a variety of environments, including environments natural for the patient.

Environmental Compensation. At any stage of recovery, adjustments may be necessary in a patient's physical and social environment, as well as in staff and family expectations, so that the patient can function adaptively despite significant deficits.

Personal Compensation. Patients with residual cognitive deficits— at the level of component processes or functional-integrative behaviors— may be able to compensate deliberately for those deficits that remain despite targeted practice.

Text continued on page 236.

Table 8-1. Aspects of Cognition and Stages of Recovery

Aspects of Cognition	Early Stages
I. Component Processes	
ATTENTION: holding objects, events, words, or thoughts in consciousness. *Components:* span, selectivity, filtering, maintaining, shifting, dividing.	• Severely decreased arousal or alertness • Minimal selective attention, focusing, shifting • Attention may be primarily to internal stimuli
PERCEPTION: recognition of features and relationships among features; affected by context (figure-ground) and intensity, duration, significance, and familiarity of stimuli.	• Begins to recognize (and perhaps use) familiar objects when they are highlighted • May perceive only one feature or aspect of stimulus • Adaptation to continuous stimulation
MEMORY AND LEARNING: *Encoding:* recognition, interpretation and formulation of information, including language, into an internal code; knowledge base, personal interests, and goals affect what is coded. *Storage:* retention over time. *Retrieval:* transfer from long-term memory to consciousness.	• Comprehension progresses from minimal responses to vocal intonation and stress to recognition of simple, context-bound instructions • No evidence of encoding or storage of new information.
ORGANIZING PROCESSES: Analyzing, classifying, integrating, sequencing; identifying relevant features of objects and events; comparing for similarities or differences; integrating into organized descriptions, higher level categories, and sequenced events. These processes are presupposed by higher level reasoning and efficient learning.	• No evidence of these processes

Table continued on following page.

Table 8-1 (continued).

Middle Stages	Late Stages*
• Attention generally focuses on external events • Short attention span • Poor control of attention: highly distractible, inflexible	• Attention span may or may not be reduced • Relatively weak concentration, selective attention and fluid attentional shifts • Attending problems may reflect weak organizational processes, absence of goals, or both.
• Clear recognition of familiar objects and events • Inefficient perception in context • Sharp deterioration with increases in rate, amount, and complexity of stimuli • Difficulty in perceiving whole from part	• Possibly subtle versions of perceptual problems related to rate, amount, and complexity • Possibly specific deficits (e.g., field neglect) • Possibly inefficient shifting of perceptual set • Possibly weak perception of relevant features
• Weak encoding due to poor access to knowledge base, poor integration of new with old information, or inefficient attention or perception • Inefficiently encoded information often lost after short delay • Recognition stronger than recall; receptive vocabulary superior to expressive • Disorganized search of storage system	• Possibly subtle versions of earlier problems, particularly with increases in cognitive stress • Memory problems—any combination of comprehension, encoding, storage, or retrieval deficits • Memory problems—problems recalling information related to personal experience (episodic memory) or abstracted knowledge (semantic memory)
• Weak or bizarre associations • Weak analysis of objects into features • Disorganized sequencing of events • Weak identification of similarities and differences in comparisons and classifications • Can integrate concepts into propositions; difficulty integrating propositions into main ideas • Major difficulty imposing organization on unstructured stimuli	• Possibly subtle versions of earlier problems • Difficulty maintaining goal-directed thinking • Ongoing difficulty discerning main ideas and integrating main ideas into broader themes • May easily get lost in details • Can impose organization on unstructured stimuli with prompting

*Functioning also related to age and pretrauma developmental and educational level

Table continued on following page.

Table 8-1. (Continued)

Aspects of Cognition	Early Stages
REASONING: Considering evidence and drawing inferences or conclusions; involves flexible exploration of possibilities (divergent thinking) and use of past experience. *Deductive:* Strict logical formal inference. *Inductive:* Direct inference from experience. *Analogical:* Indirect inference from experience.	• No evidence of these processes
PROBLEM SOLVING AND JUDGMENT: *Problem solving* occurs when a goal cannot be reached directly. Ideally involves goal identification, consideration of relevant information, exploration of possible solutions, and selection of the best. *Judgment:* Decision to act, based on consideration of relevant factors, including prediction of consequences.	• No evidence of these processes

II. COMPONENT SYSTEMS

WORKING MEMORY (attentional focus): Storage or holding "space" where coding and organizing occur; limited information capacity; *functional* capacity is increased by making processes automatic or by "chunking" information.	• Severely limited capacity • Progression from single to multi-modality processing of simple stimuli • Attenton to internal stimuli may exhaust attentional "space"
LONG-TERM MEMORY: Contains knowledge of concepts or words; rules, strategies, or procedures; organizational principles and knowledge frames; goals, experience, and self-concept.	• Emerging evidence of remote memory: recognition of familiar objects and persons • May assume that other contents are present but inaccessible
RESPONSE SYSTEM: Controls all output, including speech, facial expression, and fine and gross motor activity; includes motor planning.	• Severely limited; often perseverative responses • May use some gestures and speech toward end of this stage, but with motor planning problems or delayed responses

Table continued on following page.

Table 8-1 (continued).

Middle Stages	Late Stages*
• Minimal inferential thinking; may deal with concrete cause-effect relationships, particularly if overlearned • General inefficiency with abstract ideas and relationships	• Fair to good concrete reasoning in controlled settings; disorganized thinking in stressful or uncontrolled settings • Abstract thinking remains deficient
• Inability to see relationships among problems, goals, and relevant information • Inflexibility in generating or evaluating possible solutions; impulsive; trial and error approach • Inability to assess a situation and predict consequences • Severely impaired safety and social judgment	• Possibly subtle versions of earlier problems • Impulsive; disorganized problem solving • Inflexible thinking and shallow reasoning • Poor safety and social judgment may be primary residual deficits; manifested in academic and social situations
• Gradual increase in attention span to near normal, as measured by digit span • *Functional* capacity remains severely restricted due to lack of automatic organizing processes • Therefore, processing deteriorates rapidly with increases in the information load	• Often normal digit span • Inefficient organizing processes may continue to reduce *functional* capacity as information load increases
• Growing access to pretrauma contents • Recognition of strong associations (e.g., hammer-nail), basic semantic relations, and common two or three event sequences	• Recovery of access to pretraumatically acquired knowledge base stabilizes • Growth of LTM varies with type and severity of residual cognitive deficits
• Speaks or begins augmentative system • Possible motor planning problems or general slowness • Impulsiveness and possible perseveration • Motor function varies with site and extent of injury	• Generally functional communication system — usually speech • Possible motor planning problems or slowness • Possible rapid fatigue

*Functioning also related to age and pretrauma developmental and educational level

Table continued on following page.

Table 8-1. (Continued)

Aspects of Cognition	Early Stages
EXECUTIVE SYSTEM ("central processor"): Sets goals; plans and monitors activity; directs processing and operations according to goals, current input and perceptual-affective set.	• Minimal awareness of self and current condition • No apparent self-direction of behavior or cognitive processes

III. FUNCTIONAL-INTEGRATIVE PERFORMANCE

FUNCTIONAL BEHAVIOR: Performance of "real-life" tasks and activities (e.g., reading a book or conversing) Efficiency: Rate of performance and amount accomplished. Level: Developmental or academic level of performance. Scope: Variety of situations in which patient can maintain performance. Manner: Dependence or independence (need for prompts and cues); impulsive or reflective style.	• Cannot adapt to environment; activity level ranges from inactive to hyperactive; activity marginally purposeful (e.g., pulling at tubes, restraints, clothes; attempting to get out of bed); gives little or no assistance in daily care • May perform a limited range of routine tasks when prompted (e.g., brushing hair) • Profound confusion or disorientation to person, place, time, and condition • Communication severely limited, inconsistent and prefunctional; may begin to comprehend simple context-bound instructions • Minimal social interaction; little variation in facial expression; reflexive crying; may reflexively hold or shake hands • Agitated behavior at the end of this stage more pronounced in adolescents.

Table continued on following page.

Table 8-1 (continued).

Middle Stages	Late Stages*
• Growing awareness of self; poor awareness of deficits • Weak metacognitive awareness of self as thinker • Minimal goal setting, self-initiation or self-inhibition, self-monitoring, or self-evaluation	• Shallow awareness of residual deficits • Mild to severe deficits in executive functions, related in part to anterior frontolimbic damage • Metacognitive level may permit strategy training
• Performs many overlearned routines (e.g., self-care, games) in structured settings with prompts; poor retention of information from day to day; severely impaired learning of new skills • Performs simple sequential tasks (e.g., dressing) in structured setting if stimuli are controlled for rate, amount, and complexity; organization of behavior deteriorates rapidly in uncontrolled setting • Continued confusion but growing orientation to person, place, and time in structured settings and with orientation cues; gross awareness of the structure of the day • Communication: *Expressive*—usually verbal and functional (barring motor speech disorder), but often characterized by confabulation, word retrieval problems, excessive and often inappropriate output. *Receptive*—rate, amount and complexity of verbal input must be controlled to assure comprehension • Social interaction strained and often unsuccessful, due to disinhibition, inappropriateness, impaired social perception • Impulsiveness, agitation, and inability to set goals may result in minimal adaption to the environment	• Performance of pretraumatically acquired skills related to type and extent of residual deficits and ability to compensate; performance may continue to deteriorate sharply with increasing processing load; learning of new skills and strategies occurs at a reduced rate; • Performance of complex tasks requiring organization, persistence, and self-monitoring continues to be deficient; efficiency continues to be low, with slow rate and low productivity • Solid orientation to person, place, and time, but disorientation may recur with sudden changes in routine • Communication is usually conventional in form, with possible word-finding problems, expressive disorganization, and comprehension limited in efficiency; social use of language may be strained or inappropriate • Social interaction and judgment may be dominant residual symptoms, related to weak awareness of social conventions and rules, persistent impulsiveness, and poorly defined self-concept (with shallow awareness of residual deficits) • Behavior generally goal directed, but goals may be unrealistic and social and safety judgment significantly impaired; needs prompts to set goals and subgoals.

*Functioning also related to age and pretrauma developmental and educational level

Component Versus Functional-Integrative Training

Optimal functional performance is the goal for all patients, and component training can help to achieve this goal. During the middle (confused) stages of recovery, the performance of any functional task is severely impaired by limitations of processing and behavior. Engaging patients in interesting but simplified activities that place few functional demands on them directs and assists their recovery most effectively. That is, training is most productive when it provides regulated and gradual increases in processing demands while focusing on one or two variables at a time (see Chapter 11). When spontaneous recovery has slowed or ceased and the patient is no longer significantly confused, it still may be possible to improve underlying component processes (Ben-Yishay et al., 1982) by means of intensive training. If the basic processes of attention and perception can be improved by intensive training so that they become more efficient and automatic, a greater proportion of "attentional space" becomes available to the patient for learning self-monitoring and even compensatory strategies.

Furthermore, component training can provide two important types of feedback. In performing a single component task, patients can more readily observe specific deficits, such as slowness or the inability to process increasing amounts of information. The results of component exercises also lend themselves more easily to quantification, which in turn can demonstrate to patients the progress they are making.

Any given training session can alternate between components and integrative tasks. If a patient's inattention is disrupting functional-integrative activity, attentional problems can be singled out, and the patient can be trained intensively for a period of time and then reintegrated into the functional group activity.

Although the mix of treatment forms depends on a patient's age, deficits, and needs, component training usually assumes a relatively minor role in late-stage treatment. There are several reasons for focusing instead on integration and compensation during this phase. Like the research findings in related populations of brain-damaged children (Campione, 1980), our clinical experience indicates that head injured children do not automatically transfer improvements in subskills to integrative tasks, nor do they automatically generalize from the context of training to other settings. Furthermore, selection of components for specific training often requires speculation about which deficient components are in fact responsible for the breakdown of a larger functional system.

Emphasis on component training in late-stage cognitive rehabilitation programs parallels to some extent the emphasis that was once placed on remedial perceptual-motor training for learning disabled children and on the psycholinguistic skill approach to the diagnosis and treatment of language impaired children (Kirk, McCarthy, and Kirk, 1968; Rees, 1973). Extensive research into the effectiveness of this "building block" approach to the treatment of learning impaired children has shown that subcomponent training (e.g., perceptual motor exercises for reading impairments; auditory perceptual exercises for language impairments) is only marginally effective in improving the component processes and has little effect on functional-integrative skills (Kavale and Mattson, 1983). Although component training is an integral part of our cognitive rehabilitation program, primary emphasis is on functional-integrative performance in real-life situations, on compensation in the areas that do not improve with remedial exercises, and on the generalization and maintenance of both.

Patient Compensation Training

It is an unfortunate fact of rehabilitation that important cognitive functions impaired by severe head injury often do not respond to "strengthening" exercises, whether they are component training or functional-integrative training. When this failure occurs or is predicted from assessment data or when a patient simply requires a temporary "crutch" to function effectively, compensation is the only sensible alternative. Rehabilitation professionals are intimately familiar with compensatory devices and strategies for sensory or motor impairments: vision (glasses, Braille, enlarged type); hearing (aids, lip reading, sign language); gross motor (crutches, wheelchairs); speech (communication aids).

Although compensation for sensory and motor impairments has centuries of tradition behind it, relatively scant attention has been paid to compensatory devices and strategies for cognitive deficits in areas of orientation, learning and memory, organized thinking, inefficient intake of information, problem solving, or judgment. Chapter 12 (intervention at the late stage of recovery) concentrates to a large extent on this area because we believe that a very large part of late-stage cognitive rehabilitation is teaching patients to compensate for deficits by using strategies and counseling parents and teachers about issues of environmental compensation.

By compensatory strategy is meant the *deliberate, self-initiated application of a procedure to achieve a goal that is difficult to achieve because of impaired functioning.* The "deliberate, self-initiated" aspect of the definition is emphasized to distinguish this concept from "instructional strategies" implemented by the therapist or teacher as well as from "strategy" in the sense of nondeliberately organized behavior. "Desired goal" is included in the definition to underscore the extreme importance of patients' goals in their learning the use of strategies. For children, the goals must be significant to the child, not just to the therapist or the teacher.

Compensatory strategies involve one or more procedures that are either overt or covert. *Overt* procedures are "external aids," such as log books to compensate for impaired memory, or modes of behavior, such as requesting a speaker to slow down to compensate for an impairment of language processing. *Covert* procedures range from self-reminders ("pay attention") to complex mental associations or imagery schemes, all of which enhance encoding, storage, and retrieval. Chapter 12 explores this category of intervention in some depth.

Compensation training is related in several ways to both component and functional-integrative training. Patients can acquire strategies to compensate for deficits in underlying components as well as in integrative functions. Either form of practice can serve as the occasion for teaching the general concept of strategy use, including the development of metacognitive awareness. Finally, a given therapeutic activity can be classified as component or functional-integrative or compensatory training or some combination of these, depending on the goals set for that activity by the patient-therapist team and the "real-life" goals of the patient.

Three important facts about compensatory strategies should be considered. First, all people use compensatory strategies (note taking, schedule books, watches) when the limits of their unaided processing mechanisms are reached. The concept of compensatory strategies is not esoteric. Brain-damaged individuals, however, reach the limits of their processing abilities much more quickly than others and are usually less aware that these limits have been reached. Second, the acquisition of strategies will be a part of cognitive rehabilitation whether the therapist intends it or not. Relatively well-recovered patients with residual impairments will generally fashion some sort of strategy for themselves, however inefficient, maladaptive, or escapist it may be. Our job as professionals is to guide the process in an efficient and constructive manner. Third, deliberate strategy use requires attentional "space" in patients whose attentional resources may already be limited. Therefore, extensive practice in the use of a given strategy is required so that it becomes automatic and precious attentional resources can again be devoted to the mundane tasks of daily living.

Although there is little reported research on the effectiveness of compensatory strategy use with head injured children or adults, the little that does exist (reviewed by Diller and Gordon, 1981, and Levin, Benton, and Grossman, 1982) encourages further clinical exploration and research. There is a wealth of reports in the literature on special education. Campione (1980) exhaustively reviewed the literature dealing with the use of memory strategies by mentally retarded children. He concluded that retarded children can be trained to use strategies and that their performance in learning tasks improves when strategies are used. In most cases, however, these children failed to generalize and maintain the use of these strategies. However, even here, Campione gives reason for optimism if the training is conducted correctly. His brief review of variables involved in the increased use of strategies among *normal* children indicates that training might be a much more complex process than has yet been carried out systematically. The literature on learning disabilities includes a large number of recent reports of the effective acquisition of strategies to improve academic performance. Pressley and Levin (1983) present a good review of strategy research in education. This growing evidence and our clinical experience lead us to be cautiously optimistic about this mode of cognitive intervention.

Environmental Compensations

Environmental compensations are simply modifications in any aspect of the patient's environment that facilitate effective functioning despite significant cognitive deficits. These compensations are categorized in the following terms:

1. Physical environment: Spatial arrangements, equipment such as orientation cues, memory aids, and environmental controls.

2. Routines: Consistent schedules for activities, consistent formats.

3. Personnel: Consistent assignment of staff.

4. Interactions: Simplification of the rate, amount, and complexity of information; increased processing and response time for the patient.

5. Behavioral expectations: Realistic performance expectations to prevent a growing sense of failure and worthlessness.

The goal is gradually to decrease the amount of environmental compensation needed, but not at the expense of the patient's adaptive and successful functioning. Chapter 11 includes a detailed discussion of environmental compensation for cognitive deficits.

General Principles of Treatment

Our chief concern throughout the recovery process is effective functioning of patients in progressively more "normalized" life situations. It is equally important for patients to acquire and maintain a positive and productive self-concept. The seven principles outlined in Table 8–2 govern our approach to cognitive rehabilitation therapy for children and adolescents from early through late stages of cognitive recovery and, we believe, increase the probability that patients' potentials for independent and effective functioning will be realized. The table lists these treatment principles with examples of their application at the early, middle, and late stages of recovery.

Figure 8–1 presents a schematic form of the CRT program used at The Rehabilitation Institute of Pittsburgh. Placement of an individual in any aspect of the program depends on many factors, including age, stage of recovery, deficits, and a ranking of functional needs. Therapeutic procedures are discussed in Chapters 10, 11, 12. Management aspects of the program are discussed in Chapter 17.

Table 8–2. Cognitive Rehabilitation Therapy: General Principles of Treatment

There is no "curriculum" through which all patients move in a rigidly sequential fashion; pretraumatic diversity, compounded by the nature and severity of the injury and by varying reactions to the injury, require individualization and regular readjustments of treatment priorities, therapeutic activities, mixes of group and individual therapies, interactive styles of staff, and behavior management.

EARLY STAGES	MIDDLE STAGES	LATE STAGES
PRINCIPLE 1: *Success, resulting from planned compensation and appropriate expectations, facilitates progress while building a productive self-concept.*		
Environment modified to fit patient functioning; consistency in staff and routine; reduced rate of activities; simplification and repetition of stimulation and communication; orienting cues (e.g., familiar pictures, posters, objects, music).	Consistency and predictability in staff and routines; log books, maps, and schedule cards to compensate for memory and orientation deficits; orienting information given as needed; few questions asked; high density of success in therapy and daily living tasks; compensatory strategies and procedures introduced without expecting the patient to use new strategies spontaneously.	High density of success in therapy, possibly mixed with carefully planned failure experiences to help patients recognize deficit areas; mutually respectful and supportive therapeutic community; older children and adolescents given strategies to compensate for residual impairments; gradually increasing independence in learning and living environments as close to normal as possible; may require controlled and volitional cognitive processes that were once automatic.
PRINCIPLE 2: *The systematic gradation of activities can facilitate cognitive recovery and development.*		
Stimulation sessions graded along the following dimensions: single to multimodality stimulation; phylogenetically lower to higher forms of stimulation; amount of time per session; degree of patient active involvement.	Therapeutic activities graded along the following dimensions: attention span; demands on selective attention; rate of stimulus presentation; rate of response; number of simultaneous stimulus modalities; complexity of stimuli; concreteness of stimulus-response modality and of concepts; permanence of stimulus; density of cues; demands on retrieval; degree of patient initiation.	Processing and organizational demands increased until real-life forms of cognitive stress are reached; patient is given increasing responsibility to understand processing limitations and actively control input.

EARLY STAGES	MIDDLE STAGES	LATE STAGES

PRINCIPLE 3: *Habituation and generalization training are necessary for learning.*

	Large number of trials are required for skill improvement or acquisition of new information; some variety in tasks is required to avoid the acquisition of splinter skills of no functional benefit.	Large number of trials are required to improve a skill or internalize a compensatory strategy; microcomputer training appropriate for component skill improvement; context-bound skills avoided by explicitly targeting generalization: functional skill or compensatory strategy is practiced in variety of settings and training focuses not simply on target behavior, but also on recognition of conditions that require a given target behavior; highest goal is self-initiated problem solving.

PRINCIPLE 4: *Patient initiation and motivation facilitate recovery and are essential for effective and independent functioning.*

Patient is treated as *agent:* that is, physically prompted to engage in familiar activities (e.g., self-care, remote switch control of environmental events); staff members respond to patient behavior as though it were communicative.	High interest activities selected; choices are given to patient; frequent review of goals and purposes, even when the patient is processing little; immediate and consistent feedback; relationship established with patient to facilitate acceptance of goals and activities.	Specific training in self-awareness of deficits and realistic goal setting; use of motivating activities; use of supportive group therapy to help patient recognize the need for treatment; use of video therapy techniques for objective confrontation and feedback.

PRINCIPLE 5: *Integration of treatment among staff and family members facilitates the patient's orientation, learning, and generalization of learned skills.*

Stimulation program integrated among therapy staff, nursing staff, and family members.	Treatment and recreational activities integrated among all staff and family members according to level of difficulty and interest in activities, interactive style, and response to inappropriate behavior.	All staff members encourage use of consistent compensatory strategies to enhance generalization and to avoid cognitive fragmentation that results from fragmented intervention.

Table 8-2 (continued).

EARLY STAGES	MIDDLE STAGES	LATE STAGES
PRINCIPLE 6: *Chronological and developmental age must be considered in treatment design.*		
Goals same for all ages; techniques similar (rocking, holding, oral stimulation more offensive to older patients); content of communication always made age appropriate.	Goals same for all ages; techniques similar for all ages; level of activities, nature of materials, and communication style age appropriate; behavioral *expectations* increase with age, requiring greater understanding on the part of staff and family of the confused adolescent.	Goals vary with age; 1. *Independence* has different meanings at different developmental ages. 2. Developmentally young patients are not expected to internalize compensatory strategies. 3. Vocationally oriented goals are appropriate for older adolescents. Treatment goals follow a generally developmental sequence in that levels of difficulty are gradually increased and cognitive and metacognitive prerequisites are established for each new goal.
PRINICIPLE 7: *Inidividual and group treatment are both necessary to provide specificity of intervention as well as training in social cognition.*		
At the end of this stage, patients enter orientation group sessions to begin adjustment to group settings.	*Individual treatment:* 1. To create close relationship with primary therapist. 2. To carefully monitor recovery and fine tune therapeutic activities. *Group treatment:* 1. To begin to establish mutually supportive peer relationships. 2. To use peer modeling. 3. To target cognitive-social goals. 4. To develop attention and concentration skills with increased distractions.	*Individual treatment:* 1. To create close, motivating relationship with primary therapist. 2. To target sensitive issues inappropriate for groups. 3. To individualize and intensify treatment. *Group treatment:* 1. To create a mutually supportive community of patients. 2. To help patients reestablish appropriate and meaningful social and communicative interaction. 3. To use peer modeling, coaching, encouragement. 4. To teach self-monitoring and self-coaching through group role-playing activities.

Figure 8-1. Cognitive rehabilitation therapy program.

EARLY STAGES OF RECOVERY	**MIDDLE STAGES OF RECOVERY**	**LATE STAGES OF RECOVERY**
FOCUS: sensory and sensorimotor stimulation	*FOCUS:* milieu therapy to reduce confusion; retraining of cognitive components	*FOCUS:* functional integration of components; compensatory strategies

---

FAMILY EDUCATION AND COUNSELING

Information regarding the nature of head injury, stages of recovery, and forms of rehabilitation; concrete guidance on family participation in rehabilitation at each stage of recovery; group and individual support or counseling

---

STIMULATION PROGRAM

Arousal; alertness, recognition of environmental events; emerging adaptive responses

INDIVIDUAL COGNITIVE REHABILITATION THERAPY

Therapeutic relationship with primary therapist; objectives can include any of those being pursued in group therapy, but in a more carefully controlled, precisely targeted, intensive, and socially nonthreatening context

---

ORIENTATION GROUP

Orientation to person, place, time, and current condition or needs; group behavior: attention and appropriateness

SOCIAL COGNITION GROUP

Social awareness; social appropriateness; communicative-interactive effectiveness

---

ATTENTION-CONCENTRATION GROUP

Attention span; selective attention; simple perceptual processing; direction following; parallel play

PERCEPTUAL GROUP

Higher level perceptual motor organization or efficiency; treatment of specific residual perceptual deficits

---

STRUCTURED ACTIVITY GROUP

Direction following; planning or organizing; cooperative group behavior through simple group tasks

STRUCTURED ACTIVITY GROUP

Task analysis or synthesis; cooperative play; planning and organizing; memory; problem solving through complex tasks

---

THOUGHT ORGANIZATION GROUP

Concept organization; language comprehension-memory-organized expression; cognitive flexibility and self-monitoring

THOUGHT ORGANIZATION GROUP

Verbal comprehension-organization-memory-expression; problem solving and reasoning; self-monitoring and impulse control

---

COMMUNITY REENTRY GROUP

Community mobility and safety; knowledge of community resources; social and safety judgment; community problem solving

---

SELF-AWARENESS GROUP
(Adolescents)

Awareness of deficits and their implications; adjustment to revised goals; improved "executive" functioning

---

SPECIAL EDUCATION PROGRAM
(School-age children)

Prevocational or vocational program (adolescents)

REFERENCES

Bandura, A. (1977). *Social learning theory.* Englewood Cliffs, NJ: Prentice-Hall.

Ben-Yishay, Y., Rattok, J., Ross, B., Lakin, P., Ezrachi, O., Silver, S., and Diller, L. (1982). Rehabilitation of cognitive and perceptual defects in people with traumatic brain damage: A five year clinical research study. In *Working approaches to remediation of cognitive deficits in brain damaged persons* (Rehabilitation Monograph No. 64). New York University Medical Center: Institute of Rehabilitation Medicine, pp. 127–176.

Brown, A. L. (1979). Theories of memory and the problems of development: Activity, growth, and knowledge. In F. I. M. Craik and L. Cermak (Eds.), *Levels of processing and memory.* Hillsdale, NJ: Lawrence Erlbaum Associates.

Campione, J. C. (1980). Improving memory skills in mentally retarded children: Empirical Research and Strategies for Intervention Technical Report No. 196. Cambridge, MA: Bolt, Bernek, and Newman.

Ceci, S. J., and Howe, J. A. (1978). Age-related differences in free recall as a function of retrieval flexibility. *Journal of Experimental Child Psychology, 26,* 432–442.

Chi, M. T. H. (1976). Short-term memory limitations in children: Capacity or processing deficits? *Memory and Cognition, 4,* 559–572.

Chi, M. T. H. (1978). Knowledge structures and memory development. In R. S. Siegler (Ed.), *Children's thinking: What develops?* Hillsdale, NJ: Lawrence Erlbaum Associates.

Diller, L., and Gordon, W. (1981). Interventions for cognitive deficits in brain-injured adults. *Journal of Consulting and Clinical Psychology, 49,* 822–834.

Dodd, D., and White, R. M., Jr. (1980). *Cognition mental structures and processes.* Boston: Allyn and Bacon.

Flavell, J. H. (1977). *Cognitive development.* Englewood Cliffs, NJ: Prentice-Hall.

Fowler, W. (1977). Sequence and styles in cognitive development. In I. C. Uzgiris and F. Weizmann (Eds.), *The structuring of experience.* New York: Plenum Press.

Gitomer, D. H., Pellegrino, J. W., and Bisanz, J. (1983). Developmental change and invariance in semantic processing. *Journal of Experimental Child Psychology, 35,* 56–80.

Gordon, F., and Flavell, J. (1977). The development of intuitions about cognitive cueing. *Child Development, 48,* 1027–1033.

Hagen, C. (1981). Language disorders secondary to closed head injury: Diagnosis and treatment. Topics in Language Disorders, 1, 73–87.

Hagen, J., Barclay, C., and Schwethelm, B. (1982). Cognitive development of the learning disabled child. *International review of research in mental retardation* (Vol. II). New York: Academic Press.

Hagen, J. W., Jongeward, R. H., Jr., and Kail, R. V., Jr. (1975). Cognitive perspectives on the development of memory. In H. W. Reese (Ed.), *Advances in child development and behavior (Vol 10).* New York: Academic Press.

Hall, R. (1980). Cognitive behavior modification and information processing skills of exceptional children. *Exceptional Educational Quarterly, 1,* 83–88.

Harter, S. (1978). Effective motivation reconsidered: Toward a developmental model. *Human Development, 21,* 34–64.

Hallahan, D. P., Hall, R., Ianna, S., Kneedler, R., Lloyd, J. Loper, A., and Reeve, R. (1983). Summary of findings at the University of Virginia Learning Disabilities Research Institute. *Exceptional Education Quarterly, 4,* 95–114.

Hebb, D. O. (1949). *The organization of behavior.* New York: John Wiley & Sons.

Kail, R., and Bisanz, J. (1982). Information processing and cognitive development. In H. Reese (Ed.), *Advances in child development and behavior (Vol. 17)*. New York: Academic Press.

Kail, R., and Siegel, A. (1977). The development of mnemonic encoding in children. In R. Kail and J. Hagen (Eds.), *Perspectives on the development of memory and cognition*. New Jersey: Lawrence Erlbaum Associates.

Kavale, K., and Mattson, P. (1983). "One jumped off the balance beam": Meta-analysis of perceptual-motor training. *Journal of Learning Disabilities, 16*, 165–173.

Keogh, B. K., and Glover, A. T. (1980). The generality and durability of cognitive training effects. *Exceptional Education Quarterly, 1*, 75–82.

Kirk, S., McCarthy, J., and Kirk, W. (1968). *Illinois test of psycholinguistic abilities* (rev. ed.). Urbana, IL: University of Illinois Press.

Kneedler, R. D. (1980). The use of cognitive training to change social behaviors. *Exceptional Educational Quarterly, 1*, 65–73.

Levin, H., Benton, A., and Grossman, R. (1982). *Neuobehavioral consequences of closed head injury*. New York: Oxford University Press.

Lodico, M., Ghatala, E., Levin, J., Pressley, M., and Bell, J. (1983). The effects of strategy monitoring training on children's selection of effective memory strategies. *Journal of Experimental Child Psychology, 35*, 263–277.

Loper, A. B. (1983). Metacognitive development: Implications for cognitive training. *Exceptional Children Quarterly, 1*, 1–8.

Luria, A. R. (1963). *Restoration of function after brain injury*. New York: Macmillan.

Markman, E. M. (1979). Realizing that you don't understand: Elementary school children's awareness of inconsistencies. *Child Development, 50*, 643–655.

Meichenbaum, D. (1977). *Cognitive behavior modification: An integrative approach*. New York: Plenum Press.

Meichenbaum, D., and Goodman, J. (1971). Training impulsive children to talk to themselves: A means of developing self-control. *Journal of Abnormal Child Psychology, 77*, 115–126.

Miller, N. E., and Dollard, J. (1941). *Social learning and imitation*. New Haven: Yale University Press.

Nelson, K. (1978). Semantic development and the development of semantic memory. In K. E. Nelson (Ed.), *Children's language (Vol. 1)*. New York: Gardner Press.

Piaget, J. (1983). Piaget's theory. In W. Kessen (Ed.), *Handbook of child psychology. Vol. 1, History, theory and methods* (pp. 103–128). New York: John Wiley and Sons.

Pressley, M., and Levin, J. R. (1983). *Cognitive strategy research: Educational applications*. New York: Springer-Verlag.

Rees, N. (1973). Auditory processing factors in language disorders: A view from Procruste's bed. *Journal of Speech and Hearing Disorders, 38*, 304–315.

Roblinsky, S., and Cruse, D. (1981). The role of frameworks in children's retention of sex-related story content. *Journal of Experimental Psychology, 31*, 321–331.

Rutter, M. (1981). Psychological sequelae of brain damage in children. *The American Journal of Psychiatry, 138*, 1533–1544.

Sanborn, D. E., Pyke, H. F., and Sanborn, C. J. (1975). Videotape playback and psychotherapy: A review. *Psychotherapy: Theory, Research and Practice, 12*, 179–186.

Siegler, R. S. (1983). Information processing approaches to development. In W. Kessen (Ed.), *Handbook of child psychology. Vol. 1, History, theory and methods* (pp. 129–211). New York: John Wiley and Sons.

Skinner, B. F. (1969). *Contingencies of reinforcement*. New York: Apple–Century-Crofts.

Stevenson, H. (1983). How children learn—the quest for a theory. In W. Kessen (Ed.), *Handbook of child psychology. Vol. 1, History, theory and methods.* New York: John Wiley and Sons.

Teasdale, G., and Jennett, B. (1974). Assessment of coma and impaired consciousness: A practical scale. *Lancet, 2,* 81–84.

Tenney, Y. I. (1975). The child's conception of organization and recall. *Journal of Experimental Child Psychology, 19,* 100–114.

Wellman, H. M. (1977). Tip of the tongue and feeling of knowing experiments: A developmental study of memory monitoring. *Child Development, 48,* 13–21.

Chapter 9

Comprehensive Cognitive Assessment

Ronald Baxter, PhD,
Sally B. Cohen, MEd, and
Mark Ylvisaker, MA, CCC/Sp*

In this chapter, the assessment of head injured children and adolescents is related to cognitive rehabilitation and educational programming. Our experience has primarily been with patients whose injuries were sufficiently severe to require a program of rehabilitation following their acute-care hospitalization. Many of the issues discussed in this chapter, however, apply also to individuals with milder head injuries, which are receiving increasing attention (Boll, 1983; Rimel, Giordani, Barth, Boll, and Jane, 1981). There is a growing conviction that careful assessment of and special attention to school programs are also important for this second group of children.

THE IMPORTANCE OF COGNITIVE ASSESSMENT

It is now well established that cognitive and psychosocial sequelae are more debilitating for head injured patients as a group than are motor deficits (Levin, Benton, and Grossman, 1982; Lishman, 1978). Although long-term outcome has been less thoroughly studied in children than in adults, there is reason to believe that this finding is at least as true of children as of adults; the academic environment a child enters following an injury places a maximal demand on cognitive and behavioral integrity. It is all too common for children with "invisible" cognitive deficits to return

*Authorship listed alphabetically at the authors' request.

prematurely to an overly stressful educational and social environment, in which their academic performance and behavior will likely suffer.

Closed head injuries are notorious in this regard: the types of brain damage frequently associated with cognitive and psychosocial dysfunction following closed head injury may not be detected by any combination of neurologic evaluation of the sensory and motor systems, computed tomographic (CT) scan, EEG, and evoked potentials (Brooks, Aughton, Bond, Jones, and Rizvi, 1980). These types include widespread cortical and subcortical shearing lesions and perhaps mild anterior frontal and temporal lobe contusions (see Chapter 1). For example, although diffuse damage resulting from shearing lesions is not observable on CT scans of the brain, it can significantly affect a child's endurance and attentional and processing abilities, all of which are important for effective learning and social functioning. Anterior frontal lobe damage, even if mild, may affect the child's "executive functions" (see Chapter 8) but remains silent to thorough neurologic evaluation. (We cannot speak with confidence about frontal lobe damage in young children because of the inadequate understanding of brain-behavior relationships in young children [Rutter, 1981] and because of the relatively late development of the frontal lobes.)

Rehabilitation-Relevant Assessment

Although the many purposes of cognitive assessment are not mutually exclusive, each purpose does demand a particular selection of assessment tools. Research purposes include group descriptions, the determination of brain-behavior relationships, and studies of the effectiveness of intervention, for which a rehabilitation center is a natural setting. One clinical purpose of assessment is to establish a patient's eligibility for educational services.

This discussion is restricted to a model of cognitive assessment that is directly relevant to the rehabilitation process. The model includes establishing baseline levels, documenting progress, and, more importantly, formulating and modulating a coherent program of cognitive rehabilitation. With respect to cognitive rehabilitation and educational programming, an effective assessment helps clinicians with the following objectives:

- To set goals as well as specific target behaviors
- To make appropriate placements within a multifaceted cognitive rehabilitation program that includes special education
- To obtain baseline levels as an appropriate starting point for intervention and as a yardstick against which to measure progress

- To identify a pattern of assets and deficits so that areas of greatest strength are involved as much as possible in the processes of remediating or compensating for deficits.

In other words, cognitive assessment that is most effective in planning treatment ("rehabilitation-relevant" assessment—Ben Yishay and Diller, 1983) results in a thorough description of what patients can do well and of their key functional deficits, and in an integrated and efficient plan for the rehabilitation team to make patients maximally functional in their current environment and projected discharge environment.

A multidisciplinary team is best equipped to cover the entire terrain of comprehensive cognitive assessment (Fuld and Fisher, 1977; Goldman, L'Engle Stein, and Guerry, 1983). In most rehabilitation settings, as in ours, assessment is a layered process that involves several disciplines and proceeds over a considerable stretch of recovery time.

A complete assessment includes a review of the patient's medical records and pretrauma educational and social history, which will not be discussed here. The three additional sources of assessment data that must be integrated to ground a rational rehabilitation plan are covered: formal assessment, informal assessment, and diagnostic treatment.

Formal Assessment

Formal assessment includes a neuropsychological battery (discussed later in this chapter). The purposes of neuropsychological assessment are to provide a comprehensive profile of the patient's intellectual status and cognitive and psychomotor processes, as well as a more precise delineation of the components implicated in the disruption of complex functional systems.

Occupational therapists, speech-language pathologists, and educational diagnosticians add the following components to neuropsychological assessment:

- Levels needed for individual and group therapy or classroom placement
- Baseline data for specific goal areas
- Specific discipline-related testing of hypotheses that remain unresolved by the neuropsychological assessment.

Therapists should choose only tests that will influence planning of rehabilitation by providing answers to questions that have not been satisfactorily answered by previous testing. Discipline-related testing should, in this sense, be highly flexible both in the choice of test instruments for a given patient and in the possible modification of the administration of a test. The goal is to resolve unanswered questions about the patient's abilities and deficits, not to accumulate test scores.

Informal Assessment

Family interviews and structured observation of patients during testing sessions and in more natural settings provide information that is difficult to obtain by means of formal testing alone (Hartlage and Telzrow, 1983). A structured family interview is valuable to the treatment team because family members may see the child's best functioning in a sheltered, familiar home environment. More commonly, however, family members will see problems that do not appear in formal testing sessions, especially those of safety and social judgment, self-initiated problem solving, endurance, and persistence. Family interviews also provide valuable reports of pretraumatic functioning, particularly for preschoolers for whom school records are not available.

In their observations, clinicians should note the patient's abilities in the following areas, some of which are measured by neuropsychological tests.

1. Attention span, quality of attention, and distractability.
2. Flexibility in task orientation and shifting.
3. Use of strategies observed during testing.
4. Awareness of strategies used (e.g., answers to questions such as "How did you help yourself do that?").
5. Ability to improve performance with strategy suggestions.
6. Awareness of deficits (e.g., accuracy of responses to questions such as "How do you think you did?" — applicable to children roughly 7 years old or older).
7. Response to stress, whether self-imposed or imposed by the demands of a given test.
8. Initiation, appropriateness, and adaptability of functional behaviors in a natural environment, including communication.
9. Spontaneous problem solving in less structured environments without cues or environmental supports.

Diagnostic Treatment

Often a patient's learning ability and style are not fully understood before trial therapeutic intervention or classroom teaching begins. This difficulty is compounded with very young children, since it may not be known what knowledge and skills they possessed pretraumatically. A child's rapid acquisition of knowledge or skills in therapy or in the classroom may lead professionals to be optimistic about long-term outcome. This progress may, however, represent reacquisition of pretraumatic levels of knowledge, whereas the patient's ability to learn essentially new material may and often does fall dramatically.

Assessing these variables within a context of diagnostic treatment involves systematic exploration of factors which affect learning and general adaptive behavior, such as the following:

- Learning environment: level of activity, type and amount of distractions, pace of activities, structure and consistency, level of teacher-peer pressure
- Endurance, persistence, and initiative of the patient
- Alternative cuing systems
- Types of tasks presented and their relation to the patient's motivation and ability to understand them
- Explicitness of rules and instructions, amount of success, and types of reinforcement
- Acquisition of compensatory strategies and the ability to generalize and maintain use of them

Integration of Assessment Data

Two inherent dangers of multidisciplinary assessment are overtesting and failing to integrate all aspects of assessment into a coherent and rational rehabilitation plan that a therapist can adjust quickly as the patient changes. How assessment results translate into rehabilitation planning after all the assessment data have been integrated remains a thorny issue that the professional community has not yet resolved. The actual integration of assessment data at our facility occurs in a series of regularly scheduled treatment planning meetings. At these meetings members of the cognitive rehabilitation team as well as education staff compare formal and informal assessment results and make ongoing adjustments in goals and treatment procedures based on the patient's response to treatment. Chapter 17 includes a discussion of this process.

NEUROPSYCHOLOGICAL ASSESSMENT

Background

It is now commonly understood that neuropsychological assessment is concerned with the measurement and description of brain-behavior relationships in individuals who have sustained some type of cerebral lesion. Early investigations focused on establishing the validity of neuropsychological evaluation as a basis for inferring brain damage in adults. Such procedures have long since demonstrated their effectiveness in providing a noninvasive basis for differential diagnosis. Furthermore, in the hands of experienced neuropsychologists, the data obtained have also provided information on the lateralization, localization, and causes of cerebral lesions. Controversies persist, however, in the area of pediatric neuropsychological assessment, since specific brain-behavior relationships have not been clearly established in children (Rutter, 1981).

The increasing rate of survival of head injured individuals has placed new demands on the field of rehabilitation. In the past (Golden, 1978), brain damaged patients were not regarded as candidates for rehabilitation efforts except insofar as motor and communication functioning could be improved. Recent work, however (Craine and Gudeman, 1981; Diller et al., 1974), suggests that systematic and intensive retraining of head injured adults improves cognitive functioning. As a consequence, neuropsychological assessment has come to play a larger role in rehabilitation planning.

Neuropsychological Assessment in a Rehabilitation Setting

Unlike the long-standing medical practice models in which diagnosis translates directly into treatment, the rehabilitation model for the head injured person is still in a stage of infancy. Rehabilitation professionals are not concerned with differential diagnosis in the usual sense, since treatment is predicated on the fact that the patient has sustained a brain lesion. What these professionals need is an assessment that will identify the full range of cognitive assets as well as cognitive deficits. It is not surprising, therefore, that a multidisciplinary approach to assessment has evolved in most rehabilitation facilities.

The neuropsychological assessment of head injured patients serves four basic purposes within the framework of rehabilitation:

1. It provides a baseline description of all skills and abilities that depend upon cortical functioning.
2. It aids in formulating a prognosis.
3. It aids in formulating a cognitive rehabilitation treatment plan.
4. It helps monitor patient progress over the course of the rehabilitation program

Baseline Description. Since adequate descriptions of methods for gathering neuropsychological assessment data appear elsewhere (Golden, 1978; Lezak, 1976), the merits of standard as opposed to flexible neuropsychological test batteries will not be explored.

Treatment Implications. The work of Luria (1966, 1973) and more recently of Golden (1978) has had a profound impact in directing the course and focus of treatment for head injured patients. The extent to which the assessment data provide a basis for cognitive rehabilitation of adults is most apparent in the work of Craine and Gudeman (1981). In order to be useful, assessment data must be considered from the perspective of a frame of reference in which cognitive functions and their interrelationships can be understood. Such a framework is presented in Chapter 8, and Chapters 11 and 12 present concrete treatment suggestions.

Monitoring Progress. If baseline data have been thoroughly established and treatment implications adequately drawn, the effectiveness of subsequent rehabilitation efforts can be measured. The enormous costs associated with rehabilitation make these considerations of effectiveness imperative. Neuropsychological reevaluation is one way to monitor patients' progress, although many effects of the rehabilitation process can be evaluated only by descriptions of functional behaviors from actual life situations. Patients may acquire compensatory strategies, for instance, that may not be reflected in assessment scores.

Prediction. For the most part, children and adolescents are expected to return to their school environment. School psychologists, teachers, and school administrators have traditionally used test results to recommend appropriate placements or programs of instruction. In addition, psychological tests have come to be regarded as having long-range predictive value for any given student's future achievement. Unfortunately, educators are too often mired exclusively in an approach to test interpretation that is based on level of performance. Our experiences as well as those of others have shown that level of performance alone predicts extremely poorly the progress of head injured patients (Jennett and Teasdale, 1981; Reitan, 1974; Ylvisaker, 1981).

Rationale for Comprehensive Neuropsychological Assessment

Lesions resulting from typical closed head injuries include widespread diffuse damage that disrupts or seriously impairs a wide range of abilities at both basic and higher cognitive levels that depend upon cortical integrity.

A meaningful rehabilitation program can be formulated only through a complete identification of cognitive assets as well as deficits. As Craine and Gudeman (1981) have noted, far less information would suffice if the sole purpose were to make a differential diagnosis.

However, since brain functions must be understood as the activity of an enormously complex interrelated set of systems, describing and measuring them fully requires a battery of related tests and procedures that sample the broadest possible range of skills and abilities. It has been pointed out (Boll, 1981; Golden, 1978) that this approach to assessment provides a basis for a multiple-inference approach that takes account of level and pattern of performance and pathognomonic signs, and compares the ability of one side of the body to the other.

Assessment Content

The social and emotional as well as the cognitive aspects of a patient's functioning are all taken into account in any thorough assessment. For the purposes of this chapter, however, discussion is limited to cognitive assessment.

Every effort should be made to obtain data about the patient's pretraumatic cognitive functioning. Sources of information include clinical interviews with parents and other family members, school records, grade placements, achievement test results, IQ scores, hobbies, interests, extracurricular activities, and peer group associations, among others. We cannot overemphasize the value of such data to the treatment of head injured children.

A neuropsychological evaluation battery should sample the following areas of cortical functioning:

- Organizational skills
- Intellectual functioning
- Sensory and perceptual functioning
- Language comprehension and expression
- Attention, concentration, and alertness
- Problem solving and judgment
- Flexibility of thought processes
- Academic functions, such as reading, writing, and arithmetic
- Memory and learning
- Rate of information processing in any modality
- Effects of feedback on performance
- Sequencing ability

- Temporal and spatial abilities
- Fatigue
- Motor functioning

Although not exhaustive, the list covers areas that are included in the two most widely used neuropsychological test batteries— those associated with Halstead and Reitan (Reitan, 1974) and those associated with Golden (Golden, Hammeke, and Purisch, 1978). An age-appropriate Wechsler test of intelligence and an achievement test are usually also included as part of the formal assessment procedure.

The extensiveness of such a battery provides an overall description of a patient's cortical assets and deficits. Although none of the tests measures *subcortical* functioning, information concerning cortical activity contributes significantly to the establishment of baseline levels of functioning.

Assessment Procedures

Wechsler Intelligence Test: Cautions

The Wechsler Intelligence Scale for Children–Revised (WISC-R) has probably become the most widely used individual test of intelligence. Its strengths lie in its capacity to measure performance levels as well as to establish a profile of patterns of those performances. However, it has been convincingly shown (Siemensen and Sutherland, 1974) that by itself it lacks predictive value in the assessment of brain lesions. Head injured children often show significant processing and learning disorders despite normal Full Scale IQ values, comparable Verbal and Performance Scale results, and no significant subtest scatter.

Unfortunately, school psychologists and teachers place such heavy reliance on WISC-R results alone that many errors of omission and commission have resulted from the evaluation of both normal and brain injured children. Additionally, this test instrument has been used inappropriately to infer not only the presence of cerebral impairment but also the lateralization and localization of such inferred impairment. The use of the WISC-R alone for making inferences about cortical functioning is irresponsible because the test measures cerebral functioning incompletely. The fact that some subtests (e.g., Coding) are comparatively more "sensitive" to the effects of cortical impairment than others does not endorse the use of the test except as part of a complete neuropsychological test battery.

Neuropsychological Test Batteries

A complete description of the most widely used neuropsychological test batteries is beyond the scope of this chapter. However, Table 9-1 presents a comparative summary of the Halstead-Reitan and the Luria-Nebraska batteries. It should be kept in mind that each test or series of test items in the table is intended to measure both simple and complex skills and abilities and that no single test or single series of test items was designed to measure all aspects of cognitive function. The tabled values represent an average of the ratings of the different tests as measures of the cognitive functions that psychologists at our facility gave.

Luria-Nebraska Tests. The test items are divided in such a way that composite scores can be obtained for each of 11 scales of functioning: Motor; Rhythm; Tactile; Visual; Receptive Speech; Expressive Language; Writing; Reading; Arithmetic; Memory; and Intellectual Processes. Items within each scale are designed to measure, in both simple and complex forms, more than the particular ability suggested by the name of the scale. Items from each of the 11 regular scales are used to generate two additional sets of scales, one of which provides a basis for inferring the lateralization and localization of cortical lesions, whereas the second provides more highly specific information on such basic skills and abilities as visual acuity and naming, phonemic discrimination, and simple tactile sensation, plus 27 additional areas of cognitive function. Patients' scores are compared to a Critical Level determined on the basis of age and education.

The Luria-Nebraska batteries represent efforts to translate directly Luria's theories (Luria, 1966, 1973) of brain-behavior relationships into a standardized test procedure. Whether or not this translation has been successful remains a controversial issue (Adams, 1980; Spiers, 1981; Stambrook, 1983).

Halstead-Reitan Tests. By contrast to the theoretical underpinning of the Luria-Nebraska batteries, the Halstead-Reitan batteries are more empirically based. The Halstead-Reitan set of batteries has been far more extensively validated than the Luria-Nebraska tests on patient populations with known cerebral lesions. These tests were devised by Ward Halstead, and development has been continued by Ralph Reitan. In its current form the battery consists of five tests (Category Test, Tactual Performance Test, Speech Sounds Perception Test, Finger Tapping Test, and Seashore Rhythm Test), which are supplemented by Reitan's inclusion of an aphasia examination, a sensory-perceptual examination, the Trail Making Test (parts A and B), and a measure of bilateral grip strength. This battery, together with the age-appropriate Wechsler test of intelligence, a measure of achievement, and procedures specifically designed for very young

Table 9-1. Comparison of the Luria-Nebraska and Halstead-Reitan Neuropsychological Test Batteries

Cognitive Function	Luria-Nebraska Scales											Halstead-Reitan Tests and Allied Procedures														
	Motor	Rhythm	Tactile	Visual-Spatial	Receptive Speech	Expressive Speech	Writing	Reading	Arithmetic	Memory	Intellectual	Category	Tactual Performance	Rhythm	Finger Tapping	Speech Sounds	Dynamometer	Aphasia Examination	Trail Making	Sensory-Perceptual	Individual Performance*	Color Form*	Progressive Figures*	Target*	Marching*	Matching Pictures*	Lateral Dominance
Intelligence	0	0	0	1	1	1	0	0	1	1	2	2	1	0	0	0	0	1	1	0	1	0	1	1	0	0	0
Language Comprehension	1	1	1	1	2	1	0	0	1	1	2	0	0	0	0	0	0	2	0	0	1	1	0	0	0	0	0
Language Expression	0	0	1	0	1	1	0	0	0	0	2	0	0	0	0	0	0	1	0	0	0	0	0	0	0	0	0
Sensory/Perceptual	0	1	2	0	0	0	0	0	0	0	0	0	2	1	0	1	0	0	0	2	1	0	1	1	0	1	0
Attention/Concentration/Alertness	0	1	2	0	0	0	0	0	0	1	0	1	1	2	0	2	0	0	0	1	1	1	1	2	1	0	0
Organization	0	0	0	1	2	1	0	0	0	0	1	1	2	0	0	0	0	0	1	0	0	0	0	0	0	0	0
Problem Solving	1	0	0	0	2	0	0	0	0	0	0	2	2	0	0	0	0	0	0	0	0	0	0	0	0	0	0
Flexibility	0	0	0	0	1	1	1	1	0	0	2	2	1	0	0	0	0	0	1	0	0	2	0	0	1	0	0
Reading	0	0	0	0	1	0	0	1	0	0	1	0	0	0	0	0	0	0	0	0	0	0	0	0	0	0	0
Writing	0	0	0	0	0	1	1	0	1	0	0	0	0	0	0	0	0	0	0	0	0	0	0	0	0	0	0
Arithmetic	0	0	1	0	1	0	0	1	0	0	1	0	0	0	0	0	0	0	0	0	0	0	0	0	0	0	0
Judgment	0	1	0	0	0	1	1	0	0	0	1	0	0	0	0	0	0	0	0	0	0	0	0	0	0	0	0
Memory	0	0	0	0	1	0	0	0	0	3	1	0	1	0	0	0	0	0	0	0	0	0	0	2	0	0	0
Learning	0	0	0	0	0	1	0	0	1	2	1	1	2	0	0	1	0	0	0	0	1	0	0	0	0	0	0
Processing Rate	0	0	0	0	2	0	0	0	0	0	0	2	0	0	0	0	0	0	0	1	0	1	0	0	1	0	0
Feedback on Performance	0	0	0	0	0	1	0	0	0	0	1	0	1	0	0	0	0	0	0	0	0	0	0	0	0	0	0
Sequencing	1	0	0	0	1	0	0	0	0	1	1	0	2	0	0	0	0	0	2	0	0	2	0	2	0	0	0
Temporal	0	1	0	0	1	1	0	0	0	0	1	0	0	1	0	0	0	0	0	0	1	0	0	0	1	0	0
Spatial	0	0	0	2	0	0	0	0	1	0	0	2	1	0	0	0	0	2	0	0	0	2	0	1	0	0	0
Fatigue and Stress	0	0	0	0	0	0	0	0	0	0	0	0	0	0	1	1	1	0	0	0	0	0	0	0	0	0	0
Motor	2	0	0	0	0	0	0	0	0	0	0	0	2	0	2	0	2	1	1	0	0	1	0	0	2	0	0

Key: 0 = weakly measures
1 = moderately measures
2 = strongly measures

*Special tests for ages 5-8

children (ages 5 to 8 years) represents what most often is administered under the umbrella of a Halstead-Reitan neuropsychological test battery (Table 9-1).

COGNITIVE-LANGUAGE ASSESSMENT

Traditional aphasia syndromes can occur following closed head injuries that result in focal lesions in the language centers of the brain. These syndromes, however, are not common in either adults (Heilman, Safran, and Geschwind, 1971) or children (see Chapter 2). Despite the relatively low incidence of specific linguistic impairments (lexicon, morphology, and syntax), language disturbances of a sort not directly associated with knowledge of the linguistic code are very common in head injured adults (Sarno, 1980) and children (Ylvisaker, 1981). Hence, this section emphasizes assessment procedures for language deficits and language learning deficits, both of which are in most cases secondary to more general cognitive dysfunction and are characteristic sequelae of severe closed head injury. These deficits, outlined in Table 9-2, often exist in patients whose speech and language appear to be superficially unaffected. Although subtle or mild, such problems can become serious in demanding academic or work environments.

Assessment of the patient's knowledge of the linguistic code is appropriate when the therapist observes aphasic symptoms. However, typical batteries for aphasia and batteries designed for children with congenital language impairments that focus on knowledge of codes (syntax, morphology, lexicon) are generally less useful for assessing the abilities of head injured patients than an assessment of the patient's current language learning potential and the ability to process, mentally manipulate, and produce language in an efficient and organized manner, particularly under some form of stress. The goals of cognitive-language assessment, combined with neuropsychological assessment, are the following:

1. To determine a language profile: strengths and deficits.
2. To identify factors responsible for the disruption of complex language functions.
3. To establish goals for cognitive-language therapy.
4. To provide family and treatment team members with information on the child's language processing, organizational, and expressive limits, and on how to communicate effectively with the child and to facilitate communication recovery.

In Table 9-2 the key areas of cognitive-language assessment are outlined. Within each of these areas the left column lists crucial questions

Table 9-2. Cognitive-Language Assessment

Area	Assessment Focus	Possible Assessment Procedures
Receptive Language	1. Establish vocabulary level; compare with comprehension as affected by (a) increased length of utterance (b) increased complexity of utterance (c) increased rate of verbal input (d) increased amount of information (e) increased environmental interference (f) conversational demands *Key Questions* 1. What is the level of the patient's language knowledge base (vocabulary)? 2. How is language comprehension affected by varied and increasing processing demands? *Comment:* With children, the demands of *new* concept formation and language learning may cause vocabulary levels to deteriorate, relative to age, over the long run post trauma.	1. *Peabody Picture Vocabulary Test:* L or M (Dunn and Dunn, 1981) (a) and (b): *Children's Token Test* (DiSimoni, 1978); insensitive at upper range (c) *Token Test* commands spoken rapidly (tape recorded at approximately 200 words/minute) (d) Paragraphs or longer passages from reading tests or graded readers used informally to assess auditory comprehension. *Free recall* (story retelling) more informative than cued *recall* (objective questions). For well-recovered older patients, reading and summarizing a chapter or more of age and interest appropriate material may reveal subtle language comprehension or integration problems. (e) *Informal:* Assess comprehension with background recorded conversation as interference. (f) *Informal:* Observe comprehension of ongoing conversation; does patient detect and correctly interpret contextual cues and speaker's suprasegmental and nonverbal behavior?
Expressive Language	1. Expressive vocabulary level. 2. Word retrieval under varying forms of stress. 3. Expressive organization of increasing amounts of information. 4. Conversational competence.	1. *Expressive One-Word Picture Vocabulary Test* (Gardner, 1979) 2. *Rapid Automatized Naming Tests* (Denckla and Rudel, 1976): time pressure with easy vocabulary and picture cues; *Word Fluency* from *Neurosensory Center Comprehensive*

Table continued on following page.

Table 9-2 (continued).

Area	Assessment Focus	Possible Assessment Procedures
	Key Questions 1. What is the patient's unstressed expressive vocabulary level? Compare with receptive vocabulary. 2. How do varying forms of stress affect word retrieval? 3. Can the patient organize large amounts of information for clear and coherent expression? 4. Is the patient's conversation competent and appropriate in unstructured situations? *Comment:* Word retrieval problems are common following head injury, and different forms of stress can have different effects. Even mild word retrieval or language organizational problems may be handicapping in a busy classroom or stressful social situation.	*Examination for Aphasia,* children's norms in Gaddes and Crocket (1975): Time pressure, no visual cues. Category naming also useful. *Informal:* observe efficiency of word retrieval in conversation. 3. Complex picture description (e.g., "The Cookie Theft" from *Boston Diagnostic Aphasia Examination,* Goodglass and Kaplan, 1972); explanation of complex game; written summary of age and interest appropriate chapter. Analyze for: *main idea, presupposition, organization, expansion, accuracy, detail.* 4. *Informal:* Analyze unstructured conversation for *initiation, relevance, topic maintenance, turn taking, logical topic shifting, "rambling," inhibition, social appropriateness.*
Integrative Language and Verbal Reasoning	1. Cognitive-semantic system with increasing semantic complexity or abstractness. 2. Concept formation and cognitive-semantic flexibility. 3. Verbal reasoning and problem solving. *Key Questions* 1. What is the patient's level of language processing? How well organized is the semantic system? Can the patient detect subtleties of meaning? 2. Can the patient efficiently form new verbal concepts and flexibly readjust the concept scheme?	1. *The Word Test* (Jorgenson, Barrett, Huisingh, and Zachman, (1981): Associations, Synonyms, Antonyms, Definitions, Semantic Absurdities, Multiple Definitions. *Detroit Tests of Learning Aptitude* (Baker and Leland, 1967): Verbal Absurdities, Likeness and Differences. Analogy tests may yield inflated results since the analogies are often automatic; requesting an explanation of the analogic principle yields more useful results. 2. Concept Formation subtest of the *Woodcock-Johnson Psychoeducational Battery: Tests of Cognitive Ability*

Table 9-2 (continued).

Area	Assessment Focus	Possible Assessment Procedures
	3. Can the patient use language to engage in higher level abstraction and reasoning processes? *Comment:* Success with structured abstraction or problem-solving measures is no guarantee that the patient will maintain an abstract and problem-solving attitude in the real world.	(Woodcock and Johnson, 1977)—particularly useful for cognitive flexibility and ability to reorient in response to changing task instructions. 3. *Ross Test of Higher Cognitive Processes* (Ross and Ross, 1976). *Informal:* story or paragraph *discussion* format to assess patient's ability to detect main ideas, draw inferences, construct interpretations or explanations, flexibly construct multiple interpretations or explanations, engage in organized verbal problem solving.
Verbal Memory and New Learning	1. Immediate recall of unrelated and of semantically connected verbal material. 2. Delayed recall. 3. Verbal learning with feedback. 4. Functional recall of daily events. *Key Questions* 1. Immediate recall tasks: what is the patient's level of attention or concentration and "space" in working memory? 2. Can the patient store and retrieve new information over extended periods of time? 3. Does the patient make effective use of feedback in learning verbal information? Does the patient spontaneously use strategies to aid learning and retention? 4. Does the patient efficiently store and retrieve daily events (episodic memory)? 5. What variables appear to be particularly related to memory efficiency: interest level? attention? perceptual	1. Digit span; immediate recall of short story or paragraph (e.g., Logical Memory subtest from *Wechsler Memory Test* for older adolescents, Wechsler, 1945). 2. Thirty minute delay norms for *Wechsler Memory Scale* paragraphs (Russell, 1975). *Informal:* for younger children, use story retelling procedure: immediate versus 30 min delay versus 24 hour delay. 3. *Selective Reminding Task* (Buschke and Fuld, 1974; unpublished norms from H. Levin). Involves verbal learning over several trials with feedback. The "consistent long-term retrieval" measure is a good indication of the ability to learn rote material. Auditory-Visual Learning subtest of *Woodcock-Johnson Psychoeducational Battery: Tests of Cognitive Ability*—involves new learning of a symbol system with feedback; useful indication

Table continued on following page.

Table 9-2 (continued).

Area	Assessment Focus	Possible Assessment Procedures
	modality? familiarity? inherent organization? context? personal importance? mnemonic strategies? *Comment:* If memory performance is poor, it is difficult to distinguish *inefficient processing or encoding* from *inefficient storage or retrieval* or from *inefficient executive direction.*	of new learning rate and strategies. 4. Informal probes.

that evaluators should ask about the language functioning of head injured patients. The specific assessment procedures that are listed in the right column are less important than the questions therapists ask to make their assessments. A rehabilitation-relevant language assessment should be a procedure of testing hypotheses about a given child's breakdowns. These hypotheses derive from pathophysiologic data, neuropsychological assessment results, knowledge of typical head injury sequelae, informal communication with the patient, and the patient's response to initial intervention.

The assessment procedures outlined in Table 9-2 assume that the speech mechanism is adequately intact and also that the academic evaluation includes reading and writing.

EDUCATIONAL ASSESSMENT

Purpose of Assessment

Head injured patients in a rehabilitation center can benefit from a program that integrates cognitive rehabilitation therapy with educational programming. Educational assessments help to determine appropriate classroom placements. In addition to identifying academic levels, they evaluate the patient's ability to integrate skills to perform complex, cognitive tasks. *Assessment should indicate what patients know as well as what they do not know.* Teaching should begin where learning breaks down and should incorporate styles and strategies that were found to be effective during the assessment.

Since formal and informal evaluations provide complementary information and since diagnostic, prescriptive teaching is a form of evaluation, it is important to note whether a student's performance in a busy classroom differs from performance in the more formal, controlled testing situation.

Selection of Assessment Instruments

Speech-language and neuropsychological assessment results help the educational diagnostician select instruments with appropriate comprehension levels and response requirements and thus avoid overtesting. Educational evaluations translate these findings into the graded teaching process. In addition, reports describing pretraumatic functioning help the examiner and teacher distinguish between newly acquired and pretraumatic behaviors (Fuld and Fisher, 1977) and plan school programs with realistic expectations.

Basic Skills

Head injured individuals often have difficulty integrating skills that are necessary for everyday activities and school tasks. The classroom is an effective environment in which to develop specific cognitive components and skill integration.

Skills basic for learning should be evaluated separately and also in the context of more complex, academic tasks. Basic learning skills include visual and auditory discrimination, sequencing, and memory; fine motor planning for manipulating objects or doing paper-pencil tasks; gross motor and fine motor skills; orientation and organization; and concrete and abstract levels of language comprehension and expression. Evaluators should also assess social skills in the context of peer-group interaction (see Chapter 15).

Test Variety

Head injuries can produce a wide range of impairments (see Chapter 2). Since one purpose of assessment is to have individuals *demonstrate what they know,* it is necessary to have evaluation materials that require a variety of response modes and that have content presented in different formats. The nonspeaking individual can respond by pointing, gesturing, or using eye-gaze. The person who has difficulty recalling information can demonstrate comprehension by selecting multiple choice responses (printed or oral) or by referring to material for answers. The person with impaired writing can demonstrate visual memory by pointing to or describing items that were shown. The visually distracted individual can demonstrate a comprehension level by responding to material presented orally or to small amounts of visual material. Patients can provide evaluators with reading comprehension levels by reading one sentence silently and pointing to a response (Peabody Individual Achievement Test, Dunn and Markwardt, 1980), by completing a sentence orally that they read silently (Woodcock Reading Mastery Tests, Woodcock, 1973), by reading a short paragraph orally or silently and answering oral questions from memory (Diagnostic Reading Scales, Spache, 1981), or by reading a short paragraph silently and referring back to the context to select and underline a printed multiple choice answer (Group Diagnostic Reading Aptitude and Achievement Tests, Monroe and Sherman, 1966).

When selecting evaluation instruments, reviewing test performance, and planning educational programs, evaluators must attend to the following factors:

| *Stimulus* | *Content* | *Response* |
| (method of presentation) | (test or task items) | |

Test directions can affect performance significantly. Evaluators should note whether the length, level, and mode of presentation of directions are appropriate, whether directions are clear visually and linguistically, are printed or pictured and can be used for reference, are oral and require intact memory skills, have a familiar or pictured format that requires no explanation, provide practice items, or have time requirements that can be stressful.

When reviewing the content of test items, evaluators should recognize that successful completion of an item can require the use of skills other than the one(s) the item was designed to test (Torgeson, 1979), for example, directions for a visual-motor test are often oral; visual-memory tasks may involve language skills (oral response) or fine motor and spatial orientation-organization ability (written response); the material can be meaningful or nonmeaningful; some material requires well thought out responses whereas other material may require rote responses; the length of items, the complexity of the language of the test, and the required degree of skill integration can influence attention, comprehension, and performance.

Patients can respond to tests by pointing, manipulating objects, writing or drawing, moving about the room, and talking. When using tests with multiple choice responses, examiners should consider whether guessing could be a factor.

Examiners should compile individualized assessment batteries by using subtests from different levels and different instruments that have appropriate stimulus-response variations in comprehension, communication, and cognitive abilities. A head injured student may have good visual-motor skills and be able to decode or "word-call," but language *comprehension* may be poor. To obtain a comprehension level at which the teacher can start to rebuild the patient's language skills, the examiner may need to use assessment materials that test skills at levels far below those at which the patient functioned before the injury.

Conditions of Testing: Standardized Procedures Versus Adaptations of Test Materials

If the directions, format, and required responses of standardized instruments are not appropriate for particular patients, examiners may need to do the following:

1. Allow the patient to use different response modes, such as saying, pointing to, or looking at an answer instead of underlining or writing it.
2. Change the directions and content of test items: make them shorter, less wordy or more concrete (by adding print or pictures), or present them orally instead of in writing or vice versa.
3. Give examples to clarify the tasks.
4. Substitute multiple choice responses (oral or written) for those that involve recalling information from memory.
5. Enlarge the print of the tests.
6. Decrease the amount of printed material per item or per page.
7. Obtain timed and untimed scores.

It is important that assessment reports describe all adaptations of standardized tests so that the specific conditions under which a patient performs are known. Otherwise, those receiving the reports will assume that standardized procedures were used, will probably misinterpret students' abilities, and, at least initially, will plan inappropriate programs. Table 9–3 presents a list of educational assessment instruments that we have found useful in evaluating head injured students.

Observing Behavior

Cognitive problems of severly head injured students include poor organization of thoughts and the inability to generalize, to solve problems, to remember or retrieve information, and to understand material that

Table 9-3. Educational Assessment Instruments
    The following is a list of some assessment instruments that are useful when evaluating head injured students. Specific subtests are designated occasionally, but other parts of these tests may also provide valuable information for individual students. Subtest selection will depend upon the content of the test instruments in the total battery.

Preschool-Kindergarten Level:
    Learning Accomplishment Profile—Diagnostic Edition (Le May, Griffin, and Sanford, 1977). Translates easily into program goals; separate receptive-expressive language sections; good analysis of basic cognitive skills. (6 months to 72 months)
    Kraner Preschool Math Inventory (Kraner, 1976). Evaluates pre-math and language concepts as well as number concept and beginning computation; picture and printed presentation; includes relatively abstract concepts (e.g., a square with a dot in the center represents a "ball in a box"); mostly pointing response. (3½ to 6½ years)
    The Developmental Resource, Volume I (Cohen and Gross, 1979). Tracks development in major developmental areas. Excellent breakdown of skills, especially for neonate to 2 year level. Good descriptions of behaviors. Includes review of the literature. (Neonate through 6 years)
    Assessment in Infancy (Uzgiris and Hunt, 1975). Good analysis of skills from birth to 2 years.
    Early-Lap (Glover, Preminger, and Sanford, 1978). Developmental checklist with specific procedures for task presentation and conditions for mastery; good for classroom evaluations. (Birth through 36 months)
    Yellow Brick Road (Kallstrom, 1975). Evaluates skills basic for learning; mostly pointing response; directions relate to Wizard of Oz theme and may need to be rewritten to clarify the task. (3 to 6 years)
    Inventory of Early Development (Brigance, 1978). Must be used selectively; detailed subtests can supplement information obtained with other instruments; good for classroom evaluations. (Birth through 6 years)
Formal Academic Levels:
    Revised Pre-Reading Screening Procedures (Slingerland, 1977).
    Slingerland Screening Tests for Identifying Children with Specific Language Disorders: Form A (Grade I and Beginning Grade II), Form B (Grade II and Beginning Grade III), Form C (Grades III and IV), Form D (Grades V and VI) (Slingerland, 1970, 1974).
    Specific Language Disability Test — Grades 6, 7, 8 (Malcomesius, 1967). The Slingerland and Malcomesius tests provide information on perceptual skills and integrative processing. Directions are oral, can be complex, are similar to those in academic materials, and are usually difficult for head injured students; on-task behavior, overload, and flexibility can be monitored; drawing and writing are involved in many tasks.
    Diagnostic Reading Scales (Spache, 1981). Provides sight vocabulary lists and comprehension scores for oral or silent reading and listening; short-term memory required for open-ended questions; passages get progressively longer and print gets smaller; head injured students may score less well on this test than on tests in which they can refer back to content or in which there are multiple choice answers (Grades 1.4 to 7.5)
    Group Diagnostic Reading Aptitude and Achievement Tests— Intermediate Form (Grades 3 to 9) (Monroe and Sherman, 1966). Silent reading of short paragraphs with multiple choice responses; integrative processing evaluated with meaningful or nonmeaningful content; written spelling; mathematics computation only; copying; timed requirements.
    Peabody Individual Achievement Test (Dunn and Markwardt, 1970). Subtests: Reading Comprehension; Mathematics; Spelling. Silent reading relates material (one sentence) to

Table 9-3 (continued).

a choice of pictures; short-term memory required; word problems only in mathematics; pointing response; spelling presented orally with printed multiple choice format that requires pointing response. (Grades 1.5 to 12)

Woodcock Reading Mastery Tests (Woodcock, 1973). Subtest: Passage Comprehension. Silent reading (one or two sentences) presented with pictures; word recall and concept closure required for oral responses; students can refer back to material. (Grades 1 to 12.9)

Key Math Diagnostic Arithmetic Test (Connolly, Nachtman, Pritchett, 1971). Language and mathematics skills are combined; can reveal memory and retrieval problems; material presented visually, auditorially, and in different formats indicates processing and integrative abilities. (Mid-kindergarten to Grade 9.5)

Detroit Tests of Learning Aptitude (Baker and Leland, 1967). Subtests: Number 1, Pictorial Absurdities; Number 6, Auditory Attention Span for Unrelated Words; Number 7, Oral Commissions; Number 9, Visual Attention Span for Objects; Number 13, Auditory Attention Span for Related Syllables; Number 18, Oral Directions. These tasks evaluate visual and auditory processing of meaningful and nonmeaningful material, judgment (Number 1), sequencing and memory (Numbers 6, 7, 9, 13, 18), flexibility and skill integration. Subtest Number 18 corresponds to school-related tasks. (Mental Age: 3 years to 19 years)

Gates-McKillop Reading Diagnostic Tests (Gates and McKillop, 1962). Subtest: Spelling (oral). (Grades 1.6 to 9.0+)

Inventory of Basic Skills (Brigance, 1977). (Kindergarten to Grade 6)

Inventory of Essential Skills (Brigance, 1981). (For secondary students with special needs)

Comprehensive Inventory of Basic Skills (Brigance, 1983). (Kindergarten to Grade 9)

Brigance materials are good for supplementary information and for classroom evaluations; must be used selectively.

---

increases in length and complexity. In the testing situation, it is as important to discover how these individuals arrive at their answers as it is to note what the answer is. In this regard, the examiner should observe the following:

- attention, distractibility, and orientation in relation to the kind of task presented
- flexibility: adjustment to changes in content, format, and response modes
- perseverative responses
- ability to work under stress: tolerance for the testing situation in general and for timed tests in particular
- performance rate related to type of task and type of response
- response to content that is familiar or unfamiliar, concrete or abstract, visual or auditory
- differences in oral, written, and gestured and manipulative responses
- fatigue and its possible medical, emotional, attentional, or task-oriented causes

- anxiety reactions: excessive yawning, inappropriate or off-task comments, unpredictably delayed responses, repeated requests for assistance or clarification, resistance or refusal to respond
- confusion of past and present, reality and fantasy
- delayed responses that represent either effective processing time or generally slow performance patterns
- purposeful or nonpurposeful repetition of information
- associations to information that indicate comprehension, lack of comprehension, or poor attention
- inadequate responses or responses not given and the potential for using different modes of presentation that might elicit more appropriate answers
- ability to retain and use information learned in the testing situation
- indications that information not known now was known previously (e.g., refusing or resisting tasks, or statements such as "This is easy," or "I used to know that")
- awareness of present capabilities
- samples of conversation and language expression that are appropriate, confabulatory, disruptive, or evasive
- consistent or inconsistent performance
- spontaneous use of strategies

Of course the examiner should integrate the foregoing information with all other aspects of test performance.

Misuse of Test Information

As indicated earlier in this chapter, evaluation scores are often thought to indicate levels of academic and cognitive functioning and to predict potential to perform in these areas. Students who do well on reading comprehension tests when they read *short* paragraphs are expected to be able to comprehend at the same level school assignments that are *several pages long.* In addition, students who complete one kind of task on an evaluation are considered to be capable of doing similar tasks in other situations.

Test scores of head injured students, however, cannot be interpreted in this manner. These students may be able to read and comprehend a short paragraph at a fourth grade level, but their comprehension may decrease dramatically with more complex and lengthier material. Many of these individuals have difficulty generalizing, and the fact that they may have done one type of task on a test does not mean that they will be able to do similar tasks in the classroom. These varied performance levels can be partly the result of severe and fluctuating processing problems.

Educational diagnosticians must understand normal development to interpret assessment data accurately and to identify behaviors that need to be established or remediated. If evaluations are to be used to plan appropriate school programs, *examiners must review test items as well as test scores.* The test performance of head injured students does not indicate that they can do tasks other than those presented in the examination; it should not be assumed or predicted that these students can do anything other than the assessment tasks.

Uneven performance levels may also reveal some skills that remain relatively unaffected by the injury as well as others that are impaired, a discrepancy that can lead evaluators to assume that overall recovery is greater than it actually is. It is thus clearly inappropriate to place students at a given educational level on the basis of the more advanced skills. Information about translating test scores and test performance into effective teaching programs is discussed in Chapters 15 and 17.

Interpreting Test Performance to Families

Family members often feel that head injured patients who can walk and carry on sensible conversations should be discharged from the rehabilitation program and returned to their previous school settings. Recommendations from neuropsychologists or cognitive rehabilitation therapists may have little meaning for the patient or the family. However, when educational tests reveal that the 12 year old who was an average student before the trauma is now comprehending reading material at a third grade level, parents and the patient begin to realize that performance *has* changed and that rehabilitation services would be beneficial. The educational diagnostician can help families understand the purposes and results of educational assessments and can explain how cognitive and behavioral problems influence everyday functioning and school performance.

SPECIAL ISSUES IN HEAD INJURY ASSESSMENT
The Perils of Prediction

There is a growing recognition in the literature (Jennett and Teasdale, 1981) of a theme that has long been appreciated by practicing clinicians: Interpretation of test data, relying exclusively on level of performance, most often yields highly unrealistic predictions regarding a patient's academic achievement or social and vocational adjustment. This is particularly true if the tests used are not sensitive to characteristic head injury sequelae, are not interpreted by an experienced clinician, and are unaccompanied by relevant informal observation (Klonoff, Low, and Clark, 1977; Ylvisaker, 1981).

Purely formal assessments may establish conditions that compensate for the patient's most functionally impairing deficits:

1. A neat, quiet and isolated test environment may compensate for attention or concentration problems.
2. A series of short testing sessions may compensate for reduced endurance and persistence.
3. Extremely clear test instructions may compensate for poor task orientation and flexibility and for a lack of initiation and spontaneous problem solving.
4. Test items that do not include real-life *amounts* of information to be processed or *rate* of delivery may compensate for weak integration and generally reduced efficiency of information processing.
5. Independent test sessions may compensate for weak long-term storage and retrieval of new information (from day to day).
6. A supportive and encouraging examiner may compensate for an inability to cope with interpersonal stress or perception of demands.
7. Tests that tap pretraumatically acquired knowledge or skills may generate false optimism regarding new learning.
8. Even the best tests may fail to elicit the notorious difficulty of a head injured child to generalize a newly acquired skill to a novel context.

Taken together, these possibilities require professionals to exercise great caution in predicting school or work performance based strictly on test results. We have worked with large numbers of head injured children whose recovery and response to intervention were excellent, whose IQ scores returned to average or above average ranges without significant subtest scatter, but who continued to require partial or full-time special education services (Fuld and Fisher, 1977) for many years post trauma. Caution in interpretating assessment results is underscored by the fact that none of the assessment instruments mentioned in this chapter has been validated specifically for use with closed head injured children.

Introduction of Formal Assessment in the Sequence of Recovery

Informal assessment of cognitive functions is an ongoing process that begins with the patient's emergence from coma. The Glasgow Coma Scale

(Teasdale and Jennett, 1974) is useful to chart recovery during the very early acute stages. Behavioral recovery scales, most notably the Rancho Los Amigos Levels of Cognitive Functioning (Hagen, 1981) are often used to track recovery during the rehabilitation phase, particularly with older children and adults. Patients are rated on this scale by observing behaviors in the areas of orientation, attention or concentration, recent and remote memory, general information processing efficiency, organization, appropriateness, and goal-directed behavior.

A patient's appropriateness for formal assessment is based chiefly on three considerations. First, the patient must not be seriously confused. If the patient is unable to orient to the task and remain so oriented, interpretation of results will be virtually impossible. Second, the patient should have an attention span of 30 min or more to allow for meaningful testing sessions. Third, if the patient is in a period of rapid recovery, extensive testing is not indicated. Brief screening instruments can be used to establish levels of functioning for program planning and the patient's treatment plans can be modified based on response to intervention. If it is likely that a patient's levels and profile will change quickly, comprehensive assessment results will soon be dated and hence of marginal usefulness.

Assessment of Very Young Children

Very young children present a special challenge to the total assessment undertaking. Although it is valuable to determine if an apparent deficit is a result of the head injury, data about pretraumatic levels of cognitive ability of both preschool and young school-age children are often incomplete or occasionally even misreported (Fuld and Fisher, 1977). The wide variability of development in this age range (Rutter, 1981) also adds to the difficulty of assessing the effects of the head injury. Furthermore, there is as yet no standardized neuropsychological test battery for preschoolers. Thus, establishing a rudimentary baseline of pretraumatic abilities requires careful and thorough interviewing of parents as well as collecting information on testing and school experiences the children may have had.

Interpreting the behavior of preschoolers for family members is particularly difficult. A greater variety of behavior is acceptable for very young children, and parents may choose to believe that their child will outgrow behaviors that professionals identify as symptoms of learning problems.

Our experiences with very young children have shown that problems such as (1) seemingly mild impairments of attention, (2) subtle disorders of language and information processing that are related to the amount or complexity of the material or to the rate of its presentation, (3) weak behavioral organization and flexibility, and (4) a mildly slow rate of learning may have few if any functional consequences until the child faces the demands of the classroom environment. For this reason very young children in the 2 to 6 year age range should be most carefully monitored through the early grades to rule out the need for cognitive rehabilitation or special education services. Diagnostic treatment in a therapy or classroom setting, using representational play and social interaction with increasing cognitive and social stress, often reveals deficits of organization, planning, and retrieval that would not otherwise be apparent. This issue is discussed in greater detail in Chapters 12 and 15.

REFERENCES

Adams, K. M. (1980). In search of Luria's battery: A false start. *Journal of Consulting and Clinical Psychology, 48,* 511-516.

Baker, H. J., and Leland, B. (1967). *Detroit tests of learning aptitude.* Indianapolis: Bobbs-Merrill.

Ben-Yishay, Y., and Diller, L. (1983). Cognitive deficits. In M. Rosenthal, E. R. Griffith, M. R. Bond, and J. D. Miller (Eds.), *Rehabilitation of the head injured adult* (pp. 167-183). Philadelphia: F. A. Davis.

Boll, T. J. (1983). Minor head injury in children — out of sight but not out of mind. *Journal of Clinical Child Psychology, 12* (1), 74-80.

Boll, T. J. (1981). The Halstead-Reitan neuropsychology battery. In A. B. Filskov and T. J. Boll (Eds.), *Handbook of clinical neuropsychology* (pp. 579-604). New York: John Wiley and Sons.

Brigance, A. H. (1977). *Inventory of basic skills.* Woburn, MA: Curriculum Associates.

Brigance, A. H. (1978). *Inventory of early development.* Woburn, MA: Curriculum Associates.

Brigance, A. H. (1981). *Inventory of essential skills.* Woburn, MA: Curriculum Associates.

Brigance, A. H. (1983). *Comprehensive inventory of basic skills.* Woburn, MA: Curriculum Associates.

Brooks, D. N., Aughton, M. E., Bond, M. R., Jones, P., and Rizvi, S. (1980). Cognitive sequelae in relationship to early indices of severity of brain damage after severe blunt head injury. *Journal of Neurology, Neurosurgery, and Psychiatry, 43,* 529-534.

Buschke, H., and Fuld, P. A. (1974). Evaluating storage, retention, and retrieval in disordered memory and learning. *Neurology, 24,* 1019-1025.

Cohen, M. A. and Gross, P. J. (1979). *The developmental resource: Vol. I. Behavioral sequences for assessment and program planning.* New York: Grune and Stratton.

Connolly, A. J., Nachtman, W., and Pritchett, E. M. (1971). *Key math diagnostic arithmetic test.* Circle Pines, MN: American Guidance Service.

Craine, J. F., and Gudeman, H. E. (1981). *The rehabilitation of brain functions: Principles, procedures, and techniques of neurotraining.* Springfield, IL: Charles C Thomas.

Denckla, M. B., and Rudel, R. (1976). Rapid "automatized" naming (R.A.N.): Dyslexia differentiated from other learning disabilities. *Neuropsychologia, 14,* 471-479.

Diller, L., Ben-Yishay, Y., Gerstman, L. J., Goodkin, R., Gordon, W., and Weinberger, J. (1974). *Studies on cognition and rehabilitation in hemiplegia.* New York: Behavioral Science Institute of Rehabilitation Medicine.

DiSimoni, F. (1978). *The token test for children.* Boston: Teaching Resources Corporation.

Dunn, L., and Dunn, L. (1981). *Peabody picture vocabulary test — revised.* Circle Pines, MN: American Guidance Service.

Dunn, L. M., and Markwardt, F., Jr. (1970). *Peabody individual achievement test.* Circle Pines, MN: Amercian Guidance Service.

Fuld, P. A., and Fisher, P. (1977). Recovery of intellectual ability after closed head-injury. *Developmental Medicine and Child Neurology, 19,* 495–502.

Gaddes, W. H., and Crocket, D. J. (1975). The Spreen-Benton Aphasia Tests: Normative data as a measure of normal language development. *Brain and Language, 2,* 257–280.

Gardner, M. F. (1979). *Expressive one-word picture vocabulary test.* Novato, CA: Academic Therapy Publications.

Gates, A. I., and McKillop, A. S. (1962). *Gates-McKillop reading diagnostic tests.* New York: Teachers College Press, Columbia University.

Glover, M. E., Preminger, J. L., and Sanford, A. R. (1978). *Early learning accomplishment profile.* Winston-Salem, NC: Kaplan School Supply Corporation.

Golden, C. J. (1978). *Diagnosis and rehabilitation in clinical neuropsychology.* Springfield, IL: Charles C Thomas.

Golden, C. J., Hammeke, T. A., and Purisch, A. D. (1978). Diagnostic validity of a standardized neuropsychological battery derived from Luria's neuropsychological tests. *Journal of Consulting and Clinical Psychology, 46,* 1258–1265.

Goldman, J., L'Engle Stein, C., and Guerry, S. (1983). *Psychological methods of child assessment.* New York: Brunner/Mazel.

Goodglass, H., and Kaplan, E. (1972). *Boston diagnostic aphasia examination.* Philadelphia: Lea and Febiger.

Hagen, L. (1981). Language disorders secondary to closed head injury: Diagnosis and treatment. *Topics in Language Disorders, 1,* 73–87.

Hartlage, L. C., and Telzrow, C. F. (1983). The neuropsychological basis of educational intervention. *Journal of Learning Disabilities, 16,* 521–528.

Heilman, K. M., Safran, A., and Geschwind, N. (1971). Closed head trauma and aphasia. *Journal of Neurosurgery, Neurology, and Psychiatry, 34,* 265–269.

Jennett, B., and Teasdale, G. (1981). *Management of head injuries.* Philadelphia: F. A. Davis.

Jorgenson, C., Barrett, M., Huisingh, R., and Zachman, L. (1981). *The word test.* Moline, IL: Lingui Systems.

Kallstrom, C. (1975). *Yellow brick road.* Austin, TX: Learning Concepts.

Klonoff, H., Low, M. D., and Clark, C. (1977). Head injuries in children: A prospective five year follow-up. *Journal of Neurology, Neurosurgery, and Psychiatry, 40,* 1211–1219.

Kraner, R. E. (1976). *Kraner preschool math inventory.* Austin, TX: Learning Concepts.

LeMay, D. W., Griffin, P. M., and Sanford, A. P. (1977). *Learning accomplishment profile — diagnostic edition.* Winston-Salem, NC: Kaplan School Supply Corporation.

Levin, H. S., Benton, A. L., and Grossman, R. G., (1982). *Neurobehavioral consequences of closed head injury.* New York: Oxford University Press.

Lezak, M. D. (1976). *Neuropsychological assessment.* New York: Oxford University Press.

Lishman, W. A. (1978). *Organic psychiatry.* Oxford: Blackwell Scientific.

Luria, A. R. (1966). *Higher cortical functions in man* (2nd ed.) (B. Haigh, Trans.). New York: Basic Books. (Original work published 1962).

Luria, A. R. (1973). *The working brain* (B. Haigh, Trans.). New York: Basic Books.

Malcomesius, N. (1967). *Specific language disability test.* Cambridge, MA: Educators Publishing Service.

Monroe, M., and Sherman, E. E. (1966).   *Group diagnostic reading aptitude and achievement tests.* Bradenton, FL: C. H. Nevins Printing Company.

Reitan, R. M. (1974).   Methodological problems in clinical neuropsychology. In R. M. Reitan and L. A. Davison (Eds.), *Clinical neuropsychology: Current status and applications* (pp. 19–46). Washington: V. H. Winston and Sons.

Rimel, R. W., Giordani, M. A., Barth, J. T., Boll, T. J., and Jane, J. A. (1981).   Disability caused by minor head injury. *Neurosurgery, 9,* 221–228.

Ross, J. D., and Ross, C. M. (1976).   *Ross test of higher cognitive processes.* Novato, CA: Academic Therapy Publications.

Russell, E. W. (1975).   A multiple scoring method for the assessment of complex memory functions. *Journal of Consulting and Clinical Psychology, 43,* 800–809.

Rutter, M. (1981).   Psychological sequelae of brain damage in children. *American Journal of Psychiatry, 138,* 1533–1544.

Sarno, M. T. (1980).   The nature of verbal impairment after closed head injury. *Journal of Nervous and Mental Disease, 168,* 685–692.

Siemensen, R. J., and Sutherland, J. (1974).   Psychological assessment of brain damage: The Wechsler scales. *Academic Therapy, 10,* 69–81.

Slingerland, B. H. (1970).   *Slingerland screening test for identifying children with specific language disorders — forms A, B, C.* Cambridge, MA: Educators Publishing Service.

Slingerland, B. H. (1974).   *Slingerland screening tests for identifying children with specific language disorders — form D.* Cambridge, MA: Educators Publishing Service.

Slingerland, B. H. (1977).   *Revised pre-reading screening procedures.* Cambridge, MA: Educators Publishing Service.

Spache, G. D. (1981).   *Diagnostic reading scales.* Monterey, CA: CTB/McGraw-Hill.

Spiers, P. A. (1981).   Have they come to praise Luria or bury him? The Luria-Nebraska controversy. *Journal of Consulting and Clinical Psychology, 49,* 331–341.

Stambrook, M. (1983).   The Luria-Nebraska Neuropsychological Battery: A promise that may be partly fulfilled. *Journal of Clinical Neuropsychology, 5,* 247–269.

Teasdale, G., and Jennett, B. (1974).   Assessment of coma and impaired consciousness: A practical scale. *Lancet, 2,* 81–84.

Torgeson, J. K. (1979).   What shall we do with psychological processes? *Journal of Learning Disabilities, 12,* 514–521.

Uzgiris, I. C., and Hunt, J. M. (1975).   *Assessment in infancy.* Urbana, IL: University of Illinois Press.

Wechsler, D. (1945).   A standardized memory scale for clinical use. *Journal of Psychology, 19,* 87–95.

Woodcock, R. W. (1973).   *Woodcock reading mastery tests.* Circle Pines, MN: American Guidance Service.

Woodcock, R. W., and Johnson, M. B. (1977).   *The Woodcock-Johnson psychoeducational educational battery. Part one: Tests of cognitive ability.* Hingham, MA: Teaching Resources Corporation.

Ylvisaker, M. (1981, October).   *Cognitive and behavioral outcomes in head injured children.* Paper presented at the International Symposium on the Traumatic Brain Injured Adult and Child, Boston.

Chapter 10

Cognitive Rehabilitation Therapy: Early Stages of Recovery

Gloria J. Smith, OTR/L, and
Mark Ylvisaker, MA, CCC/SP*

The program of sensory and sensorimotor stimulation is designed for medically stable patients in the early stages of recovery (Chapter 8, Table 8-1). At the lower range the program includes patients emerging from deep coma whose responses to environmental events are minimal and not specifically related to the stimuli presented (e.g., extensor pattern in response to touch, bright lights, loud noises, and so forth). At the upper range are patients whose responses are stimulus specific (e.g., they localize to sound or track objects visually) and who may demonstrate functional use of some objects and comprehension of routine simple instructions, as well as make some attempts at expressive communication. Although many of the stimulation techniques may be applicable to patients with no apparent responses to stimulation, the therapist must exercise great care due to the variety and importance of the medical concerns that may contraindicate stimulation therapy (see Chapter 5). Additionally, the rationale, principles, and techniques discussed in this chapter apply to patients who are in a period of spontaneous neurologic recovery, and may not apply to the patients whose state of unresponsiveness is prolonged and is a result of widespread, irreversible, bilateral cortical damage (Plum and Posner, 1972).

From the point of view of cognitive rehabilitation, the general goals of stimulation are increased arousal and alertness, increased recognition of environmental events, and an expanded range of adaptive and functional behaviors. In practice, the cognitive dimension of the stimulation program is intimately tied to feeding therapy, nursing care, and early restoration of motor abilities.

*Authorship listed alphabetically at the authors' request.

This chapter briefly reviews the neurophysiologic rationale for early stimulation therapy as well as the evidence (based largely on inferences from animal studies) of its effectiveness. A stimulation program is outlined, procedural guidelines and activity suggestions are provided, and communication with minimally responsive patients is discussed. Although the stimulation program described here is aggressive in that it provides patients with planned and carefully monitored stimulation several times a day, in comparison with the dramatic coma stimulation programs that have received public attention in recent years (e.g., Dimancescu, cited in Lasden, 1982) it is conservative in its selection of types of stimuli.

STIMULATION TREATMENT: RATIONALE

Brain plasticity is the capacity of the central nervous system to "modify its own structural organization and functioning" (Bach-y-Rita, 1980b). The precise mechanisms responsible for spontaneous neurologic recovery following severe head injury have not been fully identified, but several possibilities exist: recovery from neural shock (diaschisis), neural substitution, neural redundancy, compensation, and the unmasking of suppressed neural pathways (Bach-y-Rita, 1980a). Whatever combination of factors is instrumental in this process, spontaneous recovery does occur in most cases. The rate and ultimate degree of recovery vary, depending on age and the severity of the injury, among other factors (see Chapters 1 and 2).

Environmental enrichment and carefully modulated sensory stimulation can accelerate this recovery process and at the same time inhibit the long-term negative effects of extended inactivity and sensory deprivation. Since there are no published reports of controlled studies of the efficacy of stimulation programs for patients in the early stages of recovery from head injury, this claim will be supported with three types of indirect evidence.

Brain Lesion Studies: Stimulation Following Brain Injury

Because the study of sensory stimulation of brain injured human subjects presents methodological and ethical problems, in writing this chapter we have drawn support in part from studies of the effects of stimulation on animals with brain lesions. In his review of a large number of studies, Will (1977) concluded that stimulation improved both the rate and the amount of functional recovery. An enriched sensory and social environment benefited animals regardless of their age at the time of lesion or at the point after trauma at which they began to receive stimulation. Postlesion stimulation has been found to improve motor recovery, perceptual recovery, and learning ability, and to result in neuroanatomic and histochemical changes in the brain. Several studies (Will, Rosenzweig, and Bennett, 1976; Will, Rosenzweig, Bennett, Herbert, and Morimoto, 1977) have noted that an increase in both cerebral weight and RNA to DNA ratio occurred in lesioned rats receiving enriched environmental stimulation. These rats also exhibited improved problem-solving scores on the Hebb-Williams maze. Studies by Yu (1976) and Black, Markowitz, and Cianci (1975) noted the beneficial results of postsurgical training in the recovery of motor function. Black and co-workers reported that surgically lesioned rats improved faster and regained more function when training was initiated early. In two separate studies, structural and functional recovery was noted in animals that were visually deprived and then reexposed to visual stimulation (Chow and Stewart, 1972; Kalil, cited in Walsh and Cummins, 1976).

Sensory Deprivation Studies

In the absence of a stimulation program, a comatose or semicomatose patient experiences severe sensory deprivation. A number of deprivation studies have established the value of a rich sensory environment. Rosenzweig (1966) and Rosenzweig, Krech, Bennett, and Diamond (1962) reported increased dendritic growth in animals raised in an enriched environment, compared with normal controls and a deprived group. It should be noted that increased sensory stimulation does not always result in a beneficial change. Dogs deprived of sensory stimulation showed overarousal and an inability to filter information in a new environment (Melzak and Burns, cited in Bach-y-Rita, 1980b). A related study with human subjects concluded that kinesthetic and proprioceptive stimulation during isolation decreased to some extent the anticipated deprivation effects (Zubek, 1963). Zubek (1969) summarizes additional sensory deprivation studies.

Neurophysiology of Arousal

The reticular activating system (RAS) is a collection of nuclei located in the brain stem, midbrain, and thalamus. This system generates overall cortical alertness, arousal to sensation, and modulation or screening of the sensory information. The senses send information to the midbrain and thalamic reticular activating system, which also has connections to motor pathways. The system is vulnerable to anesthetics, sleep and pain medication, changes in sleep patterns, and sensory deprivation (Moore, 1980). There is some reason to believe that the RAS is involved in the activation of the central nervous system, which results from controlled sensory stimulation. Farber (1982) postulates that the threshold of activation of reticular neurons may increase because of the sensory deprivation a head injured patient experiences, either from the injury itself or from the medical precautions taken to prevent further damage (see Chapter 5). One aim of controlled and structured sensory stimulation may thus be to lower the activation threshold of these reticular neurons, a reduction that may result in increased cortical activation.

From these sources of evidence, the following conclusion can be drawn: A program of organized and systematically introduced stimulation is important for medically stable but minimally responsive patients.

STIMULATION TREATMENT: GUIDELINES

The guidelines listed in the following paragraphs are based on inferences drawn from animal lesion experiments, principles of neurophysiology and normal development, and our own clinical experience with head injured patients. The program is similar to those in place at leading adult head injury rehabilitation centers (e.g., Cervelli and Berrol, 1982). Since, however, direct research in this area of rehabilitation is scant, the procedural guidelines are offered tentatively and in a spirit of experimentation.

Phylogenetic Sequence

Stimulation treatment begins with the subcortically integrated senses of touch, movement, and olfaction before it progresses to more cortically oriented systems of vision and hearing. The phylogenetically older, subcortically integrated senses of movement, touch, and smell appear to be more plastic, to have a greater number of multisensory connections, and to have greater redundancy and bilateral representation in the central nervous system. In addition, these phylogenetically older systems may not be as damaged by the trauma as are the more cortically located systems

(Moore, 1980). It may thus be valuable in the very early stages of recovery to focus treatment on tactile, vestibular, and olfactory stimulation before progressing to higher cortical levels.

Modulation of Stimulation

The overall purpose of sensory stimulation is to increase the patient's level of arousal and attentiveness to the environment and in turn to improve adaptive responses to environmental events. Because each patient can tolerate only a certain range of stimulation, exceeding or falling short of the range can cause disorganized responses or habituation to stimuli on the part of the patient (Hebb, 1955).

Because patients become habituated to repetitive or continuous stimulation, extended stimulation may have steadily decreasing effects on neurophysiologic activation. Stimulation sessions should thus be relatively brief, and particular forms of stimulation should be changed frequently. Hours of continuous television viewing or radio listening serve no useful purpose.

Stimulation that far exceeds the patient's ability to process—either in being too intensive or in combining several sensory modalities—may be equally counterproductive. Animal lesion studies (Gotsick and Marshall, 1972) suggest that a gradual and systematic increase in stimulation is preferable to immediate, intensive stimulation and handling. The patient's inability to integrate, organize, and filter overly strong or varied stimuli may result in a decrease in alertness. It is thus generally preferable at an early stage of recovery to isolate one sensory modality at a time in treatment. Multisensory stimulation can be introduced gradually as an increasing number of stimulus-specific responses indicate improvement in alertness and processing ability. The rationale for advancing to multisensory stimulation is based in part on the structure and activity of the nervous system. Multisensory (convergent) neurons, which exist throughout the central nervous system, coordinate, filter, and integrate sensory messages, which they must receive from several sensory systems (Guyton, 1982; Jung, Kornhuber, and DaFonseca, 1963) to reach the threshold for activation. Stimulation should thus be multisensory but *focused* in that all aspects of the sensory field (e.g., what is seen, heard, and felt) converge on a single, meaningful experience or activity.

Inhibition-Excitation. Certain types of stimulation tend to be facilitative (e.g., stimulation that varies in rate, direction, intensity, or duration, or is especially meaningful to the patient), whereas others are inhibitory (e.g., stimulation that is slow, gentle, and rhythmic). The facilitative or inihibitory effects of a given stimulus may depend upon the patient's age and sex, the site and extent of damage, and the current status of the emotional or autonomic nervous system. According to Farber (1982), the purpose of the multisensory approach is to promote homeostasis of the autonomic nervous system. If patients are lethargic, hypotonic, and inactive, treatment should avoid stimuli that may further depress or inhibit the central nervous system. Treatment should likewise avoid facilitative stimulation with patients whose central nervous systems may be in a state of excitation or dominated by the sympathetic nervous system. Inhibitory or facilitative stimuli may have detrimental effects on the patient's physiologic status (e.g., heart rate, blood pressure, or respiration). Ayres (1972) and others have cautioned against the potentially harmful effects of using vestibular stimulation without close monitoring, which is especially vital for the patient with central nervous system trauma. Movement stimulation is introduced gradually and conservatively with continual monitoring of the patient before, during, and after stimulation. Generally, any stimulus that is intense in nature, noxious, or painful to the patient should be avoided, even if these stimuli result in increased arousal. Therefore, the therapist should carefully observe the patient's emotional and physiologic status (blood pressure, heart rate, respiration, skin color and temperature, muscle tone, postural reflexes, active movements, vocalization, and facial expression) before, during, and following stimulation to select the most appropriate stimulation activity. Farber (1982) explores these intervention parameters in detail, including indications and contraindications for specific sensory and sensorimotor stimulation activities.

Familiarity

For purposes of orientation as well as arousal, the world into which a head injured patient reawakens should be as familiar as possible. The personal meaningfulness of a stimulus to a patient can contribute to cortical activation (Hebb, 1955). For this reason, we individualize stimulation programs, based on the patient's favorite foods, scents, music, toys, hobbies, books, and television shows. Since patients may be more responsive to stimulation provided by family members, parents are often trained to be active members of the stimulation team. Daily care and hygiene activities offer parents an excellent opportunity to provide structured sensory stimulation (see Chapter 5).

Patient Preparation

Before the therapist begins stimulation, the patient should be positioned appropriately (to inhibit abnormal muscle tone and postural reflexes; see Chapter 6), approached from the best side, greeted warmly but simply, and prepared verbally, and if possible visually, for the stimulation to come. Because of the patient's severely decreased processing abilities, the therapist should move slowly through these preparatory steps. The therapist must avoid frightening the patient with unusual equipment or sudden, unexpected movements. Ideally, stimulation sessions take place in a room that is well lighted and free of distractions, and at times when the patient is known to be most alert.

Treatment Progression

Part of the discussion in this chapter has focused on one aspect of stimulation therapy: the progression from unisensory to multisensory stimulation as patients' responses improve from undifferentiated to stimulus specific. Treatment is also concerned at the same time with moving from stimulating essentially passive patients to involving them in sensorimotor activity (e.g., self-care or play) that requires a pretraumatically familiar, functional motor response. Active participation and self-initiated purposeful activity result in greater cortical activation and integration, and may also improve motivation (Will, 1977).

Studies by Dru, Walker, and Walker (1975) and Ferchmin, Bennett, and Rosenzweig (1975) suggest that sensorimotor activity rather than passive sensory stimulation alone may be necessary to produce the desired stimulation effects. The Zubek study (1963) on the reduction of the effects of sensory deprivation by kinesthetic and proprioceptive activity also supports this claim.

Motorically impaired patients are physically assisted to perform familiar routines. For those who are cognitively capable but physically incapable of performing familiar routines, we explore the use of remote switch controls that assist patients in operating adapted toys, radios, televisions, and other devices.

The rate of progress through these early stages of recovery varies from patient to patient. Therapists should experiment widely with various forms of stimulation with those patients whose alertness and responsiveness appear to have stablized at an early stage. As mentioned in the introduction to this chapter, stimulation treatment may have no effect on patients whose unresponsiveness is a result of widespread bilateral cortical damage.

STIMULATION TREATMENT: INTERDISCIPLINARY TEAM

Because patients in the early stages of recovery may change status frequently or respond quite differently at different times of the day or under different circumstances, assessment is an ongoing process to which all rehabilitation professionals as well as family members contribute. Physicians and nursing staff monitor the patient's medical status and report fluctuations in cognitive levels over the course of the day. Physical and occupational therapists describe the patient's response to different positions and movements as well as the integrity of the patient's vestibular, tactile, olfactory, and visual sensory systems. Speech-language pathologists describe the patient's auditory, oral-motor, and communicative functioning. Family members provide necessary pretraumatic information as well as reports on the child's level of responsiveness with familiar people.

We have found it to be most efficient to assign to members of a stimulation team (speech and occupational therapists) stimulation sessions that are augmented by sessions with nursing staff and family as time allows. Patients receive two to three focused sensory stimulation sessions per day, each lasting from 10 to 30 minutes and each remaining within the patient's range of stimulation tolerance. Each patient is seen by no more than one or two members of the team. Members of the stimulation team are trained in all of the modalities of stimulation and meet regularly to discuss the patient's response to stimulation and to revise the program if necessary. They document the patient's responses to treatment on a form under the following categories: date, time, therapist, specific activity (stimulus), and specific response. They review these forms weekly and revise their plans both by concentrating on those activities that have correlated with increased arousal and adaptive responses and also by experimenting with novel activities.

STIMULATION TREATMENT: ACTIVITY SUGGESTIONS

Table 10–1 contains a sampling of stimulation activities that are categorized by stimulus modality and ranked in an order corresponding roughly to the phylogenetic sequence (from bottom to top). The table is

Table 10-1. Sensory Stimulation Program: Sample Activities

Basic Visual Perceptual Motor (VPM) Activities
1. Functional, self-care tasks: either partial or full participation (e.g., dressing, hygiene)
2. simple novel VPM tasks (e.g., puzzles, sorting, matching, sequencing, high interest simple video games, programs)

↑

Object Use Activities
1. Automatic, overlearned activities (e.g., self-care, either partial or full participation): With physical prompts if necessary, have patient use wash cloth, hair brush, toothbrush, eating utensils, pencil and paper, favorite toy
2. Nonautomatic, simple activities: With physical prompts if necessary, have patient do very simple two or three piece puzzles, simple tracing, copying, connect the dots

Communication Activities
Expressive language: help the patient to
1. indicate basic wants or needs, request food, objects, use toilet
2. indicate yes or no
3. indicate feelings
Explore various modes of communication: picture or object board, natural gestures, facial expression,
Receptive language: Help the patient respond to simple commands (e.g., "close your eyes," "squeeze my hand," "look at the _____," "get the _____,") with or without gestures or prompting

↑   ↑

Visual Stimulation Activities
1. Change in room lighting (e.g., turn lights off or on, bright sunlight)
2. Familiar objects (e.g., photographs, home movies, toys from home)
3. Familiar people (e.g., family, friends)
4. Food
5. Pen light or flashlight in darkened room
6. Brightly colored, contrasting objects or pictures — simple shapes

Auditory Stimulation Activities
1. Voice (e.g., familiar, unfamiliar)
2. Music (e.g., favorite songs, radio station)
3. Environmental sounds (e.g., sounds from patient's home — dog barking, children playing, birds chirping)
4. Contrasting sounds: loud noise (e.g., cymbals, noisemakers), soft noise (fan, soft music)

↑   ↑   ↑

Movement Stimulation
1. Position change (in bed, transfers, mat activities)
2. Range of motion
3. Slow, rhythmic movement (e.g., gentle rocking, even rate)
4. Uneven, arrhythmic movement with directional changes (anterior-posterior, side-side, diagonally)

Tactile Stimulation
1. Deep touch (holding, massage)
2. Light moving touch (e.g., feather, finger tips, slow stroking)
3. Soft or rough textures (e.g., felt, plush towel, burlap)
4. Temperature (e.g., cold, hot, neutral warmth)
5. Brushing hair
6. Environmental objects (e.g., grass, bark, flowers)

Olfactory Stimulation
1. Natural odors (e.g., coffee beans, vanilla, garlic, spices)
2. Familiar odors (e.g., favorite cologne, after shave, favorite food odors)
Gustatory Stimulation
1. Specific tastes (sweet, sour, salty, bitter)
2. Favorite tastes
Oral Stimulation
See Chapter 7.

Table 10-2. Communicating with Head Injured Patients: Early Stages of Recovery

How to talk to the patient:

1. Assume that the patient comprehends something in what you say, even if no more than the reassurance implied by your tone of voice.
2. Gently touch the patient and use his or her first name to gain attention.
3. Speak softly, calmly, and slowly to allow the patient time to process what you are saying. Use natural inflections.
4. Use short, simple, but age-appropriate sentences. Pause between each sentence.
5. Use demonstrations and physical prompts as needed.
6. Talk *to* the patient. Do not converse with the other staff members as though the patient were not present.
7. Do not ask questions unless the patient is capable of responding (in some way) and you are willing to honor the response.
8. Talk primarily about the here and now: objects or activities that the patient can see, hear, smell, taste, touch, or do.
9. Simply state what you are going to do with the patient, what you are doing, and what you have just done. As the processing of words increases, name, describe, and discuss an increasing number of features of the here and now.
10. Give frequent repetition of orienting information:
    a. *People:* "I'm Gloria from Speech Therapy."
    b. *Place:* "You're at The Rehabilitation Institute now. We're on our way to the PT gym."
    c. *The Accident:* "You were in an accident. You're here to get better."
    d. *Deficits:* "You're in a wheelchair because your legs haven't started to work well enough yet."
    e. *Routines:* "Lunch is over. It's time for PT. You always go to PT after lunch."
    f. *Relevant Time Information:* For young children— "Soon your mom will be here; then you eat supper." For older children— "It's spring. Flowers are coming up everywhere. Your birthday is coming soon." Gradually increase complexity and detail.

How to encourage the patient's communication:

1. Give the patient time to respond.
2. Be attentive to natural communicative gestures (reaching, looking, facial expression, tugging at a zipper); respond to the inferred meaning.
3. Include the patient in conversations, directing eye contact to the patient, even though there may be no response.
4. In establishing a yes-no and simple request system, try natural gestures first (e.g., head nod, reaching) before attempting to teach novel communicative gestures that are not natural and are less easy to interpret (e.g., eye blinking, finger raising). The system must be used consistently by staff members. Since yes and no, in the sense of affirming and denying information, are relatively abstract concepts, establishing a reliable yes-no system may require considerable time and patience from staff and family members.
5. Explore simple, alternate means of communication (e.g., looking at objects or photographs to select an activity).
6. For a patient who begins to talk but uses language inappropriately, simply state the facts correctly. Do not argue.

not intended to represent a rigid hierarchy, nor is it intended to be a comprehensive listing of activities. Depending on the nature of the brain damage, a patient could be more appropriately responsive to higher than to lower levels of stimulation or interaction. Organized and individualized stimulation of the most basic, subcortically integrated systems, which appear at the base of the table, may benefit minimally responsive patients most. Activities for more responsive patients may be selected from higher levels on the table or focus more explicitly on multisensory integration.

COMMUNICATION

Although we have stressed the importance of organized sensory stimulation and sensorimotor activity, it should be remembered that communication plays an important role in the patient's recovery. Table 10–2 lists principles governing appropriate communicative interaction with patients at an early stage of recovery. Under the best circumstances, all staff members will learn these principles so that communicative exchanges are frequent, natural, and even fun rather than strained and mechanical. For head injured children, there is perhaps no experience more therapeutic than communication—even if it occurs at a developmentally early level—with another human being, especially a loved one. Communication gives the patient a foothold in social reality and a growing sense of being respected and of being loved.

REFERENCES

Ayres, A. J., (1972). *Sensory integration and learning disorders.* Los Angeles: Western Psychological Services.

Bach-y-Rita, P. (Ed.) (1980a). *Recovery of function: Theoretical considerations for brain injury rehabilitation.* Baltimore: University Park Press.

Bach-y-Rita, P. (1980b). Brain plasticity as a basis for therapeutic procedures. In P. Bach-y-Rita (Ed.), *Recovery of function: Theoretical considerations for brain injury rehabilitation* (pp. 225–260). Baltimore: University Park Press.

Black, P., Markowitz, R., and Cianci, S. N. (1975). Recovery of motor function after lesions in motor cortex of monkey. In R. Porter and D. W. Fitzimons (Eds.), *Outcome of severe damage to the central nervous system* (pp. 65–83). Ciba Foundation Symposium 34 (new series). Amsterdam: Elsevier.

Cervelli, L., and Berrol, S. (1982). Description of a model care system. In *Head injury rehabilitation project: Final report, Section III.* San Jose: Santa Clara Valley Medical Center.

Chow, K. L., and Stewart, D. L. (1972). Reversal of structural and functional effects of long-term visual deprivation in cats. *Experimental Neurology, 34,* 409–433.

Dru, D., Walker, J. P., and Walker, J. B. (1975). Self-produced locomotion restores visual capacity after striate lesions. *Science, 187,* 265–266.

Farber, S. D. (1982). *Neurorehabilitation: A multi-sensory approach.* Philadelphia: W. B. Saunders.

Ferchmin, P. A., Bennett, E. L., and Rosenzweig, M. R. (1975). Direct contact with enriched environment is required to alter cerebral weights in rats. *Journal of Comparative and Physiological Psychology, 88,* 360–367.

Gotsick, J. E., and Marshall, R. C. (1972). Time course of the septal rage syndrome. *Physiological Behavior, 9,* 685–687.

Guyton, A. C. (1982). *Human physiology and mechanisms of disease* (p. 355). Philadelphia: W. B. Saunders.

Hebb, D. O. (1955). Drives and the conceptual nervous system. *Psychological Review, 62,* 243–254.

Jung, R., Kornhuber, H. H.,, and DaFonseca, J. S. (1963). Multisensory convergence on cortical neurons. In G. Moruzzi, A. Fessard, and H. Jasper (Eds.), *Progress in brain research: Vol. 1, Brain mechanisms* (pp. 207–231). Amsterdam: Elsevier.

Lasden, M. (1982, June 27). Coming out of coma. *The New York Times Magazine,* pp. 29–54.

Moore, J. C. (1980). Neuroanatomical considerations relating to recovery of function following brain lesions. In P. Bach-y-Rita (Ed.), *Recovery of function: Theoretical considerations for brain injury rehabilitation* (pp. 9–90). Baltimore: University Park Press.

Plum, F., and Posner, J. B. (1972). *Diagnosis of stupor and coma* (2nd ed). Philadelphia, F. A. Davis.

Rosenzweig, M. R. (1966). Environmental complexity, cerebral change, and behavior. *American Psychologist, 21,* 321–332.

Rosenzweig, M. R., Krech, D., Bennett, E. L., and Diamond, M. C. (1962). Effects of environmental complexity and training on brain chemistry and anatomy: A replication and extension. *Journal of Comparative and Physiological Psychology, 55,* 429–437.

Walsh, R. N., and Cummins, R. A. (1976). Neural responses to therapeutic sensory environments. In R. N. Walsh and W. T. Greenough (Eds.), *Advances in behavioral biology: Vol. 17, Environments as therapy for brain dysfunction* (pp. 171–200). New York: Plenum Press.

Will, B. E. (1977). Methods for promoting functional recovery following brain damage. In S. R. Berenberg (Ed.), *Brain: Fetal and infant* (pp. 330–344). The Hague: Martinus Nijhoff Medical Division.

Will, B. E., Rosenzweig, M. R., and Bennett, E. (1976). Effects of differential environments on recovery from neonatal brain lesions, measured by problem solving scores and brain dimensions. *Physiology and Behavior, 16,* 603–611.

Will, B. E., Rosenzweig, M. R., Bennett, E. L., Herbert, M., and Morimoto, H. (1977). Relatively brief environmental enrichment aids recovery after post weaning brain lesions in rats. *Journal of Comparative and Physiological Psychology, 91*(1), 33–50.

Yu, J. (1976). Functional recovery with and without training following brain damage in experimental animals: A review. *Archives of Physical Medicine and Rehabilitation, 57,* 38–41.

Zubek, J. D. (1963). Counteracting effects of physical exercises performed during prolonged perceptual deprivation. *Science, 142,* 504–506.

Zubek, J. (Ed.). (1969). *Sensory deprivation: Fifteen years of research.* New York: Meredith.

Chapter 11

Cognitive Rehabilitation Therapy: Middle Stages of Recovery

Juliet Haarbauer-Krupa, MA, CCC/Sp, Lorelli Moser, OTR/L, Gloria Smith, OTR/L, Deborah M. Sullivan, MEd, and Shirley F. Szekeres, MA, CCC/Sp*

The predominant characteristic of patients at the middle stage of recovery is confusion, which results from a general disruption and depressed functioning of the cognitive system. Patients at this level process information inefficiently and have shallow recent memory and poor access to their knowledge. Even small increases in the rate, amount, duration, or complexity of stimuli may result in a functional breakdown of their performance. Although these patients are disoriented to person, place, and time, they are alert and generally responsive to their environment and with cuing can demonstrate some goal-directed behaviors. Most can function in structured task-related group or individual treatment. Patients' response systems range from "yes-no" signaling to intelligible speech and from severely limited motor acts, such as pointing, to near normal ambulation. Table 8-1 in Chapter 8 provides a more complete list of typical cognitive deficits at this stage of recovery.

Pretraumatic social, emotional, developmental, intellectual, and cultural characteristics emerge gradually throughout the middle stage, and they have a significant influence on patients' responses to tasks, to the trauma, and to intervention itself. In this chapter, our general approach to the treatment of patients at the middle stage of recovery is outlined, including goals, optimal environmental structure, communicative interaction, and intervention guidelines and procedures.

*Authorship listed alphabetically at the authors' request.

The general goals of cognitive rehabilitation at this stage of recovery are the following: (1) to reduce the patient's confusion, (2) to increase adaptive behaviors and organized environmental interaction, and (3) to reestablish basic organized thinking and structures of knowledge. We believe that a structured therapeutic environment or milieu is essential to achieving these goals.

MILIEU THERAPY

The concept of milieu therapy is well known to professionals in mental health rehabilitation (Mosey, 1976) and to those in rehabilitation of head injured adults (Hagen, 1983). It is especially important to head injured children who before their accident had fewer overlearned coping skills and who thus require more environmental structure and support than the adult patients. An appropriately structured milieu provides a nurturing, organizing, and generally helpful world for head injured patients.

Factors in the Milieu

All factors of a patient's environment are considered part of the milieu, although some cannot be altered easily. A milieu comprises the following:

The Rehabilitation Living Area. The room itself and the staff and family and their interactions with the patient.

Therapy Settings. Settings that vary from one-to-one closed-door treatment to working in a gymnasium or classroom setting, a range that arises from the multidisciplinary nature of treatment; this also includes patient-therapist interaction.

Ancillary Areas. Areas not directly associated with the patient's immediate living area, such as the evening workshop, swimming pool, or cafeteria, and also the interaction of the patient and staff in these areas.

Home Setting. Including the patient's interaction with extended family and friends at home.

A milieu, then, provides head injured children with stimulation, which can either confuse them further or contribute to cognitive recovery. Therapists alter and simplify the therapeutic environment to help the child "make sense" of the new surrounding world and to promote more flexible, organized, and productive responses than would occur without external controls (Farber, 1982).

General Principles of Milieu Treatment

1. Analysis of the complexity, rate, and duration of stimuli is important for organizing the patient's external environment and for analyzing the appropriateness of the activities in which the child is expected to participate.

2. Coordinated family and staff approaches can compensate for confused children's inability to organize information or to monitor their own responses. In other words, staff and family members should attempt in similar ways to simplify the child's environment and to respond consistently to the child's behavior under all circumstances. For example, if a child walks aimlessly during therapy or on the unit, staff and family members can agree on a specific technique to redirect the patient to the desired place and to engage the patient's attention with another activity. This strategy of redirecting behavior allows therapists to bring patients back to task without creating situations of possible confrontation. In using redirection, care must be taken not to reinforce undesirable behavior (see Chapter 13).

3. Predictability and familiarity within the physical setting promotes the development of the patient's orientation. Although some aspects of this setting such as the overall size and structure of an institution and the medical equipment needed in a brain-trauma unit cannot be changed, it is possible to reduce the patient's difficulties in orientation. For example, someone can consistently accompany the patient to the cafeteria on the same elevator at the end of the same hallway for every meal.

Photos, posters, and other items from patients' homes can make their surroundings more familiar, but decoration should be kept simple because the patients' familiarity with each will lose its effect in a complex arrangement. The child's name should be at the head or foot of the bed or even on the door, depending on the child's need. Words or simple symbolic drawings can be used to label clothing storage areas. To avoid unnecessary stress and confusion, therapists should ensure that logbooks (discussed later), toys, and personal items such as radios and tape recorders are always in the same location. There should also be a large clock, a calendar, individual schedules, and a window with open drapes in the group living space, all of which encourage orientation. Treatment areas should be labeled, and the child should receive therapy in the same room and at the same time each day.

4. Routines and repetition help to structure the sequence of events and thus encourage orientation. Meals, for instance, are important and thus become points of reference. Since patients might not be as well oriented to the times of their physical therapy sessions as they are to meals, therapists

can develop this orientation by scheduling physical therapy just before lunch every day.

An accurate journal or logbook in which staff, family members, or the patient records events of the day aids the patient's orientation throughout the recovery process. This book accompanies the patient throughout the day. Therapists, nursing staff, and family members review the book with the patient several times daily, a procedure that develops the patient's orientation, memory, and organizational skills. A copy of the patient's schedule as well as a snapshot index of significant staff members attached to the logbook also help to orient him or her to the time and place of daily activities and to staff members. If the patient is confused about personal information (e.g., birthdate, age, relatives), this can frequently be reviewed as well. Several variables are considered when implementing the logbook:

- *purpose* (e.g., promote improvement in the patient's orientation and memory; facilitate communication among staff members and between staff and family members)
- *contents* (e.g., highlights of therapy or home visits; special or routine events)
- *format of recording* (e.g., pictures, printing versus cursive writing)
- *schedule of review* (e.g., hourly, twice a day, only in the evening)
- *style of review* (e.g., details or just highlights; statements or questions)

5. Communication, which is one of the most important aspects of a patient's milieu, should be simple and appropriate to the patient's current circumstances. Specific guidelines include the following:

- Make sure you have the patient's attention.
- Reduce the rate, amount, and complexity of language.
- Keep the language of instructions consistent; give them one at a time and repeat if necessary.
- Initially, use statements rather than questions when communicating with the patient.
- Explain upcoming activities and procedures by using demonstrations, physical prompts, verbal instructions, or gestures to ensure comprehension. Do not assume the patient will remember events from one time to the next.
- Allow time for processing (e.g., pause between long phrases and clauses).
- Provide consistent and necessary information for the patient to feel oriented to the present situation (i.e., to person, time, place, condition, and reason for current placement). Asking the patient questions may increase confusion and decrease the patient's sense

of self-worth; therefore, it is better to give patients information that will be orienting for them rather than quiz them.

6. Monitoring and changing the milieu through controlled gradation of environmental distractions, stress, and choices to meet the changing abilities of the child can facilitate recovery. When we see spontaneous improvements — such as patients remaining calmer for longer periods or recalling more of a logbook entry or daily routine — these improvements are interpreted as a signal to gradually increase the demands on the patient's processing mechanism; this is done in the environment as well as in therapeutic activities. For example, patients may initially take their meals in the private space of the nursing unit, later in the group room, and still later in the cafeteria as their attention and concentration improve.

7. Coordination among and integration of the various parts of the rehabilitation program enhance the effectiveness of intervention. Although time constraints sometimes limit the communication among the members of a treatment team, ample training of staff members and a common knowledge base compensate to some extent for this problem. Staff members who are all well versed in general information about brain trauma recovery, the behaviors typically seen following a severe brain injury, and the same redirection techniques communicate with each other more effectively than untrained or on-call staff. Frequent contact— whether in a scheduled meeting or through treatment on the nursing unit— will facilitate coordination of services and communication among team members.

The Agitated Patient

Consistency, predictability, and structure are especially important for those patients whose confusion manifests itself in the form of agitation (Malkmus, Booth, and Doyle, 1983). One treatment strategy is to decrease agitation and maladaptive behaviors by engaging patients in enjoyable and energy-consuming activities before introducing goal-directed cognitive tasks. There may be signs before children begin therapy that safe, energy-consuming activities would be productive. For example, the child may at first pace rapidly about a treatment room but then calm down significantly after a long walk or a period of active, directed play with a basketball. After about 15 minutes of active movement, the child may be more able to perform the targeted therapy task. We also attempt to reduce agitation by improving the patient's physical comfort in cooperation with the nursing staff.

The previous guidelines for establishing milieu therapy apply to agitated patients as well as to other head injured patients at the middle stages of recovery. Therapists should also know specific calming or redirecting techniques that do not create situations of confrontation with patients and should be aware of safety precautions. Agitation, which is only a phase of recovery, may last from a few days to a few weeks and may reappear if environmental stresses increase too rapidly or if the demands on patients are beyond their emerging coping skills. However, some patients remain agitated for extended periods of time, depending upon the site of the lesion and the extent of the damage.

THERAPEUTIC INTERVENTION

At the middle stages of recovery a significant amount of effort is directed toward retraining cognitive components and task skills within the established milieu. Even commonly overlearned functional-integrative tasks, such as tying shoes, reading a short note, or playing a simple game, may be too complex and provoke anxiety when patients confront their inability to perform. Although we concentrate primarily on environmental compensation and component retraining at this stage (see Chapter 8 for a description of these forms of intervention), we continually work toward integrating components into meaningful activities and toward laying the groundwork for learning compensatory strategies at the late stage of recovery. In all intervention it is also essential to assure patients successful experiences. The probability of success in therapy is increased by carefully structuring both communicative interaction and therapy tasks.

Communicative Interaction

General Guidelines

The therapist must compensate for the patient's decreased ability to process information by using language that is appropriate to that particular patient's level of recovery. Therapy is a part of the overall milieu and the previously discussed principles of communication apply here also. For example, therapists should automatically repeat questions and statements when the patient has not understood them. The patient may indicate this verbally ("What did you say?") or nonverbally (the patient tries to get up and leave the area). The therapy environment should be as free as possible of visual and auditory clutter; therapy should thus occur in a quiet room with only necessary materials. The therapist's demeanor must convey the appropriate attitude for the session. A work attitude can be conveyed by focusing on the task and by consistently redirecting the patient until the task is completed. A play attitude can be conveyed by telling jokes and engaging in social conversation with the patient during work time. Our decisions to adopt a given demeanor are based, in part, on such pretrauma personality characteristics as the patient's response to discipline, mode of self-expression (shy or outgoing), and performance ability in play or school tasks. It is the therapist's responsibility to encourage the patient (e.g., "You can do it") throughout the session and to arrange for successful experiences.

Specific Communication Problems

Patients in the middle stage of recovery have difficulty expressing themselves and typically require additional time to respond, especially when they are confronted. Patients may experience problems in controlling verbal output and may need redirection. The following paragraphs describe typical communication problems at this stage and suggested treatment techniques.

Initiation or Inhibition. Patients with initiation and inhibition problems have difficulty beginning or terminating behavior, including communicative interactions. Sentence completion cues are often helpful for patients with initiation problems: "We're going to brush your teeth. You need toothpaste and _____." The patient can also be given a model of the language appropriate to a given context:

Therapist: "Here comes your sister, John. Tell her hello."

John: "Hello."

Therapist: "John, let's tell your sister about your day. First you got up and ate.."

John: "Breakfast."

Patients with inhibition problems are unable to restrain their emotions, actions, or thoughts. The therapist must redirect patients to the topic or task rather than focus on their off-task behaviors: "Jennifer, here is your sandwich. You should be eating now."

Confabulation. When patients recite "information" that apparently is unrelated to reality or seems false, the therapist can either respectfully redirect the patient or make inferences about the intended meaning and give the patient the relevant information. The logbook can be one source of this information:

Patient: "I went to physical therapy today and he said my left leg is missing and I can't walk."

Staff Member (based on facts from logbook): "You worked on your walking in physical therapy today. Your left leg feels numb and it's hard to put your weight on it."

Expressive Disorganization. The patient has trouble remaining on a topic of conversation and gives information in bits and pieces rather than in coherent form. The therapist should give the patient models of organized descriptions.

Patient: "Today I did everything. I went with her to the room and watched it for a while. Then I'm going home tomorrow and we're having that thing in a box."

Staff Member: "You went to occupational therapy today with Susan in the small gym. Tomorrow you will be going home. Maybe your family will have pizza since you like it so well."

Word Finding Problems. When patients are experiencing difficulty thinking of words to fit their ideas, one or more of the following cues may be helpful:

- *Sentence completion:* "You need toothpaste and a _____." "You write with a _____."
- *Association cues:* "Think of what it goes with"; "bread and _____."
- *Description of use or characteristics:* "Tell me what it looks like or what it does."
- *Gestural cues:* "Show me what you mean with your hands."
- *Graphic cues:* "Draw a picture to show me what you mean."
- *First sound cues:* "S _____."

Inappropriateness. Patients often have a reduced ability to monitor their behavior and may express thoughts that were previously restrained. Swearing is particularly common. The therapist should not respond strongly to or laugh at irrelevant or inappropriate remarks that the patient makes but should rather redirect the patient. Example:

Staff Member: "What's the weather like today?"

Patient: "It's raining meatballs."

Staff Member: "It's cloudy and it's starting to rain."

As the patient improves, more assistance is needed in examining others' reactions to their inappropriate comments:

Patient: "I hate working with you and these things are dumb!"

Staff Member: "It's hard for you to work on tasks that used to be easy. You should tell me that what we're doing is too easy and you want more difficult work."

Or at a later stage:

Jim (patient): "Can you hurry up and answer my question? I'm tired of waiting."

Joe (patient): "I just can't think of the words I want to say."

Staff Member: "Jim, Joe is having some trouble finding his words. It's hard to wait for him, but you hurt his feelings by saying that you're tired of waiting for him. Let's help him think of the words instead."

Poor Ability to Convey Affective States. Patients may convey emotional states in an extreme manner (e.g., crying or sobbing about home) or in a robot-like way (e.g., telling about their accidents with a straight or slightly smiling face). When working with the patient, the therapist should model natural expressions of emotion, such as smiles when patients are talking about home, and subdued tones when patients are talking about their accidents.

Initiation of Individual and Group Cognitive Rehabilitation Therapy

There are special factors to consider when initiating therapy with the child in the middle stages of recovery who has been through a frightening experience and is becoming aware of a totally new environment, perhaps even without a familiar adult present. The therapist should place as few demands as possible on the patient during the first session; reading to the child and talking about family pictures from home are appropriate activities. Therapists should work with patients near their "home base" in the nursing living unit and gradually introduce them to the therapy room. Therapists should likewise use patients' names and, in appropriate language, tell them where they are and why they are there. Younger children may be especially comforted by physical handling but if patients are fearful of such handling, they should remain in their wheelchairs for the therapy sessions. In general, therapists should set success as their highest priority for the first session and select activities accordingly.

One critical factor of successful therapy is that patients must be interested and willing to participate in their programs. It is the therapist's responsibility to maintain the child's interest by choosing appropriate activities and materials and by frequently explaining the purpose of the therapy in terms of a goal that is meaningful to the child. The therapist should keep both the patient and the family informed of the patient's progress so that families can reinforce their child's sense of success and can encourage him or her to remain in therapy. At this stage, basic activities focus on increasing the patient's attention and concentration. Individual treatment in a room without distractions may be necessary.

The patient can begin in group cognitive rehabilitation therapy when certain criteria are met in individual therapy:

1. The patient can control bizarre and interruptive behavior or those behaviors can be environmentally controlled, if only for short periods (e.g., a 10 to 15 minute period in which the patient can complete a task).

2. The patient has at least a marginally functional communication system.

3. The patient is able to complete a very simple task.

Introducing the child to group therapy is a trial process in which the therapist uses tasks that the patient performed well in individual therapy. Participation in group therapy that focuses on structured activities helps the patient to relearn old skills and begin to learn new skills. Initially therapists give much individual attention to the patient and subsequently reduce the amount of attention gradually. For example, as their group behavior improves, patients may be expected to wait longer for a turn to speak with the therapist or others in their group. Our clinical experience has shown that preschoolers may be more comfortable in group therapy than in individual therapy because they are motivated by other children and because the group reduces the pressure to perform that direct confrontation produces. Pre-school age children can participate in a group activity rather than respond directly to the therapist's request. Older children, however, may be more distracted by the presence of others.

Specific Goals in Treatment

At the middle level of recovery, there are broad possibilities of treatment because confusion and maladaptive responses are the result of general disruption of cognitive functions (see Table 8-1). Therapists must be concerned with patients' access to knowledge so that they can better receive and interpret incoming information; with patients' current functional state or performance; with their ability to perform simple tasks; and with their familiarity with the staff.

As pointed out in Chapter 8, cognitive functioning in even the simplest of functional-integrative activities involves complex interactions of cognitive processes and systems. For example, orientation is a complex concept involving attentional, perceptual, and memory processes. Therapists can, however, focus the patient's attention on functional orientation by means of task designs, feedback, and reinforcement—a focus that may incidentally foster growth of involved cognitive processes and structures. Establishing treatment groups and labeling them according to a specific cognitive focus (e.g., "thought organization group") helps also to develop the patient's metacognitive awareness. Treatment goals at the middle stage emphasize improvement in the following areas of cognition. In all of these goal areas, therapists may work toward improvement of the patient's level, efficiency, scope, or manner of performance (see Chapter 8).

Orientation

- Orientation to time, place, personal data, significant others, condition, purpose

Attention and Concentration

- Attention to physical environment, people, task
- Selective attention and attention span

Memory and Learning

- Encoding, storage, retrieval of information; semantic and espisodic; visual and auditory; short-term and long-term
- Acquisition of new information
- Relating new information to old information and formulating new concepts

Perceptual-Motor Abilities

- Accurate perception of auditory, visual, and tactile stimuli
- Perceptual-motor integration

Organizing Processes

- Input organization (imposing organization on incoming information) and output organization (organization of information for verbal and nonverbal responses)
- Organizing processes: analysis, synthesis, categorization, association, integration of information, identification of relevant features of objects and events, comparison of objects, events, and people for similarities and differences

Concrete Reasoning and Problem Solving

- Recognition of concrete event relations (e.g., cause and effect)
- Making inferences and drawing conclusions

- Flexible exploration of possible explanations for common events and possible solutions to problems as they occur
- Identification of materials and procedures needed to complete a familiar task

Social Cognition

- Parallel work and play (i.e., solitary work or play in the presence of others)
- Cooperative work and play (e.g., sharing, turn-taking, accepting supervision)
- Appropriate social interaction

Judgment

- Prediction of consequences
- Safe use of material and equipment
- Decreased impulsivity

Therapeutic Approaches

In this section, two widely applicable approaches that we use extensively at the middle stage of recovery are discussed: structured activities and verbal thought organization.

Structured Activities

Engaging patients in highly structured concrete activities has been found especially useful in treatment at the middle stage of recovery. Because patients at this stage lack organizational skills, they function more effectively if the components of an activity have been analyzed and arranged for them so that they may successfully participate in and complete the activity. The treatment principles and techniques described here apply to both individual and group sessions.

Activities are designed according to the level of the patient's cognitive and perceptual skills. Activities for patients who are just entering the middle stage should be commensurate with their current cognitive abilities and should not stress or overtly challenge them.

The therapist should be aware of the child's visual, auditory, and sensory-perceptual strengths and weaknesses. Concentrating on perceptual strengths in an activity can improve the child's performance in a number of cognitive areas. If the treatment team has noted, for instance, that the child processes visual instructions more readily than auditory instructions, team members should use written instructions or gestures when they interact with the patient.

As the patient progresses through the middle stages of recovery, therapists systematically add cognitive, perceptual, and psychosocial demands within the tasks (see Table 11-1). Since each additional demand increases the stress that the patient experiences and consequently interferes with information processing and organized response, these increments must be carefully introduced to guarantee that the patient maintains successful performance.

Activities that are appropriate for treatment include visual-perceptual motor activities (sorting, matching, doing puzzles), easy video games (such as Atari bowling), crafts, meal preparation, board or card games, community outings, and self-care tasks. These activities can be graded along a continuum, moving from simple, concrete activities to more complex, abstract tasks. Table 11-1 illustrates this continuum. The level of difficulty outlined in the column on the left is appropriate for patients who are just entering the middle stage of recovery, whereas the level of difficulty outlined in the column on the right may be appropriate for patients who are in transition to the late stage. All variables are influenced by gradations of rate, complexity, and amount of information that a task requires.

The therapist structures an activity first by assessing the patient's cognitive level and then by actively choosing and structuring activities that are therapeutically useful. Structured activities are designed for remediation of the cognitive, perceptual, and psychosocial deficits that result from head injury. Although therapists should also consider the effect of a given activity on motor ability, they should be aware that physical rehabilitation is not the primary focus of these structured activities.

Important factors in selecting an activity for the therapy session include the age and developmental level of the child. Since a preschool child has had far more experience playing than sitting at a desk, tasks for children at this age should be as much like play as possible. A school-age child can work with pictures and pencil-paper tasks at a desk, sort category cards, or even use simple computer programs. Tasks should also have closure that is obvious to the child: therapists can develop a patient's ability to attend and concentrate by selecting tasks that have an observable beginning, middle, and end. A play task with an obvious end, such as

Table 11-1. Variables for Grading Structured Activities: Middle Stages of Recovery

Variable	Gradation		
Cognitive Variables			
Attention span and endurance	Activity completed within one short treatment session	Activity completed within one extended session or several short sessions	Activity requires many sessions to complete
Familiarity of the activity	Familiar enjoyable activity	Semi-familiar activity	Unfamiliar activity requiring new learning
Sequential organization	Activity involves no sequential organization	Activity involves sequentially organizing steps with external cues	Activity involves sequentially organizing steps independently
Organizing and planning	Activity involves simple replication of a model	Activity involves some organizing and planning with external cues	Activity involves independent organizing and planning
Language comprehension	Activity involves simple instructions with picture cues	Activity involves simple instructions with no picture cues	Activity involves complex or multistep instructions
Memory (storage)	Activity does not require storage and retrieval of information	Activity requires storage and retrieval; cues and memory aids provided by staff members	Activity requires storage and retrieval; patient encouraged to initiate use of memory aids or ask questions
Response to time stress	Activity has no time requirements	Therapist encourages patient to work faster	Activity has specified time limit
Cognitive flexibility	Activity is repetitive and routine	Activity involves some novel materials or procedures	Activity involves frequent changes in materials, procedures, personnel, or location
Initiation	Activity does not require patient to initiate action or conversation	Activity requires patient to initiate action or conversation with cues	Activity requires patient to initiate action or conversation independently

Table 11-1 (continued).

Variable	Gradation		
Self-evaluation	Activity does not require patient to evaluate product (outcome of activity)	Activity requires patient to evaluate product with cues	Activity requires patient to evaluate product independently
Decision making and problem solving	Activity does not require decision making or problem solving	Activity requires patient to choose among several presented options	Activity requires patient to generate possible solutions to problems as they arise in the activity
Safety judgment	Activity does not require the use of potentially harmful tools or equipment	Activity requires supervised use of tools and equipment	Activity requires independent use of relatively safe tools and equipment
Perceptual Variables			
Sensory-integrative requirements	Activity focuses primarily on one sensory modality		Activity focuses on integrated multisensory processing
Environmental distractions	Activity occurs in a nondistracting environment; may require one-to-one treatment	Small group treatment; visual and auditory distractions are gradually introduced	Group treatment with naturally occurring visual and auditory distractions
Visual complexity	Activity involves sorting, matching, or tracing using perceptually simple materials	Activity involves materials of increasing visual complexity	Activity involves visually complex materials with a visually distracting background
Psychosocial Variables			
Success	Therapist manipulates activity to guarantee patient success		Activity includes the possibility of some failure
Interpersonal relations	One-to-one treatment requiring little interaction	Small group treatment; evolution from separate, independent activity to interactive activity	Group treatment requiring cooperation among patients with guidance of therapist

building a miniature road or feeding a baby doll, is useful for preschool children. Tasks for school-age children can be defined by the number of items in the task or by a finished product. For instance, the therapist can ask the patient to sort ten cards into two different categories, to write numbers from one to ten, or to do ten sentence-completion items on the computer. Available toys and games (e.g., Simon, Memory, Finders Keepers, simple video games, and other high-interest computer software) can also be used. The various cognitive, perceptual, and psychosocial factors, and physical considerations in the cognitive treatment of head injured patients are summarized in the next paragraphs.

Cognitive and Task Variables. Therapists must consider cognitive variables when they are grading an activity for a patient. One important factor is to limit the focus of an activity to the development of one or two behaviors or skills. For example, it is possible to improve a patient's attention span by using a timer to increase the time spent in an activity without expecting an increase in the patient's level of performance. The gradation of cognitive variables is illustrated in Table 11-1.

Perceptual Variables. Therapists must be aware of the processing requirements of an activity, whether they be auditory-perceptual, auditory-verbal, visual-perceptual, or visual-motor. Head trauma can produce generalized perceptual deficits, such as hypo- or hyperresponsiveness (e.g., tactile or auditory defensiveness) to certain stimuli. More specific types of perceptual deficits, such as diplopia, hemianopsia, and visual neglect, are frequently observed. Therapists should also be aware of the effect of confusion and of deficits of attention and concentration on the patient's ability to process or filter sensations selectively. These patients may be diagnosed incorrectly as having specific visual-perceptual or auditory-language deficits when their overall confusion and inability to attend may be the major interfering factor. We often observe that sensorimotor functioning improves when patients are engaged in a structured activity that is simple and highly motivating in an environment that is not confusing or stressful. Specific variables of perceptual performance and ways of grading these variables are listed in Table 11-1.

Psychosocial Variables. As patients progress through the middle stage of recovery, the focus on improving cognitive and perceptual functioning may need to be widened to include psychosocial concerns. Patients at this stage may frequently experience failure when they are engaged in activities that were once basic and routine. The gradual realization that his or her life has changed drastically may seriously affect a patient's sense of self-worth and motivation. Moreover, head injured patients may be focused inward emotionally and socially, and their performance in a group setting may suffer. They may be unaware of how to interact socially and of how their behavior affects others around them (see also Chapter 14).

Cognitive rehabilitation therapists can address these psychosocial variables by choosing activities that are appropriate to patients' age, level of development, interests, and cultural and community background and by helping patients interact more appropriately in groups. In general, we believe in the importance of incorporating activities that are familiar and motivating to the patient, a point already emphasized. Table 11-1 also lists psychosocial variables that should be considered in therapy.

Physical Considerations. Therapists must also consider a patient's physical limitations if completing a task requires a motor response. Factors such as the patient's strength and endurance can affect his or her performance in both cognitive and perceptual tasks. Therapists should also observe the effect of the activity on the patient's autonomic nervous system. For example, the patient may become drowsy and lethargic during sedentary activities or overstimulated during active, movement-oriented tasks. Finally, physically handicapped patients may require special adaptations of tasks to participate successfully. Our clinical experience has shown that unless therapists take these factors into account, the therapeutic value of structured activities decreases.

Verbal Thought Organization

In the preceding section, principles and techniques for improving cognitive functioning in middle-stage patients using games, puzzles, craft projects, and other structured activities that involve manipulation of objects and completion of functional activities were described. At this stage of recovery, *language activities* are also used as a medium for improving the efficiency, level, scope, and manner (see Chapter 8) of cognitive performance. Activities are designed to improve verbal thought organization, including selective listening and comprehension; retrieval of semantic information and experiences from long-term memory; organizing processes for thinking and verbal expression; reasoning and problem solving; and self-awareness. Table 11-2 lists sample activities for improving verbal organization.

One verbal organizational procedure that is easily adaptable to varied levels of cognition is the feature analysis guide shown in Figure 11-1. This guide is presented as one sample of an organizational structure that helps patients to reestablish access to knowledge; to maintain an organized or direct search of information in storage; to focus and shift attention; to classify and organize effectively; and to develop metacognitive awareness. The demands of specific tasks, feedback, and reinforcement may, of course, bring any one of these objectives into focus.

Table 11–2. Sample Activities for Verbal Organization

Goal: To improve selective attention and comprehension
- matching pictures to sentences or paragraphs
- listening for specific information (e.g., who, what, where, when, or why)
- following spoken directions
- passing messages from one patient to another
- listening to stories (from simple, one episode events to more complex plots with a series of episodes and conclusions)
- listening to other children's reports of events and answering questions

Goal: To improve retrieval of semantic knowledge and past experiences
- naming all items of a familiar category (e.g., animals)
- telling about a familiar place or thing (e.g., zoo, school, dog), using pictures of the child's experiences as prompts
- role playing or telling scripts for common tasks or events (e.g., how to make a sandwich or brush teeth)
- setting up a familiar play theme (e.g., doll house, doctor's office) and telling about it

Goal: To improve organizing processes for thinking and verbal expression
- grouping words and pictures according to a principle or theme (e.g., superordinate category, function, temporal sequence)
- explaining why words or pictures in a set go together
- telling which picture or object in a group does not belong and why
- giving directions to others
- generating descriptions and narratives about events or pictures; retelling stories
- explaining events while role playing, playing with dolls, having a tea party, etc.

Goal: To improve reasoning and problem solving
- explaining "why _____ happened"
- solving a spontaneous or preplanned problem by participating in a *group* effort (identifying and stating the problem and goal, generating possible solutions, evaluating each alternative, deciding upon the best solution)
- predicting outcomes
- making simple inferences about concrete situations
- explaining how to set up a play theme, such as "post office" and "store," when shown the props; then carrying out these plans

Goal: To improve self-awareness
- participating in exercises in which the therapist models self-questions about feelings and ways of thinking
- answering questions about feelings and ways of thinking
- observing one another for a specific behavior (e.g., interrupting)
- making observations about one's own task performance based on an observable product of the task (e.g., number correct, number of points earned, a completed puzzle)

Initially, it is important to use a structured procedure consistently. The consistent use of such a format facilitates the patient's recognition of *procedures* of thinking and permits cooperative efforts of patients in groups. Therapists should carefully direct patients in using the feature analysis guide until they can complete an analysis with minimal cuing. The therapist can then provide opportunities for elaboration (e.g., "Who

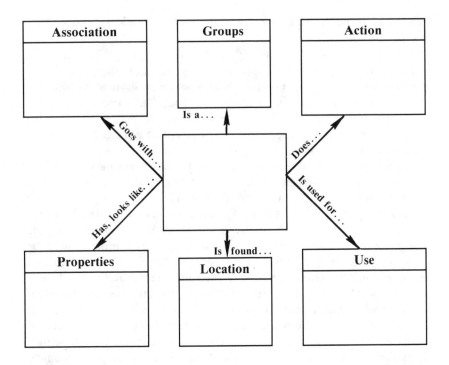

Figure 11-1. Feature analysis guide.

would use a _____?'' or ''When would you use a _____?'').

The medium of presentation of the feature analysis depends on the patient's cognitive level and age. The medium can range from a concrete level, at which patients use real objects or pictures and therapists demonstrate each feature as clearly as possible, to a more abstract level, at which patients independently analyze all features verbally. Therapists may isolate and demonstrate any feature concretely. For instance, the concept ''group'' can be demonstrated by sorting particular instances of a category (e.g., three animals, three pieces of furniture, three articles of clothing) into boxes representing their more general category (animals, furniture, clothing). Therapists can also use more natural activities to achieve the same objective (e.g., ''Let's clean up. First put the animals in their box, then the. . .''). Further, they may isolate the ''action'' feature by setting up a stage and making a toy dog jump on the stage while telling or asking the patient what the dog is doing. The boxes and the stage may be kept as prompts for the ''group'' and ''action'' features and gradually eliminated as the child learns to talk about these semantic features without props.

Therapists can also simplify the activity by exploring only one semantic feature over the course of several sessions. For example, the same props can be used consistently for a number of sessions to develop the patient's understanding of the concept of "group." The therapist can also gradually shift the emphasis of the session from the patient's knowledge of a concept, such as "dog," to a development of a *way* of thinking or retrieving information.

An important goal of this training is to develop the patient's ability to understand a concept in terms of its perceptual, semantic, and experiential features. When patients develop this ability, they are far more likely to recognize when they lack knowledge of a concept and how they can generate questions to obtain that information. When patients elaborate this procedure into a personal way of thinking, they can better describe concepts when they cannot retrieve the specific labels. Classification, organization, and reasoning require the fundamental ability to identify varied aspects of concepts systematically. If, for instance, an individual does not know one property of a shark (sharp teeth) and a characteristic action (eating flesh), he or she may swim near sharks in the ocean, not because of poor reasoning or judgment but because of missing knowledge. Organized information is an essential component of reasoning, problem solving, and judgment.

TRAINING FAMILIES AND CAREGIVERS

Families need information about cognitive recovery from head injury and about cognitive rehabilitation therapy. Therapists should spend time with the family explaining the sequence of cognitive recovery and treatment goals. For example, therapists may tell family members that the patient is at the middle stage of recovery and that he or she may be confused, disoriented, and generally disorganized, may cry for no apparent reason, and may have difficulty expressing ideas. Therapists should also give families written information concerning recovery and principles and goals of treatment. They should describe the child in terms that are familiar to the family and also clarify the terms that appear in the written information. Therapists should keep the family informed about the patient's progress, particularly about the behavioral changes that occur as a child proceeds through a particular phase of recovery. This practice is especially important for families who take their children home for weekends during the middle stages of recovery.

Part of the process of informing families about cognitive recovery is training them to recognize signs of stress due to cognitive disorganization in their children. Therapists can instruct family members on how to make the patient's environment less stressful as well as how to redirect the child when stress cannot be avoided.

The inability of many middle-stage patients to make judgments about personal safety is a combined result of a diminished ability to process information, inadequate knowledge, and weak awareness of deficits. Therapists should instruct family members on how to direct the patient. When therapists notice that patients have difficulty processing verbal directions, they can advise family members to use gestures or physical prompts. For instance, if a child climbs monkey bars and does not respond to verbal instructions, family members should gesture or use gentle physical prompts to get the patient down.

When possible, therapists should encourage parents to participate in or to observe cognitive therapy sessions so that the therapist can demonstrate techniques of interaction and redirection and suggest ways of structuring situations at home (discussed later in this chapter). The training process can be more thorough if one therapist conducts the session while another explains procedures as they occur. It is also helpful for therapists to observe the interactions of family members with the patient outside of therapy sessions so that more specific recommendations can be made based on the manner in which the family interacts with the child. For example, if therapists observe that two to three family members try to talk to the patient at the same time, causing further confusion, they should suggest that each member take turns talking with the patient.

Families often ask for specific prescriptions to keep their children occupied on weekends. Suggested activities include the following.

Television Watching. To be able to pay attention and understand, a child may need to watch television in a context free of distractions such as extraneous talking. For the sake of limiting the possibility of cognitive overload and of habituation, family members should permit the child to watch familiar television programs but only for a short period of time. In addition, family members may summarize and help interpret the content of the program for the child at every commercial and should do so in a conversational manner rather than by questioning.

Play Activities. Board or card games are suggested for older children because they provide the patient with visible structure and closure. Family members may need to redirect the patient to a game if attention wanders or change the task after 15 minutes. Parents are advised to help younger children select play activities that require very few organizational abilities, such as building a road for one toy car, feeding and bathing a doll, playing ball, and having a "tea party." We encourage families to redirect the child as much as possible, particularly to a play task, so that the child learns to concentrate on and complete tasks.

TREATING PATIENTS WHOSE CONDITIONS STABILIZE AT THE MIDDLE STAGE OF RECOVERY

Despite prolonged and intensive treatment, some patients with severe head injuries do not recover from the agitated or confused state characteristic of the middle stage. The team may decide to discharge those patients, who are many months post injury, no longer recovering spontaneously, and not responding to intensive treatment.

Once discharge is planned, the specific goals of treatment for these patients will change. Although the team continues to work on improving the patient's ability to function in real-life situations, they change the techniques, format, and goals of training to enable the patient to live as successfully, productively, and enjoyably as possible in his or her future environment. The setting in which the patient will be living determines to a large extent the target skills the team selects.

Living at home with family, attending a residential or day school, and undergoing treatment in another rehabilitation facility all demand different skills and behaviors from the patient. However, because confused patients may not be aware of their own inappropriate behaviors and responses or of possible appropriate reactions and interactions, or because they may have difficulty in inhibiting their behaviors, therapists can direct training according to a generalized scheme of developing (1) the patient's awareness of a specific situation requiring specific behaviors; (2) their recognition of appropriate behaviors; and (3) their initiation of those behaviors, including performance of specific activities. For example, if adolescent patients have a significant amount of unstructured time, therapists may decide to teach them to recognize their own boredom and ways of alleviating that boredom (e.g., by asking someone to play a game), as well as to use alternatives (e.g., being able to choose and play each of three different games). This procedure is then practiced with patients until they can initiate and complete an activity with the help of external prompts (such as printed lists of games, conversational openings, and requests). Because it is so important to the quality of life, the development of the patient's communication is considered to be the primary goal. For example, a patient who is capable of talking but who does not respond to greetings or who responds only with unintelligible vocalizations may be shunned; this patient, therefore, might be trained to respond with an appropriate and pleasant greeting and even to initiate greetings in particular contexts. At this level of recovery, patients usually require readily available written or pictorial cues in order to carry out prescribed actions even after extensive training. In addition, the confused patient cannot be expected to generalize procedures independently.

Therapists can use the principles of overlearning and behavior modification to train patients to eliminate inappropriate behaviors and to develop appropriate ones (see Chapter 13). This training can reduce, for instance, a child's aggression or tendency to be overly affectionate with strangers or an adolescent's inappropriate personal comments. The patient may also need training in specific routines to compensate for inadequate judgment (e.g., seeking a companion before going outside, asking for assistance in pouring a hot drink) as well as in the use of cues to assist him or her in completing the activities of daily living (a checklist for dressing).

Team members need also to provide directions to those people who will be in frequent contact with the patient. Family members, school staff members, and significant individuals in the patient's community should be made aware of his or her need for consistency, routine, structure, and controlled interaction. Team members should also encourage ongoing cognitive and behavioral training. Before discharging the patient, they should provide specific recommendations for appropriate activities and should support the patient and family through the phase of adjustment to new surroundings. In addition, they should conduct a follow-up inquiry at a predetermined interval (see Chapter 17).

Most patients, however, do progress through the middle stages of recovery. At some point in this progression, the patient's program may be expanded to include participation in a highly structured classroom or prevocational setting (see Chapters 15 and 16). Wherever the patient receives services, treatment incorporates the principles and guidelines discussed earlier. As the patient progresses into the late stages of recovery, therapeutic goals will shift to emphasize effective and independent functioning in increasingly normal environments and the acquisition of strategies to compensate for residual cognitive impairments.

REFERENCES

Farber, S. D. (1982). *Neurorehabilitation: A multisensory approach.* Philadelphia: W. B. Saunders.

Hagen, C. (1983). Planning a therapeutic environment for the communicatively impaired post closed head injury patient. In S. J. Shanks (Ed.), *Nursing and the management of adult communication disorders* (pp. 137–170). San Diego: College-Hill Press.

Mosey, A. C. (1976). *Activities therapy.* New York: Raven Press.

Malkmus, D., Booth, B. J., and Doyle, M. (1983, June). *Comprehensive interdisciplinary cognitive management.* Paper presented at the National Head Injury Foundation Second Annual Clinical Training Seminar (Models and Strategies in Cognitive Rehabilitation: A Comprehensive Team Management Approach to Head Injury), Boston.

Chapter 12

Cognitive Rehabilitation Therapy: Late Stages of Recovery

Juliet Haarbauer-Krupa, MA, CCC/Sp,
Kevin Henry, MEd,
Shirley F. Szekeres, MA, CCC/Sp, and
*Mark Ylvisaker, MA, CCC/Sp**

In Chapter 8, Table 8-1 lists typical cognitive sequelae of closed head injury. Although no patient's case exactly resembles the paradigms found in textbooks, it is useful to have in mind a model of the "classic" head injured patient at each of the three broad phases of recovery. In the absence of a motor impairment, deficits that patients have at the late stages of recovery are relatively hidden. Patients may *appear* to have returned to pretraumatic levels of functioning, but closer examination reveals noticeable slowness, disorganization, and inappropriate behavior. An even more careful examination often uncovers more specific residual impairments that affect general cognitive, academic, vocational, and social functioning. These impairments include the following:

- Impaired attention, concentration, and ability to shift attentional focus
- Greater than expected disorientation caused by unannounced changes in routine
- General inefficiency in processing information
- Relatively marked deterioration of comprehension caused by increases in the amount, complexity, and abstractness of information and in the rate of presentation
- Inefficient retrieval of information and of words
- Poorly organized behavior and language expression

*Authorship listed alphabetically at the authors' request.

- Inability to reason abstractly
- Impulsive and socially awkward behavior
- Disorganized problem solving
- Impaired "executive" functions: goal setting, planning, self-initiation or inhibition, self-monitoring, self-evaluation

In this chapter the categories of cognitive intervention (introduced in Chapter 8) are reviewed for children and adolescents who are beyond the stage of significant confusion and disorientation. The discussion is illustrated with case studies and a sampling of intervention techniques and activities. An exhaustive listing of therapy procedures is far beyond the scope of this chapter; the intent is only to give acceptable answers to questions such as "What are you trying to do for the patient?" (goals), "What kinds of things do you do?" (forms of intervention), and "Roughly, how do you do it?" (procedures).

GOAL OF TREATMENT

The overall goal is effective and independent functioning of the patient at a level and in an environment that approximate pretraumatic expectations of family, friends, and patients themselves. Patients' independence is viewed in terms of their daily activities in social, academic, and vocational settings. Because any particular conception of independence depends on a number of factors, patients are encouraged to achieve a level of independence that is appropriate to their age and abilities. Patients can achieve this goal through (1) improvements in cognitive processes, (2) functional integration of these processes in real-life tasks, and (3) the use of strategies to compensate for deficits that do not respond adequately to remediation.

FORMS OF INTERVENTION

In Chapter 8, four roughly distinguishable forms of cognitive rehabilitation were discussed, all of which can play a role in treatment at the late stages: environmental compensation, component training, functional-integrative training, and compensatory strategy training. Forms of intervention are selected according to the patients' functional strengths and deficits; to the constraints of their current and projected social, and educational or vocational settings; to the general principles of treatment listed in Table 8–2; and to our ongoing experience with their response to treatment.

Environmental Compensation

One important key to producing functional independence at the late stages of recovery is to *reduce* systematically the extensive environmental engineering that dominates the middle stages. Real-life forms of cognitive and social stress are introduced, and patients are taught to function in a natural environment without or, if necessary, with the aid of personal compensatory strategies. Head injured children, however, even those whose recovery has been excellent, often require some environmental compensations indefinitely. These are discussed in Chapters 8 and 11.

Component Training

Ben-Yishay and colleagues (1982) have demonstrated with head injured adults that component processes at all levels— from basic attentional to perceptual-motor to linguistic to higher level reasoning processes— can be improved by intensive and carefully designed retraining programs. Young children have a special need for intensive and systematic practice of component skills, since they lack the metacognitive ability to acquire compensatory strategies and use them independently. However, the reported evidence that intensive training can improve component processes has led many professionals to focus disproportionately on underlying component training and to concentrate uncritically on customized electronic training machines and computer-assisted retraining of cognitive components. Although training that focuses on attentional, perceptual-motor, and simple language, memory, and organizational components is useful for these patients, several reasons were given in Chapter 8 for rejecting component training as the rehabilitation keystone for patients at the late stages of recovery.

Compensatory Strategy Training

It is a hard fact of rehabilitation that some residual impairments of severely brain injured patients cannot be remedied through practice, however intensive and well conceived it may be. If these patients are at an adequate level of development, the therapist can most plausibly teach them deliberate compensatory strategies. These strategies are a principal focus of this chapter.

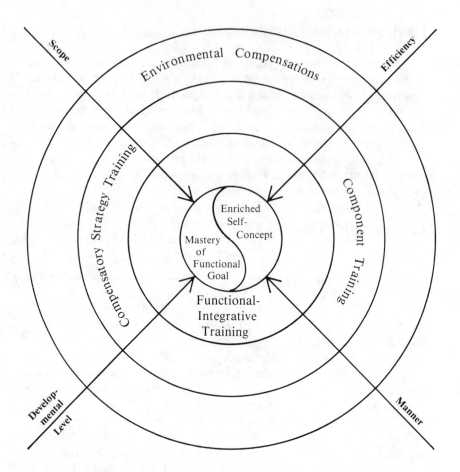

Figure 12–1. Forms of cognitive rehabilitation.

Functional-Integrative Training

Unless planned integration of cognitive components in functional tasks and practice in the real-life use of compensatory strategies are a major part of the rehabilitation program, meaningful improvement is unlikely to occur. Brain injured patients do not automatically integrate skills, generalize improvements to new settings, or maintain training over time. The emphasis at the late stage of cognitive rehabilitation is thus to have patients practice functional-integrative behaviors intensively, *in natural settings,* with or without personal compensations.

Figure 12-1 illustrates the relationship among these four forms of intervention differentially emphasized during recovery. The diagram also highlights the pervasive influence of the four performance variables (scope, efficiency, level, and manner, discussed in Chapter 8) on cognitive-social mastery.

TEACHING COMPENSATORY STRATEGIES

Strategy intervention requires three important and difficult decisions: The therapist must select appropriate candidates for such intervention, appropriate strategies for a given patient, and appropriate teaching procedures that help the patient to acquire the strategy efficiently as well as to generalize and maintain it.

Selection of Candidates

Table 12-1 lists patient variables that pertain to all three decisions. Detailed discussion of these, however, is beyond the scope of this chapter. Therapists should generally consider selecting patients according to the following attributes, which in the aggregate are those of the ideal candidate for compensatory strategy intervention:
- General intelligence within normal limits
- Metacognitive awareness (ability to think about learning and other cognitive issues) that is at least equivalent to that of normal 7 or 8 year old children (older for abstract strategies)
- Realistic goals or at least tentative acceptance of therapists' goals
- Desire to accomplish something to which strategies pertain
- Spontaneous use of concrete strategies in familiar games
- Lack of significant confusion and disorientation
- Definable neuropsychological strengths and weaknesses
- Some awareness of deficits and the need to compensate

Although deviations from this ideal type do not rule out strategy training, the therapist must consider the person who meets only a few of these conditions a poor candidate. Often a therapist can determine a patient's ability to profit from strategy intervention only by a period of trial therapy. When necessary, the first phase of intervention is directed to the patient's lack of goals, lack of awareness of deficits, or lack of intent to employ strategies.

Table 12-1. Variables to Consider in the Selection and Training of Compensatory Strategies

1. Developmental Factors
   a. Age
   b. Pretraumatic intellectual functioning
2. Environmental-Social Factors
   a. Pretraumatic social-educational-occupational status
   b. Current functional needs and environmental supports
   c. Proposed discharge setting: needs and supports
3. Cognitive Profile: Strengths and Deficits
   a. Sensory-perceptual-perceptual-motor abilities
   b. Attention: span, concentration, flexibility, "space"
   c. Memory: encoding, storage, retrieval
   d. Language abilities
   e. Knowledge (level of content and organization)
   f. Organizational abilities
   g. Reasoning and problem-solving abilities
   h. Metacognitive abilities: awareness of cognitive function (e.g., attention, memory, organization), explanation of own strategies, prediction of performance
   i. Strategic intent and spontaneous use of strategies
4. Readiness for New Learning: Degree of Confusion, Disorientation, Attentional Impairment
5. Personality and Social Control
   a. Shy-aggressive; fearful-confident
   b. Attitude toward rehabilitation
6. Motivation
   a. Presence of realistic and meaningful goals
   b. Perceived need to use a strategy
   c. Effective reinforcers
7. Executive Functions
   a. Self-awareness of deficits and their implications
   b. Self-initiation, self-direction, self-monitoring, self-evaluation
8. Cognitive Style (Pretrauma and Posttrauma): Impulsive-reflective; passive-active; rigid-flexible; indecisive-decisive; easily deterred–persistent
9. Situational Discrimination: Ability to distinguish situations that do or do not require application of a given strategy.
10. Medications: Expected positive-negative effects
11. Brain Injury: type, extent, and location

Selection of Strategies

Table 12-1 also includes factors that pertain to the selection of a compensatory strategy for a given patient. Patients who are just emerging from the confused phase of recovery or who are in the early phase of metacognitive development generally have difficulty with strategies other than external aids (e.g., memory books, reminder cards or drawings) or very concrete internal procedures (e.g., rehearsal).

Matching patients with appropriate strategies requires careful deliberation. Patients with generalized memory impairments who otherwise show skills in simultaneous visual-spatial processing that are superior to their skills in sequential linguistic processing would be candidates for visual imagery mnemonics rather than for verbal association. A shy and fearful patient would not be a good candidate for an input-control strategy involving requests for repetition, clarification, or slowing of the rate of input. Other things being equal, strategies that the patient uses or selects spontaneously are more valuable than those that the therapist selects, except in cases in which spontaneously used strategies fail or the neuropsychological data clearly predict failure.

Although other factors are also relevant, the important point is that this type of deliberation, or "head fitting," must be thorough and must take into account all of the listed variables before strategy intervention begins. Appendix 12-1 contains a pool of strategies that we have used with selected patients. Before deciding on a strategy from this list and initiating a training program, therapists should carefully consider the cautionary notes included in this and the preceding section.

Selection of Teaching Procedures

Table 12-2 outlines an intervention process with three phases, each of which has general goals, specific objectives, and selected teaching procedures. The phases are not rigidly sequential or mutually exclusive. Training head injured patients to think strategically and to be aware of their deficits, for example, may continue indefinitely, regardless of other objectives being pursued. Furthermore, generalization training can and often should begin before the patient becomes habituated to the use of a strategy in a therapy setting. Finally, whereas the procedures listed in Table 12-2 are useful and effective, they hardly exhaust the set of effective teaching techniques.

Training can take place within group or individual therapy sessions, in the classroom, or in a vocational training setting. As with all effective rehabilitation, patients need to experience frequent success and support despite the fact that therapists call attention to deficits and to patients' need to compensate. Staff members within an agency must take care not to introduce too many strategies at once or to teach similar strategies that may confuse the patient. Head injured patients with limited "attentional space" may become completely dysfunctional if that space is filled with strategy thoughts that prevent the patient from concentrating on the task

Table 12-2. Teaching Compensatory Strategies

Phase I: General Strategic Thinking
A. Self-Awareness
   Goals: Patients will discriminate effective from ineffective performance; become aware
   of deficits; recognize implications of deficits.
   Rationale: Patients do not acquire and spontaneously use strategies designed to compensate
   for deficits that they do not recognize. Given the frequency of frontolimbic involvement
   in closed head injury, self-awareness is a major concern.
   Procedures:
   1. *Objective:* Improve the patient's perception of successful versus unsuccessful task
      performance. Show the patient two video tapes (or role-play) illustrating successful
      and unsuccessful performance of a task. The task should be relevant to the patient's
      needs and goals. In both cases, analyze the tapes in sufficient detail that the patient
      can identify the features that account for successful versus unsuccessful performance.
      Young school-age children can do this with very concrete activities, such as games.
   2. *Objective:* Improve the patient's ability to perceive functional impairments. Individually,
      request the patient to make note of specific deficits of other head injured patients
      in group therapy. In individual sessions, discuss these observations with the patient.
      Discuss the effects of head injury on cognitive and social functioning.
   3. *Objective:* Improve the patient's awareness of his or her own deficits. Videotape the
      patient in an activity designed to reveal a weak area of functioning. (Alternatively, use
      role-play.) Review the tape, first without commentary. This should not be the patient's
      first self-observation on videotape. Comment on what the patient does well and, if
      required, on what he or she does poorly. Several sessions of this sort may be required.
      Gradually turn over to the patient the responsibility of stopping the tape when problems
      are noted.
   4. *Objective:* Improve the patient's understanding of the relation between deficits and
      long-term goals. Discuss in concrete detail the patient's long-term goals and expectations.
      Create a list of specific skills needed to achieve those goals. Review with the patient
      the skills that are present and those that are weak relative to this goal.
B. Value of Strategies
   Goal: Patients will agree that strategies are helpful in accomplishing their goals.
   Rationale: Head injured patients often lack strategies even when acutely aware of a
   problem.
   Procedures:
   1. Show the patient two video tapes: a person (stranger) failing in a functional task without
      a strategy and then succeeding when a strategy is used. (Alternatively, use role-play.)
   2. In group, have advanced patients demonstrate the value of a strategy or offer a
      "testimonial."
   3. Engage patients in a problem-solving discussion regarding a deficit. Orchestrate the
      discussion so that a strategy solution is initiated by the patients.
   4. Using video tape, have patients evaluate their own success on a task, with and without
      a strategy.
   5. Discuss with patients the widespread use of compensatory strategies (lists, memos,
      tape recorders, and so forth) by people without head injuries.

Phase II: Teaching the Strategy
   Procedures:
   1. *Self-Discovery:* Use "product monitoring" procedures as described above. (I. A. 1).
      Select tasks that clearly illustrate the value of a strategy (e.g., comprehension of a
      paragraph when given insufficient reading time versus comprehension when given

Table 12-2 (continued).

---

adequate reading time after making the strategic request, "May I have more time?").

2. *Modeling:* The steps in a strategy can be modeled by the therapist or a peer, by means of video tapes, puppet shows, or other media. Modeling is initially accompanied by overt verbalization of the strategy by the model. The patient then rehearses the strategy with gradually decreasing cues.

3. *Direct Instruction:* Explain clearly the purpose and use of the strategy to the patient.

Visual Aids:

   With most patients, the initial use of a strategy should be guided by visual cues: pictures, written instructions, diagrams, outlines, flow charts, game boards, and so forth. This helps to make the strategy procedures more concrete and easier to remember. Patients with significant visual disorganization may not be aided by such concrete visual representations.

Phase III: Generalization and Maintenance

Generalization of a strategy beyond the context of training is a combined consequence of the perceived utility of the strategy for the patient, specific teaching procedures designed to enhance generalization, and the inherent generalizability of the strategy.

1. *Objective:* Improve the patient's discrimination of situations that require or do not require a given strategy.
   - Use video taped scenes or role playing to illustrate the correct use of a strategy in an appropriate situation, inappropriate use of the strategy, and failure to use the strategy when appropriate. Discuss the conditions that require the strategy.
   - Use short video taped scenes to train the patient in efficient and accurate judgments as to whether a strategy is appropriate.

2. *Objective:* Increase the patient's spontaneous use of the strategy in varied situations.
   - Include family members, teachers, and work supervisors in strategy training to (1) provide varied opportunities for use of the strategy, and (2) reinforce the patient's use of the strategy in varied contexts.
   - Ask older patients to keep a log in which they record their successes and failures in strategy use. Make generalization an explicit goal.

3. *Objective:* Increase the patient's awareness of the utility of the strategy.
   - Give explicit feedback regarding the value of the strategy relative to the patient's goals.

---

at hand. A patient may have difficulty concentrating on school work, for example, if he or she is concentrating on strategies learned in physical therapy (e.g., "Keep my shoulders even"), in occupational therapy (e.g., "Look thoroughly to the right"), in speech therapy (e.g., "Breathe deeply before each sentence"), and in cognitive rehabilitation therapy (e.g., "Review the order of my thoughts before speaking").

Literature on the effectiveness of strategy intervention was reviewed briefly in Chapter 8. On the basis of clinical experience and data from studies of closely related populations, we are cautiously optimistic about this form of intervention for head injured children.

Two Case Illustrations

Case Study: Dan. Dan suffered a severe head injury (2 month coma) at age 14 years. Residual impairments included inefficiency (of rate and amount) in information processing, particularly of verbal information, and word retrieval problems. Over the course of his rehabilitation, Dan acquired a variety of compensatory strategies (among those listed in Appendix 12-1). He generalized the use of these strategies from cognitive rehabilitation therapy treatment sessions to the hospital classroom and later to his community school, where he received average grades in mainstream classes one grade below his age-appropriate grade level. The success of our strategy intervention with Dan appeared to result primarily from two factors. First, even during the confused stages of recovery, Dan showed active strategic intent in simple board and card games. Second, he was actively engaged in his rehabilitation, spontaneously identifying problems and participating in the selection of compensatory strategies. The combination of normal intelligence, metacognitive maturity, and personal initiative made Dan an excellent candidate for strategy training.

Case Study: Susan. Susan was 7 years old (18 months post trauma) when she participated in a program that used a specifically designed gameboard to improve her sequencing skills, reduce her impulsiveness, and develop her self-monitoring strategies. When Susan began her program, she appeared to be a good candidate for training. She used concrete strategies in simple board games, was aware of her problems in sequencing, and had age-appropriate language skills, a positive self-image, and a supportive environment at school and at home.

Although Susan was consistently accurate in therapy in using the strategy, which included self-instructions, she did not successfully transfer its use to academic and other functional tasks, even with cuing. This failure to generalize appears to have resulted primarily from two factors. First, Susan's metacognitive development was not adequate for her to appreciate the value of a systematic approach to problems requiring sequential organization. Second, she had difficulty distinguishing situations that required the use of the strategy from those that did not.

TREATMENT GOALS AND THERAPEUTIC ACTIVITIES

Cognitive and Behavioral Organization

At some point in their recovery, all severely head injured patients from early childhood through adolescence demonstrate organizational problems;

for many, these problems prove to be residual deficits of some magnitude. Evidence of poor organizational abilities may appear in play, in daily living activities, in academic tasks, in comprehension and expression of language, in recall, in behavioral self-control, and in reasoning and problem solving. Since cognitive organization is a theme that integrates many aspects of cognitive rehabilitation, the concept of organization is discussed briefly before we proceed with proposals for specific treatment.

Disorganized information has consistently been found to be more difficult to comprehend and to recall than organized information (Dodd and White, 1980). Everyone needs organization to store and gain access to large amounts of information. Retraining or facilitating the development of organizational skills is a complex process and is especially essential for head injured children, who typically have difficulty with new learning and with increased processing loads. These children can process and integrate information more effectively and efficiently if they become more adept at organizing it.

The importance of distinguishing aspects of organization is discussed by Pellegrino and Ingram (1978). We have found the following three-way distinction to be clinically useful:

1. Organization as a *product*. Behavior, objects, or events are organized when a specifiable principle exists that defines that organization (Mandler, 1967). The arrangement or apparent principle by which a child manipulates or arranges objects can be described. For example, the child may combine all objects that are the same color or shape (perceptual similarity principle); pile all the furniture or animals together (semantic similarity principle); arrange objects in groups based on their use in an activity (functional principle); or use dolls to simulate ordinary activities, such as eating breakfast or going to work (themes or experiential scripts). These are arrangements that children typically create, but they hardly represent the total number of possible arrangements. The notion of organization as a product implies that a principle inheres in a given arrangement of elements. Some important principles are degree of a property (e.g., size, shape, hardness), chronological order, serial order, temporal sequence, possession, spatial location, strong associations from the real world (e.g., horse and saddle), or logical order within discourse, reasoning, and problem solving.

2. Organization as *conceptual structure*. From a number of observations of the arrangements imposed on stimuli and of improvements in comprehension and recall when the patient arranges stimuli according to certain organizational principles, assumptions can be made about the organization of knowledge in long-term memory and about the specific organizing principles the child has developed. Tulving (1972) discusses the fit between the organizational structure of knowledge and the

organizational structure of the stimuli ("head fitting"), which Brown (1979) has emphasized as important in intervention.

3. Organization as a *process*. If people do not perceive a meaningful structure in stimuli, they may deliberately arrange the stimuli to achieve a goal. Organization can then be an active process an individual carries out while assimilating and encoding information (input organization), retrieving information, and organizing it for expression, structuring behavior, or arranging objects in the environment (output organization). Organizing is a complex activity involving the entire cognitive system. For instance, the individual has a purpose, scans the environment, perceives relevant elements, generates action to carry out the arrangement, and monitors or evaluates the product in terms of the goal. Specifications for the arrangement are the result of the individual's specific goal and the types of knowledge structures and organizational procedures that he or she can devise or retrieve from long-term memory.

To help the patient to develop organizational skills, we have created many forms and visual illustrations, some of which appear in Chapters 11 and 12. On the one hand, these forms and illustrations represent concretely to patients their environmental interactions and thinking processes. On the other hand, they help therapists to establish common and consistent procedures and clinical vocabularies, which serve and reinforce patients' progress and their ability to work with each other. Appendix 12-1 includes some strategies that can help patients compensate for organizational impairments.

Deficits in Processing Information

The primary goals of developing information processing skills may be grouped under three major headings: regulation of input; the processes of encoding, storage, and retrieval; and regulation of output. Deficits in these areas frequently limit the efficiency, scope, and manner of functional-integrative performance.

1. Regulation of input includes the following abilities:
   - to comprehend information at the *rate* at which it is presented
   - to comprehend adequate *amounts* of information
   - to maintain comprehension for adequate periods of time
   - to suppress distracting stimuli
   - to comprehend information at formerly successful levels of *complexity* and *abstraction*
   - to cope with information *overload*

2. Encoding-storage-retrieval includes the following abilities:
   - to *rehearse* information, either to maintain it in short-term storage or to *elaborate* it (expand in personally meaningfully ways) sufficiently for transfer to permanent storage
   - to devise or use *organizing procedures* in order to structure input, such as recalling similar scripts, schemata, or experiences already stored in permanent memory; chunking information thematically or categorically; or employing helpful forms of self-questioning for retrieving stories or conversational content (e.g., "*Who* was mentioned, *what* did they do, *where* did it happen, . . .?")
   - to distinguish *main ideas* from related details, as well as *relevant* from *irrelevant* information
   - to integrate new with old information
   - to *find words* necessary for fluent self-expression
3. Regulation of response includes the following abilities:
   - to *self-monitor* adequately in order to check confabulation, the poor generation of sequences, or needed topic closure or constraint
   - to *plan* complete and organized responses, whether for verbal or nonverbal output
   - to discern, attend to, or request necessary *feedback* that pertains to verbal and or nonverbal output

Intervention for Processing Deficits

A list of strategies from which the clinician may draw in formulating plans to treat processing deficits is included in Appendix 12-1. We reemphasize our belief, however, in the plausibility of teaching functional-integrative behaviors in their natural environments as soon as possible. Because we recognize the pervasiveness of the above-mentioned functional deficits and believe in using remediation techniques that "cover the most ground," we intensively train patients to use strategies that are generally applicable to those processing deficits.

1. Strategies for controlling input include teaching patients the following skills:
   - to recognize the rate, amount, duration, distractability, and complexity levels at which they can comfortably and efficiently succeed, and to request necessary adjustments directly from the provider of information, such as through the use of simple questions:

a. "Please say that in different words."
b. "Say that slower, please."
c. "Please repeat that."
d. "Let me think about that for a minute."

Requests of this type — which patients are taught to deliver with self-assurance — help to control the above-mentioned input variables and allow patients to process what they did not process the first time.

• to relax prior to anxiety-producing situations by means of guided imagery or self-instructional techniques

2. Strategies for controlling processes of encoding and retrieval include teaching patients the following skills:

• to select experiences from permanent memory that are similar to or triggered by the new input. The coupling of new information with a deeply rooted memory strengthens the patient's ability to retain it. The attention a patient devotes to the new material in this process also increases the likelihood of retrieval.

• to use visual imagery, particularly for patients with relatively intact visual-perceptual skills. These images should be vivid, novel, and action based.

• to rehearse and elaborate subvocally (particularly those patients with relatively intact verbal skills). This includes simple repeating as well as associating semantically, formulating opinions about the information, and deciding where it will be useful.

• to take notes.

• to use the sun diagram (Fig. 12–2), emphasizing either encoding or retrieval functions or both. The diagram is an organizing schema by which patients can classify information during input and retrieve it systematically. The patient also develops the ability to distinguish between main ideas and supporting details, to listen for specific information, and to discriminate between facts and opinions.

3. Strategies for regulating response include teaching patients the following skills:

• to use the sun diagram to improve awareness of the completeness of their responses. The diagram also provides a means of organizing descriptions, conversations, and stories, and of defining closure.

• to use the sun diagram as a tool for planning activities or for heightening patients' basic awareness of all the aspects of a task to be organized.

Sun Diagram

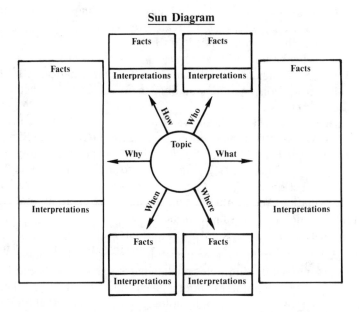

Figure 12-2. Teaching organized information processing using the sun diagram.

Deficits: Disorganized and incomplete processing of verbal information; difficulty distinguishing main ideas from details and facts from opinions.

Procedures:

1. The therapist should begin by explaining and illustrating the inherent structure of verbal information, e.g., that stories and conversations have topics (main ideas) and details (which may be classified by the six content "rays" of the diagram).

2. The therapist then introduces the sun diagram and explains the relationship between its parts and the components of verbal information.

3. Exercises in selective listening or reading are then provided to train patients to identify preselected categories of information and assign them to the corresponding parts of the diagram. Listening demands are gradually increased (first, only topics; then topics and "who"; then topics, "who," and "what," etc.).

4. When patients are successful in summarizing verbal information for all seven parts, the therapist should encourage them to generate interpretations or opinions for each of the "rays" and to distinguish between facts and interpretations of those facts.

5. The therapist then fades use of the graphic format gradually and encourages patients to use the diagram mentally during encoding.

6. The therapist provides cues and reminders as needed for using the diagram mentally in future comprehension exercises.

- to use self-instructional techniques (e.g., asking questions such as "Did I say or do what I really wanted to?", "Am I saying too much or too little?", "Am I thinking this through well?" (Meichenbaum, 1977).
- to scan a listener's facial expression for confirmation of his or her confusion or understanding, or to ask directly whether a statement is clear.

In earlier sections of this book we have emphasized the relationship of attention (Wood, 1983), perception, organization (Chase and Simon, 1973), knowledge (Brown, 1975; Schank, 1981), context (Tulving and Thompson, 1973; Waters, 1981), and goals and intention to remember (Schank and Abelson, 1977) to a person's ability to encode, store, and retrieve information. We would like now to emphasize an additional very important but deceptively simple principle: everyone, including head injured patients, retains more information more easily and for longer periods of time if they find it personally meaningful and interesting (Smirnov, 1973; Underwood and Schultz, 1960).

Social Cognition

Impaired social interaction is a primary residual deficit in severely head injured children as well as adults and is often the most devastating deficit for family, friends, and the patient. Although psychodynamic factors such as those discussed in Chapter 14 may be involved, problems of social interaction usually have a cognitive dimension. Some of the cognitive factors involved in interactive impairments are inadequate retrieval of rules of social interaction; poor awareness and perception of social and communicative events; reduced ability to take alternative perspectives; disorganization at the level of introducing, maintaining, and terminating topics of conversation; disinhibition and weak self-monitoring of verbal and nonverbal behavior that often result in the patient's repeating information, making inappropriate and offensive remarks, and communicating unintended nonverbal messages; reduced comprehension; and inability to organize information into main ideas and relevant details.

Many of the procedures of cognitive treatment presented in this chapter are directly applicable to social-cognitive training. As Flavell (1977) observed, "The head that thinks about the social world is the self-same head that thinks about the nonsocial world" (p. 122). Organizational strategies can be used to develop patients' verbal expression, to heighten their awareness of social interaction by means of feature analyses (see Chapter 11) of conversation, and to facilitate the use of encoding, retrieval, and problem-solving strategies in a social context.

There is an additional and important dimension of social cognition training. Personal interaction carries with it a much higher degree of unpredictability than does environmental interaction with inanimate objects. Unlike learning to perform structured academic or game activities, it requires ongoing monitoring of a constantly changing situation. Conversation is "locally controlled"; that is, there is often no predetermined topic or direction. Conversation requires that an individual monitor the flow of a topic, attempt to "read" what the other person is thinking or feeling, and maintain the information that was gained during an interaction. Memory disturbances often interfere with storing new information about a communication partner, and mistakes made once are often repeated in subsequent interactions.

Interpersonal Process Recall is an established treatment procedure designed for remediation of deficits in these areas (Kagan, 1969). Targets can include any of the areas listed earlier and can be as specific as improving eye contact and posture during conversation, shortening the length of conversational "turns," and increasing the use of polite forms and of requests for clarification. The technique basically comprises structured analysis of videotaped interactions between patient and clinician, identification of problems, mutual problem solving, and intensive and heavily coached practice of more appropriate and effective interactive behavior. Helffenstein and Wechsler (1982) found this technique effective with head injured adults. We use modifications of the technique with children as young as early grade schoolers.

Impulsiveness and a general lack of self-control also impair the behavior of young, school-age children. One established technique for improving self-control of behavior is cognitive behavior modification (CBM) (Meichenbaum, 1977), which basically teaches children to control their behavior by means of self-monitoring and self-instruction. The specific progression for acquiring these self-instructional skills is as follows: therapist modeling, imitation by the patient, and overt self-instruction by the patient, gradually proceeding through whispered to fully covert self-instructions.

In teaching self-instructional strategies to children, a response-cost reinforcement system has been found to be effective (Nelson, Finch, and Hooke, 1975). This system can be established quickly, provides direct and concrete feedback on problems, rules, and solutions, and encourages self-monitoring and self-evaluation. Table 12–3 outlines a program for teaching behavioral self-control by means of CBM techniques. However, these techniques are inappropriate for children whose behavior is attention-seeking rather than impulsive, since the attention that they receive following the undesirable behavior is likely to increase rather than to decrease the frequency of its occurrence (see Chapter 13).

Table 12-3. Teaching Self-Instruction, Self-Monitoring, and Impulse Control to Children

Deficits: Impulsive and poorly monitored behavior; reduced initiation

Goals: Improve behavioral control through self-instruction and self-monitoring

*Possible Target
Behaviors:*   Remaining in seat; raising hand to ask questions; asking for help when
            confused

Procedures:
1. Each child has a point card that specifies target self-control areas.
2. Each child is given five points per area and asked to define what area he or she will be
   addressing, based on areas in which points were lost the previous session.
3. The therapist removes a point for each failure to maintain the target behavior and asks
   questions relevant to that behavior (e.g., "What is your job?", "Where should you be?").
   At a later stage of treatment, the children are expected to ask themselves the questions
   when the points are removed.
4. The therapist then models the appropriate self-instruction (e.g., "Stay in your seat") and
   requests overt self-instruction from the child. In subsequent sessions, the child's self-
   instructions become whispers and later fully covert.
5. The session ends with a recitation of successful performance and areas requiring work
   (i.e., areas in which points were lost).
6. As needed, the therapist gives the children job explanations, behavior models, self-
   instruction models, reminders to attend to the point card, and praise for improvement
   and successful performance.
7. Video tapes may be used to give concrete, objective feedback.
8. The system is integrated into other settings by instructing children to keep their point
   card "in their heads."

Activities: This system works best in a small group but can also be used in individual
            sessions. It can be used with many different types of activities, e.g., games,
            craft projects, planning community outings.

Although the sequelae of head injury in young children are similar
to those in older children and adolescents, intervention techniques differ
because children think concretely and are metacognitively immature.
Preschoolers and children in the early grades focus primarily on the
observable features of tasks and events in general and are less able to reflect
on cognitive variables, such as attention, memory, organization, and self-
control (Loper, 1980). The likelihood of a young child's appreciating the
importance of active cognitive behavior does increase, however, as the
task increases in importance, familiarity, and concreteness.

Reasoning, Problem Solving, and Judgment

Improved problem solving, or practical reasoning, may be the highest
goal of cognitive rehabilitation for head injured adults and older children.

We give it this lofty ranking because adequate problem-solving abilities enable a patient to assume a self-coaching role and to achieve independence more quickly. It is particularly important to train head injured patients to solve problems because of the variety of new problems that their injuries will create and because of the high incidence of damage to the anterior frontal lobes, which are involved in problem solving (see Chapter 1).

As with all "focusing" procedures (Richman and Gholson, 1978), the systematic problem-solving strategy discussed first in this section assumes that the child is able to think hypothetically (a major feature of the formal operational stage of cognitive development), and thus the strategy is inappropriate for children at earlier stages of cognitive development.

Organized problem solving is a multistage process involving several distinct types of reasoning (see Table 12-4): isolation of main ideas (I, II); divergent (flexible, lateral, creative) thinking (III, IV); reflection on the relevance and adequacy of information (III); categorization of information (III); evaluative reasoning (V, VIII); analogical reasoning (V); convergent reasoning (VI); executive goal setting (II); planning and organizing (VII); and monitoring (VIII).

These components could be and typically are exercised in workbook fashion through multitrial practice sessions that focus separately on distinct reasoning components. We prefer to integrate remedial reasoning exercises within the context of real-life problem solving. Specific components (e.g., divergent thinking or sense of relevance) that interfere disproportionately with effective problem solving can be singled out for intensive component training.

On the one hand, the problem-solving guide presented in Table 12-4 could be considered a strategy that a patient may use deliberately to compensate for shallow or disorganized practical reasoning. In this case patients are taught to proceed systematically and independently through the steps of this guide when they are thinking about important problems in their lives. Patients generally need a written outline to be able to do this. On the other hand, the outline could simply be considered a basis for functional-integrative reasoning exercises in therapy sessions. In either case, the integration of reasoning components is not left to chance, and since the focus of the practice is on patients' own problems, they can perceive the utility of improved reasoning more readily than if the problems have nothing to do with their own lives.

Therapists can use this outline as a guide to exercises for older children and adolescents in group or individual sessions, responses being recorded on a problem-solving form. Older adolescents can use the guide to complete problem-solving exercises independently as homework; less mature

Table 12-4. Problem-Solving Guide

Deficits: Impulsivity; lack of initiation or organization in problem solving; inflexible, shallow thinking

Goals: Improve efficiency and organization of problem solving; improve reasoning; improve judgment

Problem-Solving Outline:
  I. Problem identification ("Briefly, what is the problem?")
  II. Goal identification ("What will you gain by solving this problem?")
  III. Relevant information ("What do you need to know in order to solve the problem?")
  IV. Possible solutions ("What could you possibly do to solve this problem?")
  V. Evaluation of solutions ("What's good or bad about each of these possibilities?") Consider: effective? enough time? able to do it? like to do it? break any rules? have solutions like this been useful in the past? what are the effects on yourself? others? the environment?
  VI. Decision ("What's the smartest thing to do?")
  VII. Formulation of plan ("How do you plan to accomplish this?")
  VIII. Monitoring and evaluation of results ("Did it work? Are you satisfied? Any new problems?")

---

adolescents and children as young as 10 or 11 will require the therapist's assistance. Simplified and more concrete procedures must be used with younger children (Richman and Gholson, 1978).

Like head injured adolescents and adults, head injured children from 6 to 12 years old often lack the degree of problem-solving skill that is expected at their developmental level. The deficit may involve any combination of the following: difficulty in setting goals and in relating current behavior to established goals; generally disorganized or impulsive behavior; inflexibility in considering alternative courses of action; and shallow evaluation of proposed plans. While working on improved planning and problem solving, the children can simultaneously use the techniques outlined in Table 12-3 to improve behavioral self-monitoring and self-control. Table 12-5 outlines a program for improving problem-solving abilities; other cognitive goals can easily be included in the same activities (e.g., improved attention, task organization, and organized verbal expression).

Children in this age range frequently have difficulty organizing tasks and appreciating the value of organization. Table 12-6 presents sample activities that we use to improve head injured children's organizational abilities.

Our experience suggests that generalization and maintenance of gains in these areas may occur spontaneously but are more likely to occur if teachers and parents are simultaneously eliciting and reinforcing the same behaviors. However, even with the most effective teaching, impulsive

Table 12-5. Teaching Problem Solving to Young Children

Deficits: Disorganized problem solving; weak task organizing and planning

Goals: Improve problem solving, organizing, and planning

Procedures:
1. During the first phase, the therapist clearly models the following skills: (a) problem identification; (b) listing of relevant information; (c) listing and evaluating possible solutions; (d) creating a plan of action.
2. During the next phase, the children execute their own plans and solve their own problems, even if this involves obviously inefficient plans and solutions. The children receive feedback from the results of their activity or directly from the therapist. Ideally, segments of the activity are video taped and jointly analyzed by the children and therapist to determine the efficiency of the plans and the efficiency of the problem-solving process.
3. The therapist then guides the children in the formulation of more useful (from the childrens' point of view) ways to solve problems (e.g., simplified versions of the outline in Table 12-4).
4. Written or pictured reminders of the agreed upon problem-solving procedure for a given activity are then posted in the room. As needed, the children's attention is called to these reminders as they face problems in their group activities.

Activities: Use a variety of interesting group projects that are loosely structured, requiring group planning and decision making; for example, writing a play, making the props, and performing it, or creating a game (including rules and materials) and playing it (emphasizing social rules and cognitive strategies).

behavior and disorganized problem solving typically recur in novel or in familiar but stressful situations. Consequently, environmental modifications (see Chapter 11) continue to be necessary to maintain the child's highest level of self-control and general behavioral organization.

Impaired judgment and failure to identify and to respond to social and environmental cues make head injured children vulnerable in unsupervised settings. An essential part of head injury rehabilitation for children therefore is training in physical and social safety procedures and in the use of community resources. Table 12-7 outlines sample procedures for improving functioning in this crucial area.

Cognitive Rehabilitation Therapy for Preschool Children

Many children whose injuries were sustained in the preschool years (ages 2 to 4) have shown subsequent perceptual, motor, and linguistic development in the years immediately following the injury that approximated normal limits. Our experience leads us to suspect that processing and learning problems, however, become increasingly manifest as the children face the academic demands of the early grades. Careful

Table 12–6. Teaching Organizational Skills to Children

Deficits:	Poor organizational skills
Goals:	Improve patients' awareness of the relationship between their goals and the type of organization they impose on objects; improve patients' ability to organize a task.
Features:	This technique uses the contents of the therapy room along with appropriate props for a specific activity. In these activities, the props are kept constant while the goals and arrangements are varied.

Procedures:

Task A   Shopping

1. The therapist arranges store props, at times using organized arrangements, at times using disorganized arrangements.
2. The children are sent to the "store" to find three specified items. Each trial is timed.
3. The therapist and the children then discuss why they found their items faster when the items in the store were well organized (e.g., all the candy in one place, all the cereal in another place) and slower when there was no organization.
4. The children are then asked to create their own arrangement of the items so they can find them as fast as possible.

Task B   Creating a "set"

1. Instruct the children to arrange the room to simulate specific situations (e.g., see a movie, eat a snack, play ball).
2. The therapist demonstrates and subsequently requests the children to create arrangements for the goal stated by the therapist.
3. Variations can include children giving directions to each other, planning the arrangement in advance, or drawing the arrangement.

diagnostic treatment of preschool children often reveals other problems that parallel those of school-age and adolescent head injured patients: deterioration of performance as a result of increased processing loads; disorganization in completing tasks and using language; word retrieval difficulties, especially in confrontational contexts; poor behavioral self-control when compared with peers; and reduced ability to learn new information.

These problems cause preschoolers difficulties in communicating, attending (even with interesting materials), and independently organizing tasks, even in their own play. These children may not be able, for instance, to request what they want because they have difficulty finding words, or they may move impulsively from one toy to another. Although they may use one or two objects in representational play, they cannot independently structure their play around broader themes. Subtle processing and organizational deficits create difficulties with the increasingly complex and "decentrized" social interaction expected of children as they approach the school years. These difficulties often appear as problems in turn taking.

Table 12–7. Teaching Community Skills to Young Children

Deficits: Poor safety and social judgment; decreased processing of environmental cues; poor organizational skills

Goals: Improve the patient's (1) physical safety, (2) social safety, (3) community mobility, and (4) use of community facilities

Procedures:

Area	Simulation (In Treatment)	Environment (Real World)
Physical safety (street and playground)	Provide the children with repetitive drill to remember rules, such as the following: (a) Stop-look-and-listen; (b) wait for swings to be still before climbing on; (c) don't jump off the monkey bars Provide the children with practice by means of role-playing and simulated situations.	Practice crossing real streets while reciting or using rules. Have group activities on the playground so that the therapist can coach and prompt the children in using the learned rules. Train families or staff members, or both, to cue the children in using the same rules.
Social safety	Provide the children with repetitive drill to remember rules such as the following: (a) Don't talk to strangers; (b) check the weather before getting dressed; (c) don't take candy or presents from strangers. Provide the children with practice in using the rules by means of role-playing and simulated situations, along with discussions.	Simulate potentially dangerous social situations in a natural setting, with other staff members who are unknown to the children, using the rules previously taught. Train families or staff members, or both, to cue the children using the same rules.
Community mobility	Present a map of a familiar place on a gameboard. Encourage the children to determine what the map represents. Explain the concept of *landmarks* and have the children provide examples in verbal discussion. Have the children describe how to reach various locations on the map, using landmarks.	Have the children find landmarks to add to the map. Give the children directions to find specific locations using landmarks. Have the children take turns describing and finding places using the map. Take the children to an unfamiliar place and have them lead the group back.

Table continued on following page.

Table 12-7 (continued).

Area	Simulation (In Treatment)	Environment (Real World)
		Ask families or staff members to prompt the children to look for landmarks in their daily environment.
Use of community facilities	Discuss a plan for using community facilities (e.g., stores, libraries, theaters, playgrounds). The discussion should include the following: (a) How do we use the facility? (b) What can we learn from it? (c) What kinds of questions should we ask in each place? (d) How should we ask permission to go to each place? As a group, devise a plan for a field trip to the facility using this information.	Actually visit the community facility and follow the children's plan for the visit. Ask family or staff members to provide time for the children to plan family outings or class field trips.

playing cooperatively with other children, and other social behaviors. One of the responsibilities of a cognitive rehabilitation therapy team working with preschoolers is to monitor these developmental parameters to determine the need for long-term special education or therapeutic services (see Chapter 9).

Play is perhaps the most therapeutic context of cognitive treatment for these patients. Clinicians should structure therapeutic play activities so that processing and organizational demands can be systematically increased and provide immediate and concrete feedback. The goals of therapy should change according to the developmental needs of the child. Therapy may initially concentrate on basic listening and organized play, and focus later on turn-taking, "in seat" behavior, attending to a picture task, and other behaviors that are important in a school context. Because of their developmental level and immature metacognitive functioning, these children are not expected to learn compensatory strategies. However, they are provided with practice in "organized thinking," and the therapists establish situations that require this type of thinking in therapy, classroom, and home settings.

Treatment of word retrieval deficits illustrates these points. We use semantic feature analysis (see Chapter 11) to teach children how to understand various aspects of an object, event, or person and to generate these descriptions when they cannot recall specific names. Cuing by teachers, family, or staff members helps patients in their efforts to remember and express these ideas. Specific cues for a given child should derive from the way in which he or she responds in testing and therapy; for instance, therapists cue some children to pantomine a word, whereas they cue others to tell the group to which a word belongs or to mention other kinds of familiar associations. With this type of persistent practice, children may engage in more organized word retrieval without the *deliberate* use of compensatory strategies.

Table 12-8 includes a sample of therapy goals and activities for preschool children.

Technology in Cognitive Rehabilitation

Computer Assisted Training. In recent years a certain fascination with the use of custom designed electronic training machines has appeared; more recently, great interest has been expressed in microcomputer based cognitive retraining. Among the most popular computer programs are those developed by the staff of the Head Trauma Program, Institute of Rehabilitation Medicine, New York University Medical Center, COGREHAB (Gianutsos and Klitzer, Life Sciences Associates, NYC) and a software package developed by Bracy. These programs are reviewed by Kurlycheck and Glang (1984) and Bracy (1984).

Although most forms of computer-assisted training have been done for years without electronic assistance, using computers does have certain advantages. Computers interest children and adolescents, particularly those who are veterans of video game arcades. Computers also have unlimited patience for drill and practice, which therapists do not. Of lesser importance, computers offer precision in stimulus presentation, immediate and consistent reinforcement, objective monitoring of progress, and simulation of activities inaccessible to physically handicapped patients. For some, computers represent an efficient and economical mode of treatment because they make independent drill and practice possible.

We have deliberately given relatively little attention to computer-based cognitive retraining in this volume to avoid contributing to an uncritical overuse of this type of treatment. Most of the available programs address cognitive components at basic levels, such as attention and concentration, visual-perception, and simple memory, language, and organizational skills. There is little evidence that microcomputer training by itself significantly improves real-life performance of functional-integrative tasks. Furthermore, often it is the cognitive weaknesses—as part of and

Table 12–8. Sample Therapy Activities for Preschoolers

Goal I: Improve organized representational and dramatic play

Features of therapeutic play activities:
1. The number of objects used can be systematically increased.
2. The activity has an obvious structure (beginning, middle, end).
3. The activity has a familiar theme.

Examples of play activities:

Less Complex		More Complex
Feed the baby a bottle.	Feed the baby food and a bottle.	Take care of baby; feed, bathe, and play.
Cars: Take one person for a ride.	*Cars:* Put two people in the car.	*Cars:* Build a road and take two people for a ride to the store.
Doctor's office: The child and the therapist play roles of doctor and patient, using 2 or 3 items in doctor's kit.	*Doctor's office:* The child and therapist use more items or switch roles.	*Doctor's office:* Add additional children and roles.
Store: The child tells the therapist what he or she wants from a set of pictured items.	*Store:* The "storekeeper" and the "customer" have play money. The child is a customer who comes to the store, buys, then goes home.	*Store:* Add other children and reverse roles.

Goal II: Improve sequential organization and planning

Features of therapeutic activities:
1. The format is consistent: This includes a model of the finished product, organization of materials, demonstration of the process, and explicit instructions.
2. The activity should have a concrete product as its goal (e.g., cookies, macaroni necklace).

Process:
1. Divide the task into three clear and obviously sequential units (e.g., stir ingredients; put on cookie sheet; bake).
2. Take pictures using an instant camera of the children at each of the three phases as they complete the activity. Drawings may be used as a more advanced step.
3. Review the activity by ordering and discussing the pictures sequentially.

Goal III: Improve turn-taking

Features of therapeutic activities:
1. An external feedback system (e.g., point card) is used.
2. The activity should offer obvious turn-taking cues (e.g., lotto games or simple card games).
3. The task structure can be gradually reduced (e.g., from board games with obvious turns to cooperative art projects with less obvious turns).

Process:
1. Identify the appropriate behavior for each child at every turn; "Johnny, it's your turn to talk", "Susan, it's your turn to look at Johnny and listen." Give the children obvious turn-taking cues by calling them by name and looking at them. Gradually withdraw these cues.
2. Give points for the target behavior (e.g., waiting quietly during the other child's turn).

contributory to psychosocial dysfunction—that interfere most significantly with the functioning of head injured patients. Computer based training is not an effective technique for improving these important psychosocial behaviors.

Video Therapy. Several references have been made to the value of video therapy techniques in cognitive rehabilitation during the late stages of recovery. Video feedback helps to increase a patient's awareness of deficits and strengths by means of objective confrontation, at the same time minimizing interpersonal confrontation. Video tape review provides feedback that is immediate, concrete, and objective; makes possible the microanalysis of behavior and the magnification of therapy targets by means of starts, pauses, and replays; and lets the patient assume the responsibility for stopping the tape for review or analysis.

In addition, video therapy techniques are useful for the following purposes:

- Demonstrating the value of compensatory strategies
- Modeling (positively or negatively) the use of strategies or other desired behaviors
- Practicing target behaviors, including interpersonal communication skills, and receiving clear, immediate, and objective feedback
- Facilitating generalization by means of practice in identifying conditions that require the use of a strategy or other learned skill; videotaped vignettes for multitrial drill; access to otherwise inaccessible situations
- Creating an objective record of a session to resolve disputes with the patient based on faulty memory or defensive denial and to encourage patients who do not recognize their progress by means of pretreatment and posttreatment comparisons.

Finally, the planning and production of a video taped scene can be a fun and therapeutic organizational activity for cognitive rehabilitation therapy groups.

The efficacy of video therapy has been established by a large number of studies in the fields of education, rehabilitation, and psychotherapy. Sanborn, Pyke, and Sanborn (1975) reviewed the use of video therapy in a wide variety of health-related fields. Some of their recommendations include (1) allowing patients to become comfortable with viewing themselves on the screen before proceeding with challenging tasks; (2) using short segments; and (3) using immediate playback. Helffenstein and Wechsler (1982) demonstrated that Interpersonal Process Recall, a video therapy technique designed by Kagan (1969) and used to improve pragmatic communication skills, is effective with head injured patients. Dowrick and Biggs (1983) discuss other recent therapy applications of video technology.

COGNITIVE REHABILITATION THERAPY AS RELATIONSHIP THERAPY

A positive and viable relationship with head injured patients is desirable, advantageous, and even crucial to the recovery process. The therapist-patient relationship is the necessary framework around and within which the patient most effectively explores, develops, and implements the skills therapists seek to teach. This statement is grounded in several broad and interrelated principles:

1. Clinicians generally initiate, maintain, and modify the direction of treatment; they need the patient's cooperation, which should be based at worst on a simple trusting acquiescence and at best on open acceptance.

2. Head injured children are tenuously reestablishing themselves in the world; their ability to do so and to respond self-confidently to challenge requires the warm acceptance of a strong relationship.

3. Clinicians must skillfully reinforce desirable behaviors and strengthen reemerging cognitive skills, particularly during the later stages of treatment; reinforcing behaviors in a relationship in which there is lack of trust could well prove futile and perhaps even counterproductive.

4. Substantive and durable results depend on open communication and expressions of concern between therapists and patients.

5. Interacting comfortably is simply the most enjoyable way to work closely and intensely together, and, since treatment is often intense and exacting, enjoyment is warranted and should be welcomed.

In their work with head injured adults, Ben Yishay and Diller (1983) have emphasized the importance of such techniques as excitatory exhortations, evocative metaphors, inspirational reflections, and psychodrama. Our experience has been that the use of such techniques with younger patients succeeds to the extent that the therapist and patient have established a positive relationship. These "personalized" techniques become credible and long-range treatment efforts begin to take root in a context in which therapist and patient feel affection, respect, and trust for each other. Anyone who has had the opportunity to view video tapes of Ben-Yishay at work with his adult patients quickly discerns an interactive style that transcends exhortation, inspiration, and psychodrama. He establishes a mood of warmth, encouragement, and support that helps patients to develop the confidence, security, and self-respect they need to risk personal interactions.

What is communicated and how it is communicated are of paramount importance, but the clinician's empathic abilities alone will not substitute for discipline and frankness when they are necessary. Therapists should illustrate effective means of dealing with difficult tasks even as they encourage the patient. They must be ready to give consistent feedback, even when it is painful, to encourage the patient to respond realistically and appropriately to difficulties, but they should avoid nagging and should be as tactful as possible. Responsible clinicians must also be skillful in withdrawing their support when the time for systematic weaning comes. The goals of the therapist's efforts are to improve patients' ability to cope with frustrations, to learn from a trusted adult, and generally to come to like, accept, and respect themselves better during a difficult time of life.

Part of the beauty of relationships lies in the learning and growth afforded both partners. The way patients behave and respond to treatment often teaches therapists much about guts, persistence, and resilience. And from these lessons we—as therapists and as persons—learn and grow.

REFERENCES

Ben-Yishay, Y., and Diller, L. (1983). Cognitive remediation. In M. Rosenthal, E. Griffith, M. Bond, and J. D. Miller (Eds.), *Rehabilitation of the head injured adult* (pp. 367–380). Philadelphia: F. A. Davis.

Ben-Yishay, Y., Rattok, J., Ross, B., Lakin, P., Ezrachi, O., Silver, S., and Diller, L. (1982). Rehabilitation of cognitive and perceptual defects in people with traumatic brain damage: A five year clinical research study. In *Working Approaches to Remediation of Cognitive Deficits in Brain Damaged Persons*. Rehabilitation Monograph, No. 64 (pp. 127–176). New York: New York University Medical Center, Institute of Rehabilitation Medicine.

Bracy, O. L. (1984). Using computers in neuropsychology. In M. D. Schwartz (Ed.), *Using computers in clinical practice* (pp. 245–256). New York: Haworth Press.

Brown, A. L. (1975). The development of memory: Knowing, knowing about knowing, and knowing how to know. In H. W. Reese (Ed.), *Advances in child development and behavior*. New York: Academic Press.

Brown, A. L. (1979). Theories of memory and the problems of development: Activity, growth and knowledge. In L. Cermak and F. I. M. Craik (Eds.). *Levels of processing in memory*. Hillsdale, NJ: Lawrence Erlbaum Associates.

Chase, W. G., and Simon, H. A. (1973). The mind's eye in chess. In W. Chase (Ed.), *Visual information processing* (pp. 215–281). New York: Academic Press.

Dodd, D., and White, R. M., Jr. (1980). *Cognition: Mental structures and processes*. Boston: Allyn and Bacon.

Dowrick, P. W., and Biggs, S. J. (1983). *Using video: Psychological and social applications*. New York: John Wiley and Sons.

Flavell, J. H. (1977). *Cognitive development*. Englewood Cliffs, NJ: Prentice-Hall.

Helffenstein, D., and Wechsler, F. (1982). The use of interpersonal process recall (IPR) in the remediation of interpersonal and communication skill deficits in the newly brain-injured. *Clinical Neuropsychology, 4*, 139–143.

Kagan, N. (1969). Interpersonal process recall. *Journal of Nervous and Mental Disease, 148*, 365–374.

Kurlycheck, R. T., and Glang, A. E. (1984). The use of microcomputers in the cognitive rehabilitation of brain-injured persons. In M. D. Schwartz (Ed.), *Using computers in clinical practice* (pp. 245-256). New York: Haworth Press.

Loper, A. (1980). Metacognitive development: Implications for cognitive training. *Exceptional Education Quarterly, 1,* 1-7.

Mandler, G. (1967). Organization and memory. In K. W. Spence and J. T. Spence (Eds.), *The psychology of learning and motivation* (Vol. I). New York: Academic Press.

Meichenbaum, D. (1977). *Cognitive behavior modification: An integrative approach.* New York: Plenum Press.

Nelson, W. M., III, Finch, A. J., Jr., and Hooke, J. F. (1975). Effects of reinforcement and response-cost on the cognitive style of emotionally disturbed boys. *Journal of Abnormal Psychology, 84,* 426-428.

Pellegrino, J., and Ingram, A. (1978). Processes, products, and measures of memory organization, Learning Research and Development Center Report. Pittsburgh: University of Pittsburgh.

Richman, S., and Gholson, B. (1978). Strategy modeling, age and information-processing efficiency. *Journal of Experimental Child Psychology, 26,* 58-70.

Sanborn, D. E., Pyke, H. F., and Sanborn, C. J. (1975). Videotape playback and psychotherapy: A review. *Psychotherapy: Theory, Research, and Practice, 12.* 179-186.

Schank, R. C. (1981). Language and memory. In D. A. Norman (Ed.), *Perspectives on cognitive science* (pp. 105-146). Norwood, NJ: Ablex Publishing Corporation.

Schank, R. C., and Abelson, R. P. (1977). *Scripts, plans, goods, and understanding: An inquiry into human knowledge structures.* Hillsdale, NJ: Lawrence Erlbaum Associates.

Smirnov A. (1973). *Problems in the psychology of memory.* New York: Plenum Press.

Tulving, E. (1972). Episodic and semantic. In E. Tulving and M. Donaldson (Eds.), *Organization of memory.* New York: Academic Press.

Tulving, E., and Thompson, D. M. (1973). Encoding specificity and retrieval processes in episodic memory. *Psychological Review, 80,* 352-373.

Underwood, B. J., and Schultz, R. W. (1960). *Meaningfulness and verbal learning.* Philadelphia: J. B. Lippincott.

Waters, H. S. (1981). Organizational strategies in memory for prose: A developmental analysis. *Journal of Experimental Child Psychology, 32,* 224-246.

Wood, F. (1983, March). Attention and memory. In L. Trexler (Chair), *Models and techniques of cognitive rehabilitation III,* Third Annual International Symposium. Indianapolis, IN: Hook Rehabilitation Center.

APPENDIX 12–1
EXAMPLES OF COMPENSATORY STRATEGIES FOR PATIENTS WITH COGNITIVE IMPAIRMENTS

Attention and Concentration

A. *External Aids*
 1. Use a timer or alarm watch to focus attention for a specified period.
 2. Organize the work environment and eliminate distractions.
 3. Use a written or pictorial task plan with built-in rest periods and reinforcement; move a marker along to show progress.
 4. Place a symbol or picture card in an obvious place in the work areas as a reminder to maintain attention.

B. *Internal Procedures*
 1. Set increasingly demanding goals for self, including sustained work time.
 2. Self-instruct (e.g., "Am I wandering? What am I supposed to do? What should I be doing now?"). (Written cue cards may be needed for these during training period.)

Orientation (to time, place, person, and event)

A. *External Aids*
 1. Use a log or journal book or tape recorder to record significant information and events of the day.
 2. Refer to pictures of persons who are not readily identified (carry pictures attached to logbook).
 3. Use appointment book or daily schedule sheet.
 4. Use alarm watch set for regular intervals.
 5. Refer to maps or pictures for spatial orientation; make maps with landmarks.

B. *Internal Procedures*
 1. Select anchor points or events during the week and then attempt to reconstruct either previous or subsequent points in time (e.g., "My birthday was on Wednesday and that was yesterday, so this must be Thursday").
 2. Request time, date, and similar information from others, when necessary.
 3. Scan environment for landmarks.

Input Control (amount, duration, complexity, rate, and interference)

A. *Auditory*
 1. Give feedback to speaker (e.g., "Please slow down; speed up; break information into smaller 'chunks' ").
 2. Request repetition in another form (e.g., "Would you please write that down for me?").

B. *Visual*
 1. Request longer viewing time or repeated viewings; request extra time for reading.
 2. Cover parts of a page and look at exposed areas systematically, as in a "clockwise direction" or "left to right."
 3. Use finger or index card to assist scanning and to maintain place.
 4. Use symbol to mark right and left margins of written material or top and bottom segments as anchors in space.
 5. Use large print books or talking books.

6. Request a verbal description.
7. Remove an object from its setting to examine it; then return it to the original setting and view it again.
8. Place items in best visual field and eliminate visual distractors.
9. Turn head to compensate for field cut.

Comprehension and Memory Processes

A. Use self-question (e.g., "Do I understand? Do I need to ask a question? How is this meaningful to me? How does this fit with what I know?"). Periodically look for GMCs (gaps, misconceptions, or confusion) by summarizing or explaining and checking back with speaker, a written source, or reference material.
B. Build "frames" or background for new information that is of particular significance or interest. Read summaries, general textbooks, and ask knowledgeable persons about topic of special interest (a procedure in building frames).
C. Use a study guide for extended discourse material (e.g., SQ 3R procedure—survey, question, read, recite, review).
D. Make charts and graphs of important relationships in textual material.
E. Use external memory aids (e.g., tape recorder, logbook, notes, memos, written or pictured time lines).
F. Rehearse: Covert or overt; auditory-vocal or motor (pantomine).
G. Organization: Scan for or impose some order on incoming information.
H. Mnemonics: Method of loci, rhymes, imagery (meaningful and novel associations).
I. Use diagrams or forms that facilitate deeper encoding of information and its subsequent retrieval (e.g., "sun diagram," Fig. 12–2).
J. Relate the information to personal life experiences and current knowledge. Use semantic knowledge of basic scripts (e.g., going to a restaurant, buying groceries) to help reconstruct previous events.
K. Project and describe situation in which target information will be needed or used.
L. At retrieval reconstruct environment in which information was received.
M. Verbalize visual-spatial information (e.g., "X is to the left of Y"). Visualize verbal information in graphs, pictures, cartoons, or action-based imagery.
N. Keep items in designated places.

Word Retrieval

A. Search lexical memory according to various categories and subcategories (e.g., person: family).
B. Describe the concept; circumlocute freely (talk about or around subject).
C. Use gestures or signs.
D. Attempt to generate a sentence or use a carrier phrase.
E. Search letters or sounds of the alphabet (more effective in retrieving members of a limited category, such as names).
F. Describe perceptual attributes and semantic features of the concept.
G. Draw the item.
H. Attempt to write the word.
I. Create an image of the object in a scene; then attempt to describe the scene.
J. Attempt to retrieve the overlearned opposite.
K. Free associate with image in mind.
L. Associate persons' names with physical characteristics or a known person of the same name.

Thought Organization and Verbal Expression

A. Use a structured thinking procedure (e.g., "feature analysis guide," Fig. 11-1, or "sun diagram," Fig. 12-2).
B. Use knowledge of scripts to generate real or imagined descriptions of experiences (narratives).
C. Construct a time line to maintain appropriate sequence of events.
D. Note topic in any conversation; self-question about the main point of expression; alert others before shifting a topic abruptly.
E. Watch others for feedback as to whether your words are confusing: Watch facial expression, and so forth, or directly ask listeners, "Am I being clear?"
F. Rehearse important comments or questions and listen to self.
G. Set limits of time or allowable number of sentences in any one turn.

Reasoning, Problem Solving, Judgment

A. Use a problem-solving guide (see Table 12-4).
B. Use self-questioning for alternatives or consequences. ("What else could I do?", "What would happen if I did that?").
C. Look at possible solutions from at least two different perspectives.
D. Scan environment for cues as to appropriateness or inappropriateness of a behavior (e.g., facial expression of others; signs like "No Smoking"; formality versus informality of setting).
E. Set specific times or places for behaviors that are appropriate only in specified situations.
F. Actively envision situations to which successful procedures can be generalized.

Self Monitoring

A. Use symbols or signs, placed in obvious places, or alarms that mean: "pause" or "stop" or "Am I doing what I should be doing?"
B. Use book or notebook with cards inserted at selected places with self-monitoring cues (e.g., "Summarize what you read").
C. Pair specific self-instruction with the associated emotion (e.g., "Calm down" when angry).

Task Organization

A. Use task organization checklist: materials, sequenced steps, time-line, evaluation of results. Check each when completed.
B. Prepare work space and assign space as task demands.

PART VI
BEHAVIORAL AND
PSYCHOSOCIAL INTERVENTION

Following closed head injury, behavioral, social, and emotional problems are often most disabling for patients and hardest for families and friends to understand, accept, and deal with. These problems have implications for the entire rehabilitation program, and their treatment presents an important challenge to the team as a whole and to those professionals specifically responsible for behavioral and psychosocial intervention. Treatment is complicated by the complex and incompletely understood relationships between behavioral and social impairments on the one hand and cognitive deficits and pretraumatic characteristics on the other.

In Chapter 13, Divack, Herrle, and Scott describe a number of common patterns of behavioral disturbances as they are manifested over the stages of cognitive recovery. The authors advocate a careful and consistent application of traditional principles of behavioral analysis to the behavioral problems of head injured patients, particularly those problems that interfere with a patient's participation and progress in rehabilitation. They recommend a flexible application of these traditional principles, in some cases focusing on the manipulation of *antecedent* conditions and events and in other cases focusing on *consequent* events— but in both cases taking into account the patient's medical and cognitive status and total environment. Although considerable validation for these principles exists in the management of other categories of children with behavioral disorders, research is needed to determine the most effective application of these broad principles to head injured children.

In Chapter 14, a social worker, pediatrician, psychiatrist, and psychologist combine their diverse experiences and professional orientations to address the social and emotional problems experienced by many children and adolescents following severe head injury. This collaboration underscores the significance of these problems as well as the importance of a multifaceted yet integrated approach to their treatment. In Chapter 14, Barin, Hanchett, Jacob, and Scott describe differing patterns of emotional reaction in children and adolescents, with appropriate treatment also varying with the developmental age of the patient.

With both behavioral and emotional or social problems, the authors of these chapters emphasize the importance of full staff and family involvement in treatment. In the absence of family involvement, the generalizability and durability of treatment results are questionable. Furthermore, involvement of family members in treatment is an important element in their own orientation to the altered personality that the head injury has produced in their loved one.

Chapter 13

Behavior Management

Joseph A. Divack, MSW,
James Herrle, BA, and
Mason B. Scott, PhD*

HISTORICAL PERSPECTIVE

Although a number of studies have assessed behavioral consequences in children who have sustained a closed head injury, a wide variation in assessment methodology has been used. As a result, significant disparities exist in the literature regarding the nature of these behavioral consequences. In an early study designed to investigate behavioral functioning, Blau (1936) concluded that the head injured child acquired a "posttraumatic psychopathic personality" in which overactivity, restlessness, destructiveness, aggression, temper tantrums, and delinquency were most likely to occur. These findings were supported by Richardson (1963), who found that 10 children and adolescents who were assessed in his study required a "sheltered and tolerant environment." In a study of behavioral consequences of closed head injury in a preschool-aged population, Hjern and Nylander (1964) found that only 5 of the 23 children in the study exhibited significant psychiatric disorders 6 months after the injury. The characteristics of these disorders were not described in detail. In contrast to this relatively optimistic behavioral finding, Brink, Garret, Hale, Woo-Sam, and Nickel (1970) found many personality and behavior problems in a group of 52 preschool and school-aged children who were assessed 1 to 7 years following a closed head injury that resulted in coma of at least 1 week's duration. In a follow-up study conducted by Flach and Malmros (1972), 132 children were assessed 8 to 10 years after sustaining closed head injuries of varying severity. Twenty-seven per cent of the children in that population were "socially maladjusted." The authors noted a "slowness"

*Authorship listed alphabetically at the authors' request.

in mental and motor functions, which was incongruent with the observations of hyperkinetic behavior reported in earlier studies.

Several studies have assessed factors such as age, location of injury, and severity of injury as they relate to behavioral outcome. Although Brink and co-workers (1970) report an apparent difference in the type of behavioral consequences found on follow-up according to the age of the subject, these findings were not described in detail. In contrast to this finding, Shaffer, Chadwick, and Rutter (1975) reported that age had no bearing on the frequency of behavioral problems resulting from closed head injury. Klonoff and Low (1974) confirmed Shaffer's report by finding no difference in the relative frequency of behavioral problems and only a minor variation in the rank order of problems when comparing children who were under 9 years of age at the time of injury with a group of older children. Shaffer and colleagues (1975) also reported that the severity of the injury, as measured by the duration of coma, was related to the likelihood of subsequent behavioral disturbances. However, the location of injury appeared to be inconsequential. These findings are consistent with those reported by Naughton (1971), who reported no variation in behavioral disturbances associated with left versus right hemispheric injury. Again, the severity of injury appeared to be related to the probability of later behavioral disturbances.

MANAGEMENT FUNDAMENTALS

Management of behavior problems secondary to closed head injury is most effectively accomplished thorough the use of applied behavioral analysis, often referred to as behavior management or behavior modification. This method of intervention has traditionally been applied to diverse groups of handicapped children as well as normal children with very good results (Ullman and Krasner, 1965). Historically, applied behavioral analysis has focused on the changing of behavior through manipulation of consequences (Skinner, 1953). In addition to heavy use of this principle, we also manipulate antecedent conditions, which are the events that elicit behaviors.

Members of a number of professional disciplines have traditionally been involved in the provision of behavioral consultation services. These include psychologists, social workers, and special education personnel. In this chapter, the term "behavioral consultant" is used to refer to that professional within an agency who is responsible for providing behavioral services.

Consistency

An appropriately structured environment helps to orient the patient and can serve as a background from which consistent systematic responses to patient behaviors can be applied. Patients generally receive rehabilitation services in complex medical environments. The behavioral consultant must use the structure of this environment to the best advantage of the patient.

Consistency is required to make behavioral procedures effective. In addition, an approach that is inconsistent will confuse the patient. Lack of consistency is the primary reason for the failure of behavioral programs. The need for consistency mandates team work. A good intervention plan must be feasible and well supported by the staff and must not exceed the behavioral skills of the staff.

To develop sound behavioral procedures the behavioral consultant must take a microscopic look at staff-patient interaction. Although it is clearly impossible to produce identical verbal or nonverbal responses from a group of up to 25 people who may be giving service to a patient, it is possible to bring within acceptable limits everyone's word choice, facial expression, sentence complexity, and tone of voice. To achieve optimal consistency, it is necessary to train family members to interact with the patient according to the behavioral program. In doing so, we recognize that families may still be experiencing grief and that they come to spend time with the patient rather than to be behavior therapists. Nonetheless, it is possible to help family members interact with the patient in a way that is therapeutic rather than detrimental. This early family involvement sets the stage for later generalization of appropriate behaviors to the home and community environment.

Head injured patients frequently have medical complications in addition to behavioral problems. Since medical devices and equipment are essential to the patient, it is the job of the behavioral consultant to develop programming that can be implemented without interfering with medical procedures. This goal can be achieved if the medical procedures are thoroughly understood and if the behavioral consultant is viewed as a full member of the treatment team, rather than as an outsider who comes to offer occasional advice. In the final analysis, good behavioral procedures for the patient with intensive medical management needs are part of high quality nursing care procedures.

Behavioral procedures for patients at early, middle, and late stages of cognitive recovery are discussed in this chapter. These stages are described in Table 8-1 in Chapter 8.

EARLY STAGE BEHAVIORS

As patients regain consciousness, a unique set of behaviors emerges. These behaviors may be managed effectively through a systematic applied behavioral analysis approach. Patients are in unfamiliar surroundings with a diminished ability to process information. They are confused and disoriented and respond to internal as well as external stimulation. Agitation is common in response to this heightened sensitivity to internal and external stimuli. Patients sometimes display behaviors that were common at an earlier developmental stage. They often have significant motor limitations as well as severe expressive and receptive language deficits. Patients typically cannot eat or tend to bathroom needs without special assistance.

Because patients at this level respond to both internal and external stimulation they will often exhibit behaviors for which no clear external antecedent exists. These behaviors are likely to be under internal antecedent control.

Case Illustration

> Twelve year old Mark exhibited many early-stage characteristics on admission to the head injury unit. He was often upset, exhibiting agitated behavior randomly many times during the day. On these occasions, his speech was generally unintelligible. Careful observation by the behavioral consultant failed to reveal any external antecedent condition that elicited the behavior. Therefore, Mark's pattern of agitation was presumed to be related to an internal antecedent condition. The behavioral consultant recommended that the staff members give minimal attention to the patient during agitated periods. In addition, he suggested that a high level of attention be given by the staff during nonagitated times. Finally, several time periods were identified in which the patient showed greater tolerance for medical procedures.

Medical management at this stage may include procedures to prevent the patient from pulling on the nutritional, elimination, or respiratory tubes. These procedures may include physical restraints or simply redirection through one-to-one supervised activity. Medication may also be indicated. Agitated behavior is also commonly observed in conjunction with the use of orthopedic splints. The behavioral consultant may advise the staff to systematically ignore this agitation, limiting interaction with the patient immediately after this behavior occurs. In addition, it is possible to introduce splints on a gradual basis. This involves implementation of a successive approximation procedure whereby the patient is required to wear the splints for increasing time periods. For example, a patient may be required to wear a splint for four hours a day yet be unable to tolerate this long a period. To accomplish this objective, a baseline tolerance (maximum time that splints are tolerated) is established. Initially, the splints are worn for no more than this baseline period of time. Small increments are added to the baseline in a planned sequence until the desired duration is reached. This procedure allows for a gradual increase of tolerance and is often successful in reducing or avoiding an agitated response to a medical procedure.

TRANSITION FROM EARLY TO MIDDLE STAGES

As the patient's alertness and level of activity increase, two considerations are important from a behavioral standpoint. First, it is essential to maintain appropriate control over the antecedent conditions that may elicit inappropriate behavior. Second, it is important to respond to the patient in such a way that maladaptive behaviors are not reinforced. It is desirable to adopt a low-key approach in which the patient is provided with cues in advance of initiating any procedure. It is important to establish some type of reliable yes-no communication system for the patient since this reduces the likelihood that the patient will develop inappropriate behaviors in an attempt to communicate and also reduces patient frustration. This is discussed more fully in Chapters 10 and 11.

As the patient continues to improve, systematic positive reinforcement of appropriate cooperative responses is necessary. This positive reinforcement should take the form of immediate, quiet verbal praise. Sometimes staff members make the mistake of being "overly reinforcing" by heaping intense verbal praise on the patient. This type of stimulus may be aversive to an overly aroused patient. The important consideration at this stage is that positive reinforcement be consistent and continuous.

A frequently overlooked method to help shape behavior is the control of antecedent conditions. This involves the manipulation of environmental events that precede and elicit the behavior. The patient's perceptions are often distorted at this stage. Tolerance to sensation may also be diminished. As a result, minor alterations in the environment produce important positive changes in behavior. For example, some head injured patients seem unusually sensitive to the level of illumination and ambient noise in the room, being touched by staff members in the course of daily treatment, or the texture of foods. Underarousal to normal levels of stimulation may also be a problem.

As cognitive status improves there is often a *decrease* in compliance to therapists' requests. It appears that this change is associated with greater therapy demands as well as increased attempts by patients to gain more control over their environment. A tremendous amount of staff time and attention is required during this stage of recovery. This is frequently the time when the behavioral consultant is first asked to work with the patient or staff. As the patient continues to progress, a greater variability of responsiveness is often noted. At certain times of day the patient may be better oriented, more aware, and generally more responsive than at other times. These periods of increased responsiveness may not coincide with therapy or medical schedules. It is possible to take advantage of these fluctuations by scheduling therapy times, medical procedures, and activities of daily living so that they coincide with periods of increased responsiveness. While this rearrangement often causes scheduling problems for staff members, our experience suggests that this method is effective in reducing agitation and improving tolerance to rehabilitation procedures.

Attempts to manage combative behavior are often a time-consuming and frustrating part of rehabilitation. In our experience, behavioral procedures have been only partially effective for this problem. Although behavior management can be used to modify external antecedent conditions and consequences, it cannot address internal stimulation that often elicits the combative behavior. The goal of behavioral intervention at this point should be to contain the behavior and minimize its frequency and intensity. Although combative behavior may be occurring as a result of internal stimulation, care should be taken not to inadvertently reinforce the behavior with attention. Cooperative noncombative behavior should be reinforced frequently. Physical restraints may be prescribed as indicated. Pharmacologic intervention (discussed in Chapter 14) may be advised concurrent with a behavior management approach.

Redirection of a patient from an inappropriate activity to a more appropriate behavior is often used as a management strategy at this stage. Used correctly, it can help to minimize a patient's problem behaviors. However, incorrect use can lead to inadvertent reinforcement and exacerbation of the problem. Redirection should only be used when the behavior is perseverative in nature (i.e., occurring repeatedly in response to an internal stimulus). If the behavior is occurring in response to an external antecedent event or consequence, antecedent control or extinction should be used. Extinction occurs when the reinforcer following the behavior is removed. When redirecting the patient, staff members should choose a new activity that is incompatible with the behavior to be eliminated. This new activity should be introduced in a low-key fashion, so as not to overly reinforce the perseverative behavior.

Case Illustration

Thirteen year old Elizabeth sustained severe craniocerebral trauma when she fell out of the back of a pick-up truck. Following a long stay in the neurosurgical intensive care unit, with many complications in treatment, she was transferred to the rehabilitation center. On arrival, she was grossly confused, agitated, and uncooperative for many treatment procedures. One cause of her agitation was an indwelling Foley catheter. Once this was removed, much of Elizabeth's agitation decreased and she became more cooperative. Antecedent control procedures were used to decrease agitated behavior further. This included reducing the level of auditory stimulation and making Elizabeth's environment more predictable. Staff members approached her calmly, using quiet voices, and advised her of all procedures before they were initiated. As much as possible, procedures were conducted at the same time and in the same place every day. Because of an apparent left visual field neglect, staff members were advised to approach Elizabeth from the right side. This was particularly helpful during the course of feeding. In addition, Elizabeth was heavily reinforced for all cooperative attempts. Reinforcement was by quiet verbal praise or a smile. Partly as a result of this intervention, Elizabeth's behavior gradually began to improve during the early stage and she became increasingly compliant and aware.

MIDDLE STAGE BEHAVIORS

As patients enter the middle stages of recovery, generally positive changes are noted in a large number of areas. Patients become better able to function in the structured rehabilitation setting. Their behavior becomes easier to change using a wide variety of therapeutic modalities. Most patients are able to walk and to communicate with far greater ease. Medical management becomes less intensive as the patient's medical status stabilizes. Despite ongoing confusion and disorientation, middle stage patients are actively involved in the reacquisition of previously learned skills.

As patients become more involved in formal therapy programs, noncompliance often becomes an issue. Coupled with this are fluctuating activity levels, impaired attentional functioning, and problems of impulse control. In social situations, the patient is less adept at processing cues and making appropriate judgments. As the level of neurocognitive functioning increases, therapy performance improves. However, as patients begin to be aware of deficits, motivational problems ensue. Often patients underestimate their deficits and occasionally they deny the existence of any problems.

In the middle stages of recovery, behavioral goals fall into three areas. The first area is participation in therapy. Common objectives include a decrease in the frequency of noncompliant behavior, an improvement in motivational functioning, and an improvement in selective attention. It is often the role of the behavioral consultant to help the other treatment team members identify the specific procedures and stimulus events that bring about optimal performance. In the second area, social functioning, it is important to reteach appropriate social responses. Problems of impulse control in social situations are often targeted for behavior change, as are motivational problems related to performance in social situations. The third major area, self-care, includes objectives such as increasing motivation and ability to perform activities of daily living with decreasing cues and physical assistance.

Behavioral planning is often concerned with discharge destination at this stage. If the patient is to be discharged to home, it is most important to improve social functioning and compliance to parental requests. Intensive patient training should be initiated at this stage. If discharge planning involves transfer to a rehabilitation facility, treatment goals should focus on the improvement of cooperation in therapy and tolerance to therapeutic activities. In addition, it is worthwhile to identify antecedent conditions under which the patient performs well. Examples include the presence or absence of visual or verbal cues and rate of stimulus presentation. Considerable time needs to be given to the patients in preparing them for a shift from one rehabilitation facility to home or to another facility.

Reinforcement Strategies

For middle stage patients, there is a continuation of the general behavioral strategies that were used with patients in the early stage. Attention continues to be paid to antecedents in the environment and highly structured activities. We also can make increasing use of traditional behavior management strategies that we use with other patient populations. Positive reinforcement continues to be the major tool used to increase desirable behaviors. Successive approximation techniques are also helpful. It is essential to structure therapy tasks so that the patient experiences considerable success. Psychometric and neuropsychological data are helpful in identifying the precise level at which tasks should be initiated.

For the middle stage patient, planned reinforcement practices shift gradually from primary, immediate, and continuous to secondary, delayed, and intermittent. The intent is to move toward types and schedules of reinforcement that more closely resemble those in the natural environment. In most situations the therapists will be working hard to return the patient to a school setting. It is essential that very special reinforcement systems be faded out prior to transfer back to the school setting.

Behavioral shaping and fading procedures are commonly used with middle stage patients. Gradual changes in procedures and removal of support systems are more effective than abrupt changes. Often failures occur when therapists are not willing to take the fading and shaping procedures slowly enough. It is also important to begin to work with some patients at very low levels of accomplishment. For example, with some patients it has been very helpful to begin physical therapy with sessions limited to 60 seconds. The duration of the session can be increased incrementally to the traditional 30 or 60 minute length. It is necessary to do this very gradually and over a long period of time. In addition it is helpful to increase the number of therapy sessions per day since the patient is getting little therapy time per session.

Strategies for Behavioral Excesses

One of the common problems confronted by the rehabilitation staff with the middle stage patient is that of behavioral *excesses*. This generally includes noncompliance, high levels of activity, and increases in inappropriate social behavior. Basic extinction procedures are the best approach to decrease the frequency of these behaviors. Ignoring and time-out strategies have been very effective within our facility. As a general rule we use time-out procedures when it is essential to interrupt a behavior. This includes behaviors that are potentially dangerous, self-reinforcing, or disruptive of the therapy process, or those that infringe on other patients' rights. The procedure is implemented in a consistent fashion across all therapies. We use ignoring procedures when the behavior is purely attention getting and not dangerous or highly disruptive. The effectiveness of these procedures depends on the consistency with which they are applied. The inconsistant use of procedures does not result in appreciable reduction of the behavioral excess (Krumholtz and Krumholtz, 1972). Our typical goal is 100% utilization of the extinction procedure.

Failure to Progress

Patients who reach a plateau at a middle stage of recovery present special problems to all health care facilities. These patients seem not to profit from even the most intensive rehabilitation care. They often present challenging problems from a behavioral standpoint. In order to make treatment gains, the use of overlearning procedures requiring a large number of trials is necessary. As a result, the patient often becomes weary of the repetitive nature of the therapy and develops oppositional behavior to the therapy. What can behavioral consultants add to the treatment program for patients who are severely impaired and whose conditions are apparently static?

First, the complexity of the service package should be addressed. Patients who are not progressing may not profit from highly elaborate packages of service. Part of the problem may be that too many staff members are working on too many even slightly different objectives at one time. There is a limit to how much these patients can absorb in a program day. One alternative is to change models. A suggested alternative model is to view the severely disabled and apparently static patient as a highly impaired learner. We then begin to deliver service more along the lines of a special education model, using techniques similar to those provided to severely mentally retarded persons. We drastically reduce the number of objectives, give more attention to the conditions of learning and reinforcement, provide a large number of trials, and give greater attention to the techniques of behavior shaping and fading. Changes in objectives, as progress is made, will be small, and the rate of behavior change will be slow. This may seem a bleak forecast, but this view is more optimistic than the traditional position, which characterizes such patients as impervious to change.

LATE STAGE BEHAVIORS

In the late stages of recovery most children are essentially normal in appearance, with adequate ambulation and seemingly normal language function. Many children attend school and therapy programs independently. Behavioral deficits in younger children most often include decreased attention, reduced impulse control, and noncompliance. In older children, the primary behavioral disorders include decreased attention, noncompliance, deficient social judgment, and depressed thought processes. Patients' social functioning is related to possible deficits in social perception, learning rate, information processing, and the capacity to abstract and generalize social rules. For example, children may be unable to distinguish between two similar social situations to which two very different sets of social rules apply. They may be slower in learning which social behaviors are appropriate and which are unacceptable. Other children may have difficulty in rapidly processing all of the social and environmental cues required to make a correct social response. In many cases, behavioral progress in the late stage is within normal limits and behavioral functioning is essentially unremarkable.

The goal of behavioral intervention in the later stages of recovery is to develop the behavioral prerequisites necessary for a child to function in the normal environments of home, school, and community. Intervention must be developed with a view toward the generalization of behavior into these normal settings. Therefore, it is advisable to conduct the behavioral intervention within these environments as well as in more structured therapy and academic settings.

Behavioral functioning within the family often becomes a significant issue at this stage. Children frequently spend a considerable amount of time at home and are exposed to family situations in which they may behave inappropriately. Behavioral services should focus heavily on parent training, which should address not only specific intervention strategies but also more general behavior management principles. The principles can then be applied to new behaviors or new situations as they emerge. The behavioral consultant can also help families avoid placing the child in an overly demanding situation by clarifying their expectations for the child.

Within the school setting the primary behavioral issues for head injured students are attentional functioning, compliant behavior, social functioning, and the full utilization of self-cuing techniques.

The residual social impairments following closed head injury in adults are often the most significant and long lasting sequelae (Bond, 1975). Although corresponding research has not been conducted in a pediatric population, our impression is that the degree of social impairment has a great bearing on the child's daily functioning. In this area, intervention focuses on parental expectations, the improvement of the child's ability to mediate behavior, and a reduction in impulsivity. Behavioral strategies are often highly effective in improving peer relationships. Commonly used techniques include modeling, successive approximation, antecedent management, and extinction. These techniques apply to a large variety of target behaviors, including improved play skills, decreased impulsivity, and improved "politeness." Some psychosocial deficits are not particularly susceptible to behavioral or other types of intervention. This situation may arise when control over external reinforcers is insufficient. The deficits may also be related to extreme impairment in functions, such as impulse control or learning rate. However, significant changes in behavior can often be produced by helping parents and community agencies to shape the environment to meet the patients' needs and limit the settings in which inappropriate behavior is likely to occur.

Generalization

For behavioral intervention to be effective at this stage, the generalization of a given behavior from a structured environment to the community is essential. It is important to have a specific plan for generalization rather than just to hope it occurs naturally. For behavior to be effectively generalized, the management strategies must be simple and well stated. The frequency and type of reinforcement should not be excessive. Behavior should be shaped so that it is maintained using reinforcement schedules available in the natural environment.

Optimum discharge planning begins with a careful assessment of the proposed educational program (see Chapters 15 and 17). This assessment includes curriculum content, prerequisite skills, and method and rate of presentation of material. If children are placed in classrooms that exceed their learning potential, noncompliant and other avoidance behaviors are likely to emerge. If behavioral management is recommended, the capacity of the classroom staff to implement management procedures must be considered. Special education teachers are often better trained than mainstream teachers to manage behavior problems.

The family must also be able to implement behavior management procedures adequately. For parents to be effective mediators of their child's behavior, training must start well before discharge. It is helpful to begin such training when the child is an inpatient and visits home on the weekends. Parents then have an opportunity to implement behavioral programs and discuss their progress weekly. Appropriate parental behavior can be reinforced and incorrect behavior changed. It is also important to have the siblings involved in, or at least aware of, the behavioral intervention, particularly when extinction procedures are being used.

Case Illustration

George was a very bright seven year old boy who sustained a closed head injury. He remained an inpatient for 4 months and then continued as a day patient for the following year. Prior to his discharge, the staff began to prepare him for community-based school placement. Behavioral counseling with his parents intensified. The parents had ample opportunity to observe the manner in which his behavior was managed by the staff. During this period, the parents became more aware of George's limitations in social settings. They learned that they were unable to take George into highly stimulating situations, in which he became overly excited and uncontrollable.

Knowing that George required individualized instruction and consistent behavior management, the staff observed several classrooms in the community school and chose a small learning disabilities class. Although a slight increase in inappropriateness was noted during the first 2 weeks, George "settled in" to his new routine and the behaviors acquired during rehabilitation programming generalized to his new surroundings.

SUMMARY

Application of management strategies to the behavioral sequelae associated with closed head injury in children has proved to be of great benefit to the overall course of rehabilitation. Utilization of these procedures depends on the child's developmental status and stage of recovery, as well as the nature of the presenting problem. Emphasis is placed on the manipulation of antecedent events and on the management of consequences. Consistent implementation of a well-devised, practical plan by the entire staff contributes significantly to the efficacy of rehabilitation services. Pharmacologic intervention for severe behavioral disorders is discussed in Chapter 14.

REFERENCES

Bond, M. (1975). Assessment of psychosocial outcome after severe head injury. In R. Porter and D. W. Fitzsimons (Eds.), *Outcome of severe damage to the central nervous system.* Ciba Foundation Symposium 34 (new series) (pp. 141–157). Amsterdam: Elsevier.

Blau, A. (1936). Mental changes following head trauma in children. *Archives of Neurology and Psychiatry, 35,* 327–338.

Brink, J. D., Garrett, A. L., Hale, W. R., Woo-Sam, J., and Nickel, V. L. (1970). Recovery of intellectual function in children sustaining severe head injuries. *Developmental Medicine and Child Neurology, 12,* 565–571.

Flach, J., and Malmros, R. (1972). A long-term study of children with severe head injury. *Scandinavian Journal of Rehabilitation Medicine, 4,* 9–15.

Hjern, B., and Nylander, I. (1964) Late prognosis of severe head injuries in children. *Acta Pediatrica, 155* (Suppl.), 113–116.

Klonoff, H., and Low, M. D. (1974). Disordered brain function in young children and early adolescents. In R. M. Reitan and L. A. Davidson (Eds.), *Clinical neuropsychology: Current applications* (pp. 121–167). Washington, DC: V. H. Winston & Sons.

Krumholtz, J., and Krumholtz, H. (1972). *Changing children's behavior.* Englewood Cliffs, NJ: Prentice-Hall.

Naughton, J. A. (1971). The effects of severe head injuries in children: Psychological aspects. *Proceedings of an Intervention Symposium on Head Injuries.* Edinburgh: Churchill Livingstone.

Richardson, R. (1963). Some effects of severe head injury. A follow-up study of children and adolescents after protracted coma. *Developmental Medicine and Child Neurology, 5,* 471–482.

Shaffer, D., Chadwick, O., and Rutter, M. (1975). Psychiatric outcome of localized head injury in children. In R. Porter and D. W. Fitzsimons (Eds.), *Outcome of severe damage to the central nervous system.* Ciba Foundation Symposium 34 (new series) (pp. 191–213). Amsterdam: Elsevier.

Skinner, B. (1953). *Science and human behavior.* New York: Macmillan.

Ullman, L., and Krasner, L. (Eds.) (1965). *Case studies in behavior modification.* New York: Holt, Rinehart and Winston.

Chapter 14

Counseling the Head Injured Patient

Judy J. Barin, MSW
Jeanne M. Hanchett, MD,
W. Lindsay Jacob, MD, and
Mason B. Scott, PhD*

Helping severely head injured patients accept the trauma and adjust to their new circumstances is a challenge to all professionals who work in the field of rehabilitation. In this chapter a social worker, a pediatrician, a psychiatrist, and a psychologist combine their knowledge and experiences in counseling children and adolescents with recent head trauma. We recognize that counseling is not limited to these disciplines. In practice, each person who works with head injured patients is involved in the counseling process. The "friendly ear," reassurance, and occasional confrontation taking place during rehabilitation therapies all play a role in addressing the needs of these young people that complements more formal counseling sessions.

We feel that a multidisciplinary model is useful in the provision of counseling services to patients and their families. Within our facility referral is made to the Social Service Department on the day of admission. This initial consultation is oriented to informational as well as therapeutic issues. Ongoing counseling is provided based on need, as perceived by staff or family members. Separate referral is made for behavioral management when it is needed (see Chapter 13). Psychiatric consultation is indicated in special circumstances that are identified later in this chapter.

In this chapter we discuss common psychosocial sequelae of severe head injury in children and adolescents and offer treatment suggestions. The importance of cooperation and mutual respect among members of

*Authorship listed alphabetically at the authors' request.

the rehabilitation team is implicit when the range of professions of the authors is considered. Many patients see only one or two of these professionals; some see all of them. For some of us counseling and psychosocial treatment of patients are our prime purposes whereas for others they are part of the broader patient care responsibilities. This requires frequent and effective communication among members of the rehabilitation team and a readiness to share in this aspect of the care of head injured children and adolescents.

There are excellent references on counseling children and adolescents (for example, Scarr, 1979; Schaefer, Johnson, and Wherry, 1982; Stein and Davis, 1982; Walsh 1975), but there are few resources that deal specifically with head injured young people.

EMOTIONAL RESPONSES OF CHILDREN TO SEVERE HEAD INJURY

There are common patterns in the emotional responses of young and latency-aged children with head injuries. They include (1) fear of loss through death, either of oneself or of loved ones, (2) separation anxiety, (3) fear of medical procedures and of pain, (4) anger, sadness, or unrealistic self-demands, all resulting from the awareness of deficits, (5) guilt, (6) tendencies toward aggressiveness and violence, and (7) disordered peer relationships. Each of these will be discussed in turn.

Fear of Death

One of the most common themes observed is the fear of loss of oneself or important others. As a result of the violent trauma and physical injuries experienced by these children, they are often thrust early into an awareness of death. Most know now that "very bad things" can happen to them and to others.

Most of the latency-age children are aware that they were near death. Several children have expressed fears that their parents may become involved in accidents and have reported dreams in which they see a parent killed, often in an automobile accident. Some children have actually lost an important family member as a result of the accident in which they were injured. Those with parents who are able to talk to their children about death and their own sad feelings seem to make the best adjustment.

Case Illustration

Two boys, both latency aged, described dreams in which they experienced contact with a much loved but deceased family member. One boy claimed that his dead grandfather had appeared in his dream on the other side of a bridge and had lovingly sent him back since it was not time for him to cross. These boys reacted to the thought of death with more awe and less fear than did children who experienced the dreams about accidents.

Separation Anxiety

Very young children often exhibit separation anxiety as they become more cognitively aware. They become increasingly upset as parents leave the hospital for the night or longer; their behavior ranges from whining and rejecting comfort to anger and tantrums as the separation continues. Although this behavior is difficult for parents, it is a normal response on the part of young children and a sign of improved cognitive functioning. Older children may also go through a brief period of regression in behavior as a result of separation from their parents, but they quickly shed their need for a parent's presence as they begin to feel better and are physically more active.

Fear of Medical Procedures and Pain

All head injured children express fear of additional pain. Younger children seem to be more affected than school-aged children by medical procedures, as shown by the medical themes that recur in their play. In some children the prospect of additional medical procedures renews the fear of death or more serious bodily injury. The ability of these children to understand a medical procedure on even a basic level may be limited. Children depend on a predictable external environment. Medical procedures and hospital readmissions disrupt this external organization, resulting in uncertainty and confusion. In our experience, many of these problems can be overcome by slow, careful preparation over time.

Awareness of Deficits

We have observed a variety of reactions as children become aware of their impairments. Very young children are the least aware of their deficits and least affected by them. Children older than 5 years often become angry and frustrated as a result of their inability to perform tasks that were previously easy. Only rarely do these children exhibit a true depressive reaction with anxiety about themselves and accompanying sadness. Most often children initially deny the problems or express determination to overcome them. This leads to considerable concern for their safety on the part of the adults involved. In an attempt to prove they have recovered, these children seek activities that involve a risk. Frequently they demand permission from parents and therapists to resume such activities as bicycle riding, football, or skating.

Angry and uncooperative behaviors in children aged 5 to 12 years are an indication that they are having trouble accepting changes in themselves. They rarely verbalize their feelings of loss, but instead act them out angrily. Furthermore, they often develop their own strategies for avoiding difficult subjects and activities. For example, they may change the subject or pretend that they are sleepy. Rehabilitation professionals must be skilled at correctly interpreting such behavior and at reflecting for children the inferred feelings of sadness or of lack of confidence.

The following case study illustrates the determination of these children to overcome changes in their functioning:

Case Illustration

While on vacation, a head injured boy who walked with great difficulty because of weekness in one leg repeatedly climbed a hill to come down a water slide. He stopped only when he was exhausted. He had been teased by the other children despite his successes and had ignored his parents' requests that he stop. As the parents described their son's determination, his mother was in tears and the father's voice broke.

Guilt

Occasionally older children express a sense of guilt, particularly when a close relative has died in the same accident. This feeling, also known as survival guilt, is intensified when the injured child had been careless or disobedient at the time of the accident. It may be manifested in several ways. Some children become self-abusive or, in extreme cases, suicidal. Other children become overly repentent, vowing "never to do that again." Young children often express a sense of being "bad" following a head injury, although they cannot always identify why.

Case Illustration

One 5 year old, who had been in counseling 1 year before the accident when his father left the home, regressed to feelings of being "bad and unlovable" again while recovering from his injuries. He felt that something was "wrong" with him and had caused him to be hurt so badly. In actual fact, he had pushed his younger sister out of the way of the car and was himself hit.

Violence

A few older children express themes of violence in their thoughts and conversation. Some threaten to hurt themselves. This may be a reaction to feelings of helplessness during the trauma or to the violence which they feel was inflicted on them. These children are at greater risk for self-abuse and psychiatric consultation is warranted.

Boys especially seem to express violent themes in their play and in conversation following a head injury. One boy alarmed his parents by frequent bragging about how he was going to "kill" or "beat the hell out of" the driver of the car that had hit him. Another told how he planned to "beat up" an absent father whom he had witnessed abusing his mother many years prior to the accident. It was as though his feelings of helplessness when hit by the car recalled earlier times when he had also felt helpless and threatened. Some boys fantasize about doing violent acts to themselves. One frightened his parents into seeking psychiatric help when he talked of going into the basement, taking a rope, and hanging himself.

Case Illustration

An adolescent girl who had previously been very responsible with her much younger sister began seeking opportunities to push her, much as when she had been "pushed" by the car, which sent her flying several feet through the air and caused her injuries. When she attempted to push the 3 year old down a flight of stairs, the parents sought help.

Disordered Peer Relationships

For school-aged children, peer relationships often pose special problems following a head injury. Old friends tend to drop away, forcing the child to form new relationships. Some children solve the problem by befriending younger and less demanding playmates, whereas others withdraw. Several factors contribute to the social deficits in these children. As with normal children who choose friends of similar intelligence, head injured children also seek out friends who are intellectually similar. These new friends are frequently younger or less mature than the injured child, since severe head injury usually results in reduced intellectual functioning. Frequently impulse control is also reduced after head injury, and this reduction leads to a variety of inappropriate social behaviors, such as excessive silliness, overexcitability, or aggression.

TREATMENT OF CHILDREN'S EMOTIONAL RESPONSES TO SEVERE HEAD INJURY

Treatment of children includes support by the rehabilitation staff and parents, play therapy, and therapy in small structured group situations. We consider the child's developmental level and severity of cognitive deficits when selecting and applying specific treatment techniques.

Supportive Reassurance

The presence and involvement of parents is the key to easing the emotional distress of preschoolers. Liberal visiting hours and guest house accommodations make this possible for many parents. When parents cannot be present because of jobs or other responsibilities, nursing staff members must give the child special reassurance and nurturing. For very young children, this nurturing includes social and interactive games, such as peek-a-boo and patty-cake. We help to ease the stress of separation for older children by giving them simple calendars and pointing out the days when their parents will visit. These activities may be used with individual children or small structured groups.

When young children lose a sibling or a parent as a result of the accident in which they were injured, that information should come to the child first from the family, if at all possible. Hendin's book (1973) is helpful in understanding a child's perception of death. Families need support and guidance in preparing simple and truthful explanations for the child. The therapist then supports the family and helps the child work through his or her feelings.

Play Therapy

Play therapy is quite effective for children in the age range 3 through 9 years whose cognitive function allows for some continuity of feelings and who can attend to an activity for 10 to 15 minutes. Play therapy allows children to express their fears and work them through even though they have limited verbal skills. Schaefer and O'Connor (1983) present techniques of play therapy and provide child development frameworks for assessment. The therapist guides the play from no control over a feared situation to mastery over it and from projection onto toys to some direct verbalization of concerns. For example, a child might begin by using a monster doll to repeatedly gobble up or harm other dolls. We gradually help the child to perceive the monster doll as a symbol of the car that hit him or her. When this happens, discussion of the accident, or medical procedure, can take place and feelings can be directly acknowledged. Play therapy with head injured children differs from that with normal children only in that the therapist must often structure the initial sessions and direct the play, reteaching the child to engage in imaginative play.

Case Illustrations

One young boy demonstrated a total lack of initiative with the play therapy equipment. He was able to begin responding, however, after the therapist created a play scene and played out a story for him to watch. She slowly passed control to him by asking simple questions about what should happen next in the play story. On another occasion, a child who could not engage in imaginative play was grouped with a more competent child. The competent child engaged in play with the therapist, doing such things as cooking and serving meals to the three of them. Eventually the slower child began to enter into the play and after many sessions was able to initiate imaginative play on his own.

When a child is not ready for this type of play despite cognitive recovery to an age-appropriate level, play on an earlier developmental level is useful. A simple task, such as stacking and knocking down blocks, allows some children the practice they need in doing and directing. Often we structure the play in terms of activities and themes, such as accidents or medical settings.

Case Illustrations

One girl, who tended to deny her medical ordeals and injuries, was able to demonstrate them through play when the traditional doll house was transformed into a hospital setting and adult dolls were assigned the roles of nurses. Another young child, whose mother died in the same accident, began talking about her mother's death after the therapist staged the death and burial of a toy kitten during play therapy.

Highly structured play is required when it is necessary to give information, as in preparation for a medical procedure. On other occasions we allow the child to choose the play objects, the therapist remaining nondirective and allowing the child to direct the characters and themes, perhaps verbalizing suspected issues for the child and thereby opening up communication. Equipment for play therapy is simple: a doll house with furniture, bendable life-like doll families, and a few cars and trucks. Children are generally resourceful in finding what they need; paper clips make excellent leg braces for dolls; paper tissues can be cut to resemble bath towels or bandages.

Discussion Groups

Latency-aged children more easily establish a relationship with the therapist when a game or other enjoyable activity opens the counseling session. Small group sessions are more effective than individual counseling. When children share their experiences with one another (why are you here? how did you get hurt?), these common experiences and fears help them express their feelings. It is not so bad to have "scary dreams" if the other children also have them and if the therapist says that it is normal. With children who are excessive risk takers, structured gross motor play activities can be used by the therapist to teach improved safety practices. We may, for instance, leave the building to practice safe mobility in the community, including crossing streets at intersections and waiting for the light.

Anticipating that these children will have difficulty relating to peers when they return home, the small group affords the opportunity for role playing and teaching appropriate responses to teasing. One such group developed a theme — KTK — or Kill Them with Kindness, as a way of reacting to peers who gave them a "rough time." This was a substitute for fighting, which the boys in the group initially proposed!

Behavior Management

Head trauma influences social functioning in several ways. First, children often lose previously learned behaviors and regress developmentally, which results in their bringing a diminished repertoire of behaviors to the social setting and appearing inappropriate and immature. Second, the ability of these children to acquire new information at a normal rate is decreased. They simply require more practice to relearn social behavior. Third, head injured children often have a diminished ability to process large numbers of social cues. Many children cannot "read" the situation quickly enough to respond appropriately; in addition, they may entirely overlook subtle, but important, characteristics of the setting, resulting in inappropriate or embarrassing behavior. For instance, our patients are often unable to recognize signs of disapproval in their peer group. They can become social outcasts without understanding why.

We have found that it is sometimes helpful to view social problems such as impaired peer relationships from a behavioral perspective. Careful observation and description of these behaviors leads logically to the development of treatment plans. Specific management techniques are outlined in Chapter 13.

EMOTIONAL RESPONSES OF ADOLESCENTS TO SEVERE HEAD INJURY

Attempts to establish personal identity and autonomy and the resulting rebellion against adult authority are normal developmental issues and conflicts of adolescents. The need for peer support in dealing with these issues is a hallmark of this age group; cars, alcohol, and drugs often become symbols of autonomy and rebellion. Following head injury, the normal strivings and conflicts are intensified; denial, depression, and acting-out activities are typical responses.

Interviews with families of head injured adolescents confirm that many of these patients were struggling with these issues prior to the injury. Some patients are injured while disobeying parental dictates. In some cases girls had left their homes without permission to be with boyfriends; many patients, both girls and boys, had been "out drinking" with friends when their accidents occurred. Parents frequently report that the teenager was becoming "difficult to control" prior to the trauma. One mother confessed that even without her daughter's accident and injuries, she would have had much "heartbreak" with her since "she was becoming so wild."

Following the accident some of these patients do not recover sufficiently to return to their adolescent activities. Left with deficits in cognition and judgment and occasionally with physical impairments, a very difficult time of acting out and depression may follow.

Denial and Loss

Denial is a major defense for patients who face losses and impairments. Sometimes head injured adolescents look relatively normal; this results in anger when staff members attempt to educate and warn them about safety issues. We hear comments such as "I'm sick to death of hearing about my problems," or "I'll show you." When these adolescents return to the the community, denial may persist as they experience a series of devastating losses. Most find school much more difficult; the former college-bound student may have to settle for just finishing high school, and then only with considerable help. Former school activities, such as sports, are usually no longer open to them.

Case Illustration

One young woman enrolled in a local college three times within two years following her head injury. Because of her fear of failure she withdrew the first two times before receiving any grades. The third time she was able to complete one term successfully, but at a tremendous cost of energy and stress. Finally she decided that a college degree would not be worth the effort and withdrew permanently.

In some cases denial is best understood as a psychoreactive inability to recognize and accept deficits. In our experience, however, apparent denial of deficits is most often organically based. This inability is common with right hemisphere lesions in combination with frontal lobe damage

(Fordyce, 1983). It is important for family and staff members to understand that this behavior is not willful—these patients are genuinely unaware of their problems. If treatment team members view this organically based failure to recognize deficits as willful, the patients' rehabilitation programs may suffer. Adolescents cannot be convinced to "work hard" in therapy when they believe that they are normal. Vocational counseling is unproductive when the patients' goals are unrealistic. Typically patients are offended by the vocational options presented.

A group therapy approach that combines information with confrontation is often effective for these patients. The role of the therapist is to identify specific deficit areas for the patient and, using appropriate and concrete modes of feedback, to improve the patient's awareness of these deficits. The therapist must be direct in confronting patients. During this process patients may move from anger to denial and back to anger, before they begin to understand their deficits. A reactive depression may follow this newly discovered loss.

Especially devastating to adolescents is the loss of a former peer group. Previous dating relationships usually fade during the rehabilitation stay. Peers of the same sex continue visiting for a period of time, sometimes with token politeness; when it becomes apparent that their old friend now has different personality characteristics, they gradually stop visiting. Patients attempt to form new friendships, which are usually short-lived, since head injured adolescents are often insensitive to social nuances, moody, easily fatigued, and frequently misunderstood.

Acting-Out Behaviors

Continued denial in the face of these losses leads to acting-out behavior. Poor judgment, both for safety and social concerns, makes this a particularly dangerous time. Girls are especially vulnerable sexually since they fear that they are no longer attractive. Regardless of their pretraumatic standards and behavior patterns, many young women become promiscuous for a period of time in their attempts to secure new and reassuring relationships with men. Families need help in understanding these changes and their daughter's possible need for contraception.

Most older teens had already begun drinking with peers prior to their accident. Despite warnings about the adverse effects of combining alcohol with anticonvulsant medications, many head injured patients continue to abuse alcohol until they have an unfortunate experience, such as passing out at a party.

Driving a car or motorcycle is a major concern for adolescents over the legal driving age. Frequently patients demand to be allowed to drive. When the parents or the physician refuse to grant permission, some drive anyway, using a friend's car. One girl, advised by her ophthalmologist to drive for no more than 2 hours daily in full daylight only, took her friends on vacation and drove 2000 miles with extended periods of driving.

Loss of Self-Esteem

When head injured adolescents begin to face their deficits, self-esteem typically plunges. Perceptions of basic intelligence, competence, career possibilities, and physical attractiveness are drastically revised in those who have residual deficits. Depression follows, and the patient's self-doubts may increase.

Siblings can become particularly cruel. Many adolescents report that at least one sibling has addressed them repeatedly as "retarded." When this happens, the teenage patient usually reveals it to the counselor to gain reassurance. Another indication of decreased self-esteem is increasing defensiveness when staff members attempt to test skills and progress. Excessive flirting on the part of girls and bravado and bragging about physical powers by adolescent boys also may indicate lowered self-esteem.

Suicidal Depression

Occasionally adolescents will become suicidal after experiencing several failures. In some cases, it is the patient's perception of failure rather than actual failure that elicits the strong emotion. Family, therapists, and other staff members must be alert to signs of suicidal intentions, since patients do not always confide these beforehand.

TREATMENT OF ADOLESCENTS' EMOTIONAL RESPONSES TO SEVERE HEAD INJURY

Adequate preparation of the parents is especially important in the treatment of adolescents. In no other age group will the problem of emotional lability have such an impact on the family or will the behavior problems be so blatant, dangerous, or difficult to control. It is essential to help these parents mourn the loss of the former child and become acquainted with the new one which the head trauma has brought them. Counseling of families of adolescents begins early in the rehabilitation stay and often continues for several months or longer after discharge (see Chapter 3).

There are several guidelines to remember when working with adolescent patients who have returned to a school program and to other community activities with residual cognitive and physical deficits:

1. Adolescents will resist adult limits and authority. This is especially true following a head injury, when the patient's judgment is compromised.

2. Because of poor judgment and cognitive deficits, head injured adolescents will take risks that may cause further injury.

3. A nonjudgmental atmosphere and acceptance of the patient by the counselor is the best means of establishing a therapeutic relationship with teenagers.

4. Confidentiality is an important part of dealing with adolescents. Protection of patients' rights to privacy balanced against medical concern for their safety makes this a complex area. In addition, parents' rights to i..formation and participation in decisions regarding their children are important, as are legal issues. Consideration of each of these is necessary in achieving the correct balance in confidentiality. There are clear guidelines in some cases, such as that of adolescent girls who desire contraceptive information and request that their parents not be informed; the law states that their request may be honored. A more difficult case is that of the depressed patient who expresses suicidal thoughts and does not want the counselor to share this information with family or other staff members. In this case, the need to protect the patient from self-harm overrules the request for confidentiality.

5. Despite their initial denial of deficits and refusal to discuss them, adolescents will eventually become more receptive to such discussions within a counseling setting and many even seek information about their head injury. This information, which we present simply and gradually, will help them to integrate their experience and to make more realistic decisions.

6. It is possible for effective counselors to improve the judgment and problem-solving skills of head injured adolescents. Since social relationships are often a problem, we try to simulate social situations in counseling sessions and help patients to consider alternative decisions and their consequences. We use role-playing to improve the patient's perception of social cues, such as facial expression, posture, and tone of voice. We ask patients to attend specifically to one type of social cue and then, with the therapist's guidance, interpret that behavior.

It is also useful to aid adolescents in preparing a simple list of safety rules for social situations. This technique was particularly helpful with a head injured girl who was "picking up" strangers and placing herself in extremely dangerous situations; this behavior was markedly out of keeping with her pretraumatic personality. She was able to follow simple rules, which she helped to define:

a. Do not go out with a man the first evening you meet him.
b. Make him call for a date at a later time.
c. Make him pick you up at your home and meet a family member before you leave the house.
d. Before you go out determine where he plans to take you and when you expect to be back.

7. As head injured adolescents face their deficits, they lose self-esteem. They need help in rebuilding a self-image that they can accept. Working with patients to create a list of their strengths and likeable qualities is helpful. We also find it useful to explain clearly to patients the common reactions to loss and the resulting sadness, particularly if we couple this with an assurance that they will feel better about themselves. It also helps adolescents to know that they are liked and appreciated by their therapists.

8. Birth control is a major issue for female adolescent patients. It is important for therapists to enlist family understanding and cooperation early. We remind families that the patient's upbringing and pretraumatic behavior are no guarantee that the adolescent will act responsibly again in this area. If parents are unable to cooperate and the patient requests contraceptive help, we respond to the patient's request and also maintain confidentiality in this area. This policy is consistent with federal legal guidelines regarding adolescents' rights to obtain contraception without parental consent or knowledge.

9. One of the most intense areas of conflict between head injured adolescents and their parents is the issue of driving the family car. When it is clear that the patient is physically unable to drive, parents have no difficulty in refusing this privilege. However, it is more difficult for parents to deny the request to drive when the adolescent has adequate motor skills but impaired judgment. Evaluation by the physician coupled with a driver education course for the handicapped will usually decide whether cognitive skills (including judgment) are adequate for driving. The counselor's empathic support during this time is necessary for both patient and parent.

10. Older adolescents have often been heavily involved in alcohol abuse before their accident. We cannot expect this life style to change after a head injury. Therefore, we give very direct advice about alcohol:

a. Never drink on an empty stomach; that is, eat food if you drink.
b. Never have more than two drinks in an evening.

c. Remember that anticonvulsant medications add to the effects of alcohol. If you take phenytoin (Dilantin), phenobarbital, or one of the other anticonvulsants, two drinks are like four.

We encourage teens not to drink at all; it is illegal under age 21 in our state (Pennsylvania). However, the prudent counselor is aware that adolescents do not necessarily obey the law and frequently use alcohol as a means of identification with peers and of acting out defiance of parental wishes.

PSYCHIATRIC INTERVENTION

In general a psychiatrist is not called on to assist in the counseling process unless serious or severe reactions begin to unfold. These reactions occur primarily in adolescent patients, although at times intervention may be necessary for younger children as well.

In general we avoid giving drugs in the rehabilitation of head injured children and adolescents. At times, however, the depression or agitation of these patients becomes so extreme or their emotional lability so severe that the use of medication may be a helpful adjunct in the treatment program. Medications should be used in the smallest possible amounts and for the shortest possible time.

The main reasons for consulting a psychiatrist are the following:
- To treat extreme agitation and emotional lability
- To intervene in the severe depressive reactions that may occur a few months after the injury when patients become increasingly aware of the extent of cognitive or motor deficits they have to deal with
- To motivate severely impaired patients to learn to use their residual abilities for more effective living
- To treat psychotic reactions that occur infrequently following head injury
- To deal with the problems that may arise due to the reemergence of the patient's premorbid personality.

Agitation and Emotional Lability

In dealing with severe agitation or emotional lability in adolescents, our drugs of choice for long-term maintenance therapy (several months) are the tricyclic antidepressants, such as amitriptyline (Elavil). These medications are often remarkably effective for emotional lability in small doses, such as 30 to 50 mg/day, although at times larger doses may be required (Kuss, Junkunz, and Hosboer, 1984; Schiffer, Cash, and Herndon, 1983). For agitation, a wider range of dosage is used and must be titrated for the individual patient.

When patients begin to take these medications, they may be drowsy for a few days; the drowsiness wears off, however, and improvement in their emotional lability and cognitive functioning soon follows. At the time the drug is discontinued, usually several months later, there usually is no regression in the patient's status. We speculate that after stimulating recovery, the drug serves no further purpose in the patient's inner economy. Occasionally a patient's emotional lability lasts over a period of several years or more, requiring continued small doses of this type of medication.

There are dangers in using tricyclic antidepressants. They have a significant tendency to lower the convulsive threshold and as a result may precipitate convulsions in those patients who are not receiving anticonvulsant medication (Peck, Stern, and Watkinson, 1983). In most cases of severe agitation or emotional lability, the advantages far outweigh the dangers. Consequently, the tricyclic antidepressants should be used when necessary.

To deal with isolated episodes of extreme agitation, particularly when patients appear to be in danger of hurting themselves, we use hydroxyzine pamoate (Vistaril) or one of the benzodiazepine family of tranquilizers, such as diazepam (Valium) (Bellantuono, Reggi, Tognoni, and Garattini, 1980). We avoid the antipsychotic tranquilizers, such as haloperidol (Haldol), thioridazine (Mellaril), or chlorpromazine (Thorazine) if possible. In our experience this type of medication seems to slow down the return of cognitive functioning. A deceleration in recovery from brain damage in rats following administration of haloperidol was observed by Feeney, Gonzalez, and Law (1982).

Severe Depression

In our experience the incidence of severe depression is quite high following severe head injury and may be announced by suicidal verbalizations or gestures, such as threatening to run the wheelchair down the stairs or throwing oneself out of bed. These problems are treated with both medication and counseling. Again we prefer the tricyclic antidepressants such as amitriptyline (Elavil) or doxepin hydrochloride (Sinequan). These drugs are not particularly useful in children under 12 years of age, but they usually work quite well with adolescents. The medication, which is generally given in standard dosages for severe depression, usually takes several weeks to become effective. The medication program is accompanied by intensive counseling to help patients overcome their depression and move ahead in their rehabilitation program.

Lack of Motivation

Motivational problems are usually accompanied by depression or at least loss of hope. At our facility all staff members are instructed to be gentle but firm with these patients and not overly sympathetic with their problems. In this way the staff communicates to patients that they are able to overcome their handicaps. This expression of confidence gives the patient stronger motivation. On the other hand, if staff members are overly sympathetic, the message conveyed to patients is that they may not be capable of dealing with their problems (Abrahamson, Seligman, and Teasdale, 1978). Along with living in a therapeutic milieu, patients may receive intensive counseling. In our experience, handicapped professionals are able to motivate by their example and have been effective counselors for many patients with motivational problems. If a therapeutic environment and counseling are ineffective in treating motivational problems, patients may be placed on a tricyclic antidepressant.

Psychotic Reactions

As mentioned earlier, psychotic reactions are not common following head injury. At times a patient may manifest a transient confusional psychosis in the early stages of recovery. We are, therefore, slow to use medication, preferring to observe the patient for a few weeks. Occasionally the patient will develop a mild disorganized psychosis. In this situation small doses of an antipsychotic medication are effective. We prefer to use antipsychotic medications that do not cause sedation, such as perphenazine (Trilafon), fluphenazine hydrochloride (Prolixin), or trifluoperazine hydrochloride (Stelazine).

Premorbid Personality

As time goes on in the recovery process, the patient's premorbid personality gradually reemerges. This may include attention deficit disorders or learning problems that were present pretraumatically. At times we also see the return of psychiatric problems or character disorders that were present prior to the head injury, in addition to the social and emotional problems brought on by the injury itself (Goethe and Levine, 1984). This type of problem usually surfaces in the less severely handicapped patients during the late stages of their recovery. Some of these patients may have had a pretraumatic drug or alcohol problem that may have been associated with a character disorder. As a result, the abuse of drugs or alcohol may also reemerge as the patient recovers. The treatment of this problem often includes referral to Alcoholics Anonymous or other substance abuse programs, intensive counseling within the rehabilitation facility, and strict enforcement of hospital rules regarding the possession or use of alcohol and illicit drugs. Other premorbid psychiatric problems are treated by conventional methods for the particular problem, provided that the patient is cognitively able to cooperate in these forms of treatment.

SUMMARY

In summary, we have discussed the major emotional responses of children and adolescents to severe head injury. Treatment methods are varied and are based on the patient's developmental level, stage of recovery and severity of symptoms. The techniques of group therapy, individual counseling, behavior management, and pharmacologic intervention are also presented and discussed.

REFERENCES

Abrahamson, L. Y., Seligman, M. E. P., and Teasdale, J. D. (1978). Learned helplessness in humans: Critique and reformulation. *Journal of Abnormal Psychology, 87,* 49-74.

Bellantuono, C., Reggi, V., Tognoni, G., and Garattini, S. (1980). Benzodiazepines: Clinical pharmacology and therapeutic use. *Drugs, 19,* 195-219.

Feeney, D. M., Gonzalez, A., and Law, W. A. (1982). Amphetamine, haloperidol, and experience interact to affect rate of recovery after motor cortex injury. *Science, 217,* 855-857.

Fordyce, D. (1983, March). The role of cognition as it affects psychosocial adjustment. Paper presented at the conference Models and Techniques of Cognitive Rehabilitation III, Indianapolis, IN.

Goethe, K. E., and Levine, H. S. (1984). Behavioral manifestations during early and long-term stages of recovery after closed head injury. *Psychiatric Annals, 14,* 540-546.

Hendin, D. (1973). *Death as a fact of life.* New York: W. W. Norton.

Kuss, H. J., Junkunz, G., and Hosboer, F. (1984). Amitriptyline: Looking through the therapeutic window. *Lancet 1,* 464-465.

Peck, A. W., Stern, W. C., and Watkinson, C. (1983). Incidence of seizures during treatment with tricyclic antidepressant drugs and bupropion. *Journal of Clinical Psychiatry, 44,* 197–201.

Scarr, S. (1979). Psychology and children: Current research and practice. *American Psychologist, 34,* 809–1043.

Schaefer, C., Johnson, L., and Wherry, J. (1982). *Group therapies for children and youth: Principles and practices of group treatment.* San Francisco: Jossey-Bass.

Schaefer, C., and O'Connor, K. (1983). *Handbook of play therapy.* New York: John Wiley.

Schiffer, R. B., Cash, J., and Herndon, R. M. (1983). Treatment of emotional lability with low dosage tricyclic antidepressants. *Psychosomatics, 24,* 1094–1096.

Stein, M., and Davis, K. (1982). *Therapies for adolescents.* San Francisco: Jossey-Bass.

Walsh, W. (1975). *Counseling children and adolescents: An anthology of contemporary techniques.* Berkeley: McCuthan Publishing Corporation.

PART VII
EDUCATIONAL AND
VOCATIONAL REHABILITATION

The goal of rehabilitation is to return head injured patients to a life and a level of functioning that are consistent with their pretraumatic activities, goals, and expectations. For school-aged children this includes a return to the classroom and academic learning. For older adolescents the focus is often on employment and the training necessary to obtain it. Achievement of this broad rehabilitation goal depends in part on the level of recovery that the patient reaches. It also depends, as the authors of Chapters 15 and 16 point out, on the availability of appropriate educational and prevocational-vocational programming within rehabilitation facilities and in the community. Unfortunately, such programming is often unavailable.

In Chapter 15, Cohen, Joyce, Rhoades, and Welks discuss educational programming for severely head injured children with a focus on characteristic cognitive and social deficits rather than academic teaching in a narrow sense. They advocate a gradual reintroduction into the classroom, with the program emphasis systematically changing as the student's cognitive functioning improves. Interdisciplinary teamwork (including teachers and other rehabilitation staff), the integration of teaching and ongoing assessment, and the integration of academic, cognitive, and social goals are all important parts of this process. For relatively well recovered head injured children, the authors emphasize the teaching of strategies to compensate for residual cognitive and social deficits.

Career development, according to Gobble and Pfahl (Chapter 16), includes vocational planning and training for those adolescents who are capable of some level of employment and avocational programs for those who are not. In this sense, all head injured young adults who have progressed beyond the early stages of cognitive recovery are candidates for rehabilitation services designed to aid them in achieving economic, social, and personal fulfillment. Gobble and Pfahl discuss both vocational and avocational assessment and treatment, which complement educational programming for those who continue to progress academically.

Chapter 15

Educational Programming for Head Injured Students

Sally B. Cohen, MEd,

Colleen M. Joyce, MEd,

Kathy Weider Rhoades, MEd, and

Dianna M. Welks, MEd*

A "special" education program should be a significant part of the cognitive rehabilitation of young people who are recovering from severe head injuries (Fuld and Fisher, 1977). To date, most hospitals and rehabilitation centers have not included a school curriculum in their programs for head injured patients. The cognitive rehabilitation therapy program at The Rehabilitation Institute of Pittsburgh is unique because it can extend cognitive stimulation and development into the classrooms of its special education school, which includes students from preschool through high school. Patients progress systematically from individual therapy sessions to small group therapy sessions to larger group situations in the classroom.

In school, students are expected to integrate cognitive skills that may be worked on separately in therapy. They may be asked to *listen* to a direction, *remember* it, *read* specified items on a worksheet, *think* about the material, *write* answers to questions and, throughout, screen out distractions — all this just to complete *one* task (Bryan and Bryan, 1978). Observing problems patients have in the more "normal" school environment helps therapists plan realistic and functional treatment programs.

*Authorship listed alphabetically at authors' request.

Approaches to educational programming for head injured students will differ depending on the level of recovery of the student and on the type of facility in which the school program functions. An acute-care hospital or short-term rehabilitation center (in which the average length of stay is a few weeks) will have fewer special education staff, fewer patients, and less time to carry out a program than a long-term rehabilitation center (in which the average length of stay is from 3 to 6 months). The size of the school in a rehabilitation center can determine the format of the educational program—whether, for instance, sessions are tutorial or classroom based, what the grade span is, and whether the teachers are trained to use special education techniques. Community school systems have no specific programs for head injured students and must, therefore, place these students in the existing programs (see Chapter 17).

In this chapter we describe teaching and the behavior-management approaches and psychosocial interventions that are appropriate for head injured students and compare and contrast the educational experience of these students with that of their peers in special education or mainstream settings. Specific methods of teaching academic subjects, such as reading and mathematics are not discussed; rather, we present teaching procedures that can be used in many areas of the school program. Throughout the chapter we emphasize the important relationship between prescriptive teaching and diagnostic, educational assessment. This chapter should be read along with the section on cognitive rehabilitation therapy (Chapters 8 to 12), in which issues relevant to special education, characteristics of head injured children, and principles and techniques of cognitive assessment and treatment intervention are discussed. Our focus in this chapter is on educational programming in a long-term rehabilitation center, although most of the information we present pertains to programming for severely head injured students regardless of the educational setting.

CONSIDERATIONS FOR INITIAL SCHOOL PLACEMENT

To benefit from a school experience, head injured students should be able to do the following: attend to a task for 10 to 15 minutes, tolerate 20 to 30 minutes of general classroom stimulation (movement, noises, visual distractions, use of different materials), function within a group of two or more students, engage in some type of meaningful communication (by talking, pointing, using a communication device, or—in extreme cases—using eye-gaze), follow simple directions (perhaps with written, verbal, pictured, or gestured cues), and give evidence of learning potential, however reduced in efficiency it may be.

At this point in the recovery process, students' academic levels are often significantly lower than they were before the trauma. It is important that the teacher review past school records (Fuld and Fisher, 1977; Hartlage and Telzrow, 1983) and note such things as academic or cognitive strengths and weaknesses, intellectual capacity, learning style, personal interests, and behavior and personality characteristics. Recognizing behaviors that were part of the student's pretraumatic repertoire and identifying behaviors that have been newly acquired as a result of the head injury help teachers establish reasonable goals, select motivating activities, and interact effectively with particular students. Fuld and Fisher (1977) also note that many of these students received special education services pretraumatically. Since their learning styles and problems were so "individualized," it can be difficult to recognize when they return to their previous levels of functioning.

Some head injured students who behave impulsively or irrationally in other parts of their rehabilitation program *exhibit better control and increased abilities when placed in a classroom.* They demonstrate the overlearned "school behaviors" that are automatically associated with that familiar setting and should spend more time in this controlled and familiar environment.

PURPOSE OF EDUCATIONAL ASSESSMENTS

Although educational assessments are discussed in detail in Chapter 9, it is important to say a few words about them here. The purpose of testing is to find the point at which learning breaks down, since that is the point at which teaching should begin. The scores of psychological and academic assessments administered to head injured students *must be interpreted differently* from the scores of other students. These test results reflect only that the head injured students could perform the tasks demanded by the *specific* test items; *they do not predict* future performance.

Once classroom placements are made, teachers can observe students over a period of time, and consistent learning patterns and cognitive problems can become more evident. Teachers may develop programs for these students that begin at levels slightly lower than those achieved on the assessments so that the students can adapt to the increased classroom stimulation and work successfully. Diagnostic, prescriptive teaching techniques help teachers to monitor changes in students' performance and thus link assessment and teaching procedures.

GENERAL CONSIDERATIONS FOR PROGRAMMING

Therapists and teachers must be aware of typical developmental patterns in order to target cognitive and behavioral deficits accurately. A 4 year old child with a head injury may have poor attending skills, but young children typically do not attend to one task for very long. A head injured adolescent may be very resistant to treatment that focuses on deficits, may deny having problems, and may get angry with therapists and teachers, but adolescents typically interpret receiving help as "being told what to do" and often think that "things will be better tomorrow."

To make appropriate placements, teachers must know students' developmental and academic levels, their rate of learning, and their processing abilities (see Chapter 9). Teachers may also consider chronological age and social skills; however, most students feel comfortable when they are on the same functional level as their classmates and have similar social skills even if the classmates are younger or older.

SCHEDULING

Therapists should attempt to maintain consistent therapy schedules for head injured students because predictability and familiarity decrease their confusion and anxiety and help them feel secure. Since program priorities may require many types of rehabilitation treatment (see Chapter 17), some students may spend only a short time in the classroom. It is difficult to adjust therapy schedules so that students are available when appropriate activities are taught in school, and teachers may have to adjust programs for students who can only attend two of the three reading sessions a week. As cognitive abilities improve, however, school itself often becomes a program priority.

COGNITIVE CONSIDERATIONS FOR PROGRAMMING

School programs in a rehabilitation center integrate therapy techniques from physical therapy, occupational therapy, speech and language therapy, and cognitive rehabilitation therapy. The teacher thus becomes "a little bit of everyone else" who is treating the head injured individual. It is very difficult for teachers to distinguish between cognitive and academic skills and to see value in establishing programs that do not have a strict academic focus. The goals of school programs for head injured students should emphasize thought organization, critical thinking, and social skills. Teachers should thus realize that there is nothing fundamentally wrong with students' working on limited amounts of material or with their lack of academic progress.

When students are first placed in a group, they may only be able to listen to stories, to watch activities, to look at pictures, to have staff members talk *to* them (not *with* them), and to be helped with orientation. When the group activity is to follow directions and mark a worksheet, these students may be asked to look at the teacher when their names are called, to complete the first step of a direction (e.g., to point to a specific picture in a row of others), to sit quietly with others for 20 minutes, or to raise their hands to speak instead of talking out impulsively. When presenting a task, the teacher must be aware of the type of material each student can process and the type of response he or she can give (see Chapter 9). Teachers should remember that the objectives of programs are to develop cognitive skills and thus that programs that focus on *how* students process information may be more important than those that emphasize correct responses. Some aspects and factors of processing are the following:

- attention
- ability to follow auditory and visual directions
- comprehension of concrete and abstract language concepts
- auditory and visual memory skills
- rate of processing (e.g., delayed responses)
- rate of performance in speaking, manipulating material, and writing
- comprehension of spoken language and visual information (picture or printed information)
- comprehension of rote and meaningful information
- comprehension of smaller and larger amounts of material
- decreased comprehension due to "overload"
- cued and uncued responses
- responses to statements, multiple choice answers, and open-ended questions
- presence of delayed responses
- independent performance or performance based on a model or in imitation
- identification of relearned and newly learned material
- frustration tolerance
- fatigue level

A teacher should never take silence or an incorrect, impulsive, or resistant answer at face value; these responses may reflect processing problems. Students can be taught to indicate when they are confused or need assistance and can thus improve their understanding of material, relieve their anxiety, and increase their desire to attend and communicate. The teacher can introduce compensatory strategies to aid comprehension and students' ability to perform and thus increase the likelihood of academic success (see Chapter 12) (Hallahan et al., 1983).

INFORMAL CLASSROOM ASSESSMENT

When the students are placed in the classroom, teachers should assess the changes in performance that may have occurred since the formal evaluation was administered. Teachers can use academic materials to establish students' current grade levels as well as to indicate the adaptations or cues that help students maintain those levels. It is helpful to observe students working individually and in small groups and to note if there are differences in performance. Teachers also have an opportunity to see if students can remember and carry out classroom routines and can apply them productively in other contexts. For instance, when students learn the strategy of looking for landmarks to remember their way to the classroom, can they also follow this strategy to go to the lunchroom?

Classroom materials can be used to assess processing abilities, such as those listed in the previous section. Teachers can also obtain valuable information while watching students play a game. For instance, playing a board game reveals skills in organization (setting up the game), attending (visually and auditorially), processing directions, memory (for the steps involved and the content), and interaction with peers. Of course, throughout the school day teachers can evaluate students' judgment and peer relations, both of which we discuss in detail later in the chapter.

FORMAL INSTRUCTION

- Once students' general levels have been established, classroom instruction can begin. Through the use of diagnostic, prescriptive teaching, and task analysis teachers continue to evaluate students' skills (Torgesen, 1979), to recognize improvement in some areas and difficulties in others, and, thus, to maintain appropriate educational programs. As mentioned previously, we stress the integration of cognitive skills, which is difficult for head injured students, and we often have to teach them strategies to perform more effectively.

STRATEGIES

Strategies are procedures that help students clarify, organize, remember, and express information (Clark, Deshler, Schumaker, Alley, and Warner, 1984). They structure and emphasize parts of the learning process that most head injured students previously performed automatically. (Chapter 12 includes a list of compensatory strategies that are used in head injury treatment.) Teachers often need to spend much time teaching students *how* to use these strategies and *why* they should be used. At first, teachers use strategies to structure the environment or students' behavior (e.g., blocking out everything but the sentence students are to read). Teachers then cue students to apply the compensatory strategies in specific situations. The ultimate goal is for students to use the strategies independently (e.g., to take out a marker and use it to keep their place when they are reading). Thus, *programming should progress from the point at which the teacher implements strategies to the point at which students are expected to use them independently* (Hartlage and Telzrow, 1983).

Teachers can help students evaluate their performance and recognize areas that need improvement by modeling appropriate behaviors and by having students identify others' correct or incorrect behaviors, and, eventually, their own (Kerr and Nelson, 1983; Meichenbaum, 1977). They can develop students' self-monitoring skills by having them describe and then internalize rules, procedures, and behaviors that they should learn. (This teaching process is discussed in the socialization section of this chapter.)

Table 15-1 presents some of the cognitive problems that head injured students demonstrate and strategies that can be used to compensate for them; *many strategies can be used interchangeably for various problems.* Using a strategy may be the head injured student's goal for a specific lesson.

Figures 15-1, 15-2, and 15-3 include specific illustrations of strategies and their use in classroom instruction.

CONSIDERATIONS FOR MORE COMPLEX SCHOOL PROGRAMS

As head injured students recover and cognitive abilities improve, the teacher should present tasks requiring more involved critical thinking.

Table 15-1. Compensatory Strategies for Cognitive Problems in a Classroom Setting

Key: Strategies followed by the letter T are to be implemented by the teacher. Strategies followed by T/S can be used by the teacher or student. In the latter case, the teacher may initiate the use of the strategy and later require that the student use it independently.

PROBLEM: Attending. Students are unable to attend to auditory and visual information. They may do such things as talk out of turn or change the topic, be distracted by noise in the hall, fidget, or poke others. It is important to note that students may maintain eye contact and appear to be listening and actually not be attending.

Strategies
- Remove unnecessary distractions, such as pencils and books. Limit background noise at first and gradually increase it to more normal levels. (T)
- Provide visual cues to attend (e.g., have a sign on student's desk with the word or pictured symbol for behaviors, such as LOOK or LISTEN. Point to the sign when students are off task). (T)
- Limit the amount of information on a page. (T/S)
- Adjust assignments to the length of students' attention span so that they can complete tasks successfully. (T)
- Focus students' attention on specific information: "I'm going to read a story and ask *WHO* is in the story." (T)

PROBLEM: Language Comprehension or Following Directions. Students have difficulty understanding language that is spoken rapidly, is complex, or is lengthy.

Strategies
- Limit amount of information presented — perhaps to 1 or 2 sentences. (T/S)
- Use more concrete language. (T)
- Teach students to ask for clarification or repetitions or for information to be given at a slower rate. (T/S)
- Use pictures or written words to cue students: Use a picture of a chair and the written word *sit* if you want the students to exhibit that behavior. (T)
- Pair manual signs, gestures, or pictures with verbal information. (T/S)
- Act out directions: if the student is to collect papers and put them in a designated spot, demonstrate how this should be done. (T)
- Use cognitive mapping (Gold, 1984): Diagram ideas in order of importance or sequence to clarify content graphically. This also helps students to see part-whole relationships. (T/S)

Many of the strategies listed under memory and attending can also be used to improve language comprehension.

PROBLEM: Memory. Students are unable to retain information they have heard or read. They may not remember where to go or what materials to use.

Strategies
- Include pictures or visual cues with oral information, since this multisensory input strengthens the information and provides various ways to recall it. (T/S)

Figure 15-1 suggests a method of providing visual cues to complete a mathematical process if students cannot remember all the steps.
- Use visual imagery. Have students form a mental picture of information that is presented orally. Retrieval of the visual images may trigger the recall of oral information (Clark et al., 1984; Rose, Cundick, and Higbee, 1983). (T/S)

Table 15-1 (continued).

- Use verbal rehearsal. After the visual or auditory information is presented have the students "practice" it (repeat it) and *listen to themselves* before they act on it (Dawson, Hallahan, Reeve, and Ball, 1980; Rose et al., 1983). (T/S)
- Limit the amount of information presented so that students can retain and retrieve it. (T/S)
- Provide a matrix for students to refer to if they have difficulty recalling information (Number Fact Chart). (T/S)
- Have the student take notes or record information on tape. (T/S)
- Underline key words in a passage for emphasis. (T/S)
- Provide a log book to record assignments or daily events. (T/S)
- Provide a printed or pictured schedule of daily activities, locations, and materials needed. (T/S)
- Role-play or pantomine stories or procedures to strengthen the information to be remembered. (T/S)
- Write down key information to be remembered, such as who, what, when. (T/S) See Figure 15-2.

PROBLEM: Retrieving Information that Has Been Stored in Memory.
Strategies
- Have students gesture or role-play. They may be able to act out a situation that has occurred but not have adequate verbal language to describe it. (T/S)
- Provide visual or auditory cues: "Is it _____ or _____?" or give the beginning sound of a word. (T)
- Include written multiple choice cues or pictures in worksheets. (T)
- Teach students to compensate for word-finding problems by describing the function, size, or other attributes of items to be recalled. (See Chapter 11 for semantic feature analysis guide.) (T/S)

PROBLEM: Sequencing. Students have difficulty understanding, recognizing, displaying, or describing a sequence of events presented orally or visually.
Strategies
- Limit the number of steps in a task. (T/S)
- Present part of a sequence and have students finish it. (T)
- Show or discuss one step of the sequence (lesson) at a time. (T)
- Give general cues with each step: "What should you do first? second?" (T)
- Have students repeat multistep directions and listen to themselves before attempting a task. (T/S)
- Provide pictures or a written sequence of steps to remember: Tape a cue card to the desk with words or pictures of materials needed for a lesson, then expand original written directions. For example, if the direction was "Underline the words in each sentence in which *ou* or *ow* stands for the vowel sound. Then write the two words that have the same vowel sound," change it to "(1) Read the sentence; (2) underline *ou* and *ow* words; (3) read the underlined words; (4) find the two words that have the same vowel sounds; (5) write these two words on the lines below the sentence. (T)
- Tell students how many steps are in a task: "I'm going to tell you *three* things to do." (Hold up three fingers.) (T)
- Act out a sequence of events to clarify information. (T/S)
- Provide sample items describing how to proceed through parts of a worksheet. (T)
- Number the steps in a written direction and have the students cross off each step as it is completed. (T/S)

Table 15-1 (continued).

- Teach students to refer to directions if they are unsure of the task. (T/S)

PROBLEM: Thought Organization. Students have difficulty organizing thoughts in oral or written language. Students may not have adequate labels or vocabulary to convey a clear message; they may tend to ramble without getting to the point.

Strategies
- Attempt to limit impulsive responses by encouraging the students to take "thinking time" before they answer. (T/S)
- Have students organize information by using categories, such as who, what, when, where. (T/S) (Emphasize each of these separately if necessary.) This strategy can be used in an expanded form to write a story. See Figure 15-2.
- Teach students a sequence of steps to aid in verbal organization: have the students use cue cards with written pictured steps when formulating an answer. (T/S) See Figure 15-3.
- Focus on one type of information at a time (e.g., the main idea). (T/S)
- Decrease rambling by having students express a thought "in one sentence." (T/S)

PROBLEM: Generalization. Students learn a skill or concept but have difficulty applying it to other situations (e.g., they may count a group of coins in a structured mathematics lesson but not be able to count their money for lunch).

Strategies
- Teach the structure or format of a task (e.g., *how to* complete a worksheet or mathematics problem). (T)
- Maintain a known format and change the content of a task to help students see a relationship: Two pictures are presented and students must say if they are in the same category, or have the same initial sound; a worksheet format requires filling in blanks with words or numbers. (T)
- Change the format of the task: Have students solve mathematics facts on a worksheet as well as on flash cards. (T)
- Have completed sample worksheets in a notebook serve as models indicating how to proceed. (T/S)
- Demonstrate how skills can be used throughout the day: Discuss how students rely on the clock or a schedule to get up in the morning, begin school, or catch a bus. (T)
- Role-play in situations that simulate those which students may encounter, emphasizing the generalization of specific skills taught: completing school assignments and going to the store may involve the same strategies (making a list or asking for help). (T)

Students should now be able to do the following:
- Use even more materials and begin to know which materials are used in which situations. Visual discrimination, attention, and memory come into play when students have to select the correct book or homework paper to take to the reading group.
- Do various kinds of classroom tasks that require different skills, (e.g., read and then write a response, give an oral response, listen and repeat information, follow oral or written directions, complete worksheets, build block designs following patterns, copy from the board, discuss parts of an oral story or picture story, remember a past event).
- Work independently for longer periods. Students need greater concentration, self-motivation, and understanding to complete

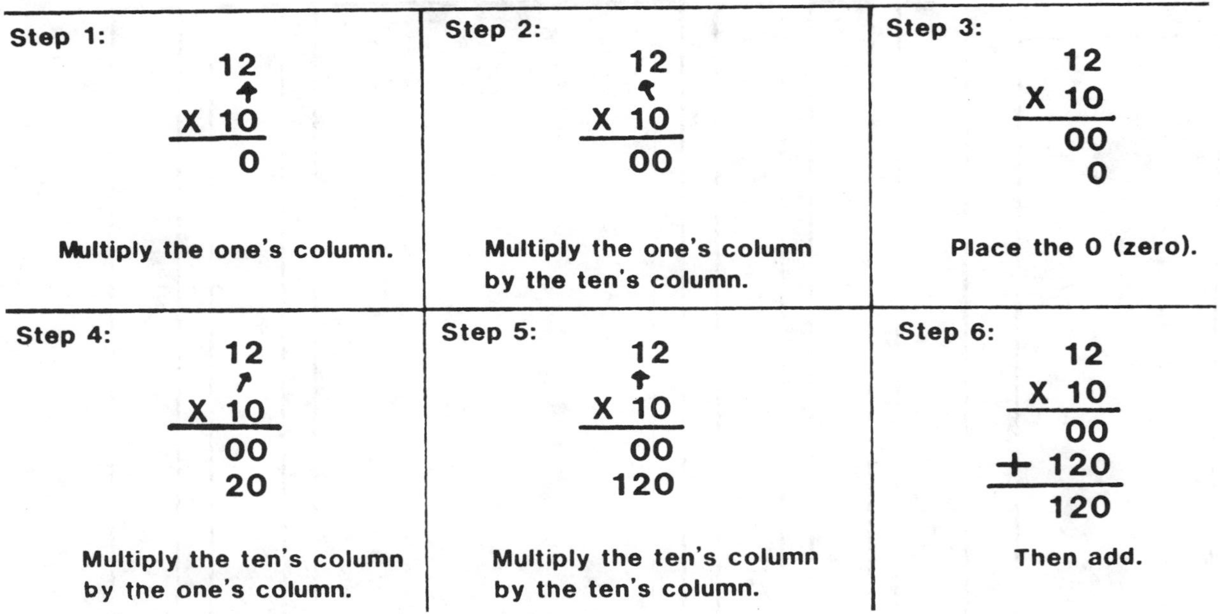

Step 1:

$$\begin{array}{r} 12 \\ \times\ 10 \\ \hline 0 \end{array}$$

Multiply the one's column.

Step 2:

$$\begin{array}{r} 12 \\ \times\ 10 \\ \hline 00 \end{array}$$

Multiply the one's column by the ten's column.

Step 3:

$$\begin{array}{r} 12 \\ \times\ 10 \\ \hline 00 \\ 0 \end{array}$$

Place the 0 (zero).

Step 4:

$$\begin{array}{r} 12 \\ \times\ 10 \\ \hline 00 \\ 20 \end{array}$$

Multiply the ten's column by the one's column.

Step 5:

$$\begin{array}{r} 12 \\ \times\ 10 \\ \hline 00 \\ 120 \end{array}$$

Multiply the ten's column by the ten's column.

Step 6:

$$\begin{array}{r} 12 \\ \times\ 10 \\ \hline 00 \\ +\ 120 \\ \hline 120 \end{array}$$

Then add.

Figure 15-1. Strategy for *sequential problem solving in arithmetic.* This strategy can be used with students who demonstrate understanding of a mathematical concept, such as two-digit multiplication without regrouping, but are inconsistent when completing problems independently. This may be due to difficulty in recalling or sequencing steps. As students' proficiency increases, the number of steps decreases. Important Note: Color coding of key aspects of each step is helpful (e.g., in step 1, the arrow and the product of 0×2 can be in red).

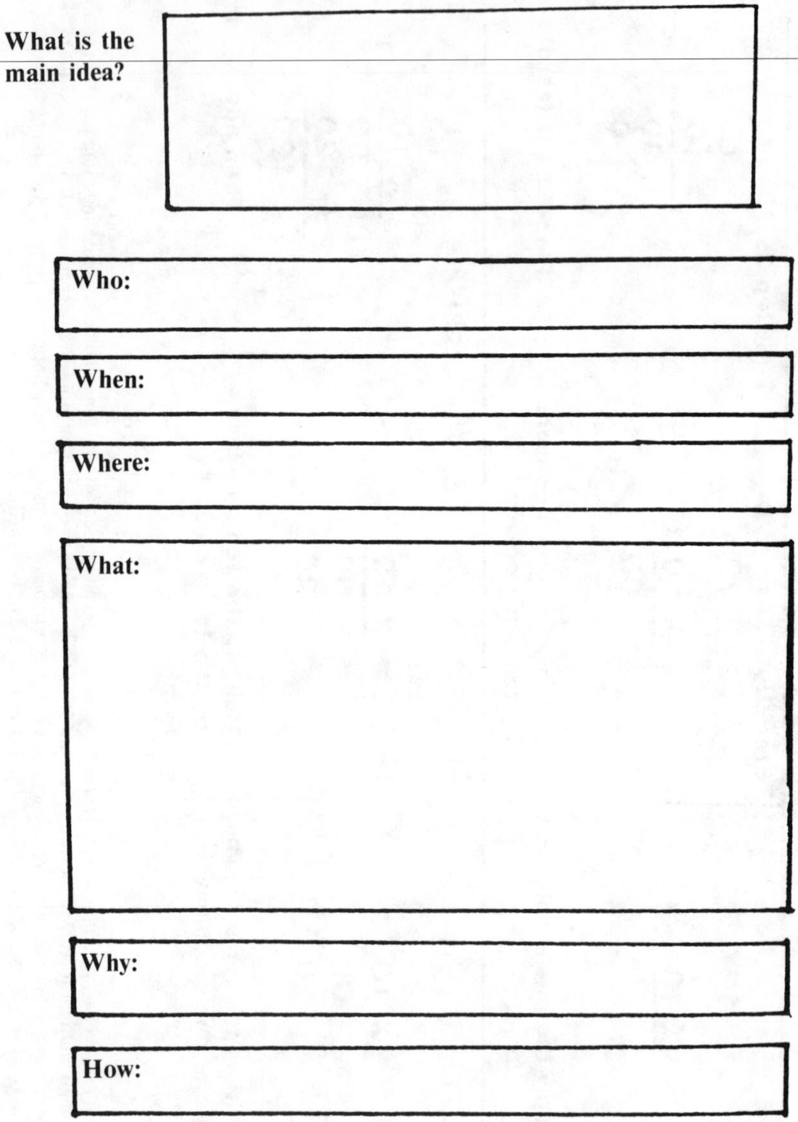

What is the main idea?

Who:

When:

Where:

What:

Why:

How:

Figure 15-2. Strategy for *organizing linguistic information*. This strategy can be used with students who have difficulty identifying key facts of the story, identifying the main idea, or summarizing the story. This can also be used to assist students in organizing information.

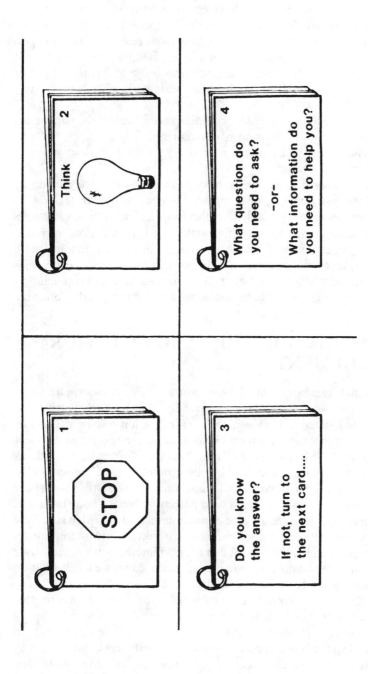

Figure 15–3. Strategy for *active processing of information.* This strategy can be used with students who do not organize their thoughts sufficiently to address a question or a problem (e.g., verbally ramble or blurt out an answer without thinking). The index cards illustrate how to organize thoughts for problem solving. Have students refer to cards as needed.

work on their own in a busy environment.
- Become more flexible: change activities, follow a schedule, complete an activity that requires one response mode (e.g., writing) and begin a second that requires another (e.g., talking), follow different procedures while completing worksheets, go to specified parts of the room for different lessons, and work with several staff members.
- Complete longer and more complex assignments if the patient can maintain comprehension of the material.
- Generalize at least simple procedures.
- Work more rapidly.
- Tolerate some stress, such as having to work more quickly, complete longer assignments, or recognize the need to use strategies.

The teacher may work with other therapists and develop new strategies to help students maintain cognitive skills, such as attention, memory, thought organization, and problem solving, while they are doing more complex tasks. Some students often need help to interact socially with classmates, and teachers must use prescriptive teaching and task analysis to teach social cognition. These techniques are discussed in the following section.

SOCIAL INTEGRATION AND BEHAVIOR MANAGEMENT

Although rehabilitation of head injured children has traditionally emphasized physical restoration, cognitive deficits have lately received the attention they deserve. However, little consideration has been given to psychosocial problems which most profoundly interfere with readjustment (Eiben et al., 1984; Rutter, 1981) to home and friends, as well as performance in school or vocational settings (Bond, 1975; Thomsen, 1974).

To be socially effective, an individual must possess insight and have the ability to "read" subtleties in communication, such as body language, facial expression, and tone of voice. Head injured students often lack these skills as well as the confidence necessary to initiate interaction and to participate in social situations. When they do interact with others, their approach may be inappropriate; they may totally dominate a conversation or not know when to terminate an exchange.

Several factors may influence their behavior. After an accident or illness, head injured individuals become the center of attention in the family and in the acute-care hospital setting; thus they have little opportunity to practice or expand more ordinary interactions with peers and adults. As a result, their behavior can become very demanding and controlling. The realization that their intellectual abilities and physical appearance have been altered by the trauma may also affect patients' behavior. Personality changes caused by the brain injury itself can further cómplicate the social behavior of head injured individuals.

Integrating Students Into Classroom Group Activities

The classroom provides head injured students with structured experiences in group interaction. Teachers can design a curriculum that addresses social and emotional recovery as well as cognitive and academic development. Since many rehabilitation centers provide therapy on an individual basis, the classroom may well be the head injured student's first exposure to group situations. This may be stressful and cause them to exhibit behaviors that can be misinterpreted as noncompliance. Because they are confused or anxious, students may act out (Rutter, 1981), refuse to participate, or be unable to follow directions. *Avoidance* behaviors, such as yawning, asking irrelevant questions, disturbing peers, humming, or playing with objects in their desks, may represent efforts to divert attention from their classroom activity and can indicate a lack of confidence in their ability to perform. These individuals may no longer know or recall expected school behaviors. In addition, *memory* and *word finding* problems often interfere with their ability to make quick, accurate replies to questions or express themselves clearly. *Overload* may also occur when the student's performance deteriorates sharply under the burden of longer sessions or increased amounts of information.

An initial period of individual classroom instruction or evaluation can ease the tension for head injured students. They can be aware of the presence of other students but not feel obligated to interact with them. The frequency and duration of these one-to-one sessions will depend on students' abilities as well as on the availability of the teacher.

The teacher should next place students in groups of two to four peers, selecting activities that assure the students' frequent success. The group goals of these students may be different from those of the others, and they may be asked to participate in only a part of the lesson. The teacher must note if students do the following:

- Maintain visual and auditory attention during periods of instruction or are distracted by objects or other students.
- Raise their hands prior to asking a question, making a response, or adding to the discussion.
- Stay on the topic or interrupt the lesson with irrelevant comments.

Table 15-2. Compenstory Strategies for Behavioral and Social Problems in a Classroom Setting

Key: Strategies followed by the letter T are to be implemented by the teacher. Strategies followed by T/S can be used by the teacher or student. In the latter case, the teacher may initiate the use of the strategy and later require that the student use it independently.

PROBLEM: Disorientation or Confusion.

Strategies
• Provide an uncluttered, quiet environment. (T)
• Provide printed or pictorial charts, schedules, or classroom maps that describe routines and rules of expected behaviors. Review these before each session and as needed throughout the day. (T)
• Maintain consistent staff, room arrangement, and materials. (T)
• Label significant objects and areas; provide name tags for staff. (T)
• Redirect undesirable behavior by focusing students' attention on tasks that are sufficiently interesting to break the pattern of disruptive or perseverative responses. (Note: Do *not* use this technique if the student's behavior is attention seeking. Consultation with a behavior psychologist may be indicated.) (T)
• Teach students to look for permanent landmarks and name the landmarks when they come to them. (T/S)
• Have students verbalize how to go to a specific place *before* starting or while moving. (T/S)
• Use a buddy system. (T/S)

PROBLEM: Transitions—changing activities (e.g., moving from a reading group to a mathematics lesson or from a "free" period to a learning session).

Strategies
• Provide verbal cues: "In five minutes it will be time for math," "After our reading lesson, we will go to lunch." (T)
• "Walk through" transitions with the students: Return the reading text to the desk, take out the math book, and move to the appropriate area for the math lesson. (T)
• Encourage students to refer to printed or pictorial schedules with changes of activities, materials, or lesson locations. (T/S)
• Have students observe peers for cues for what to do next. (T/S)

PROBLEM: Beginning an Activity. Students may not remember what to do, know what to expect, or know if they possess the skills needed to perform accurately.

Strategies
• Explain the purpose of the lesson; relate following directions to functional, everyday situations, such as assembling a model car or reading a recipe. (T)
• Review printed or pictorial descriptions of how to do a task to relieve tensions that result from the student's not knowing what is expected. (T/S)
• Talk through several examples to help individuals get started. (T)
• Review pictorial or printed rules of behavior before each lesson: "Look, listen, raise your hand." (T/S)
• Praise students once they have begun a task and remind them that they are capable of completing the activity. (T)
• Role-play or tell students what to say when they are initiating social contacts with peers. (T)

PROBLEM: Ending an Activity.

Strategies
• Emphasize closure of activities by giving students jobs such as collecting papers, cleaning up materials, or writing in their log books. (T/S)

Table 15-2 (continued).

- Encourage students to observe the behavior of others as tasks end. (T/S)
- List steps to the task and check them off when completed; emphasize where they are in relation to the final step. (T/S)
- List end-of-session behaviors: "Put papers in blue box, return to desk." (T)

PROBLEM: Impulsive Responses. Head injured students often call out answers during lessons, grab materials, begin activities before directions are provided, have difficulty taking turns, and may even leave the room or lesson without warning.

Strategies

- Place unnecessary materials out of sight or out of reach. (T)
- Discuss rules and their importance at the beginning of the lesson. (T)
- Explain how students' impulsive acts (e.g., calling out) disturb others. (T)
- Role-play appropriate responses (e.g., raising hand). Place a sign on the student's desk with a picture of a hand and point to this when the student interrupts. (T)
- Employ "stop-action" technique: Immediately stop individuals from disrupting an activity, encourage them to verbalize an alternative behavior, and have them follow through appropriately. (T)
- Provide time at the end of a session for students to tell personal stories or jokes. (T)

PROBLEM: Recognizing the Need for Help or Asking for Help.

Strategies

- Make students aware of what they can and cannot do: Expand tasks that are done successfully by adding one step that will be "harder." (T)
- Make asking for help a student goal and reinforce this heavily. (T)
- Attach cue cards to desk: "Raise your hand for help." (T/S)
- Decrease daydreaming that results from an inability to proceed by asking direct questions or by providing cue cards: "Are you stuck?" "Is that clear?" (T/S)
- Model desired behavior; role-play situations. (T)

PROBLEM: Working Independently. Head injured individuals may be hesitant to perform, even when they are able to do the task.

Strategies

- Review directions or sample items. (T)
- Provide a written sequence to follow and thus circumvent memory problems and anxiety. (T/S)
- Assure them that they *can* complete the task. (T)
- Select only a portion of the task or short assignments to be completed independently. (T/S)
- Point to a sign ("Return to work") when students stop working. (T)
- Use a timer intermittently, and reward students who are working when it rings. (T)
- Provide additional time for students who work slowly to complete tasks. (T)

PROBLEM: Self-Criticism or Perseveration. Students may erase excessively, tear up papers, redo activities in an effort to perform with pretraumatic efficiency, or refuse to participate in structured lessons.

Strategies

- Emphasize what the individuals *can* do and point out progress that they have made: Compare recent past and present work. (T)
- Chart achievement of goals to build self-confidence. (T/S)
- Limit perseverative behavior by using verbal directions ("Erase only once") or by focusing attention on less threatening tasks. (T)

- Refuse to participate, thus perhaps indicating a lack of confidence or an emerging awareness of deficits.
- Sit quietly for an appropriate amount of time.
- Demonstrate avoidance behaviors.

Head injured students may have more difficulty focusing attention in activities that involve the *entire* class. Because of increased distractions, fewer opportunities for active participation, and the need to attend to and interact with more people, they may become "saturated" and simply be unable to take in additional information. Because lack of self-confidence also influences their reactions in these situations (Rampp, 1980), avoidance behaviors may increase and become more intense.

In summary, severely head injured students reentering a classroom learning situation typically show a range of social and behavioral problems more pronounced than those of peers who have not suffered brain damage.

Behavioral Techniques

Our experience suggests that traditional behavior management techniques (rewarding desirable and ignoring undesirable behavior) (Kazdin, 1984; Kerr and Nelson, 1983; Wallace and Kauffman, 1973) are often ineffective in modifying the behavior of head injured students in the classroom. This system relies heavily on an individual's ability to pick up cues from the positive actions of others, to understand cause-effect relationships, to remember information, to generalize from one situation to another, and to control impulsive responses or reactions. All of these may be difficult for head injured students. Hence, if a teacher establishes a contingency plan by which students can earn a reward for performing a targeted behavior (e.g., hand raising), head injured students may not be able to respond appropriately because of impulsiveness, an inability to conceive the consequences of their actions, or an inability to recall the targeted response.

A more direct approach to establishing appropriate response is often effective with head injured students. If a patient (for example, a child named Todd) is continually rocking in his chair, a standard behavioral technique would be to ignore him and reinforce students who are properly seated or to reinforce Todd when he stops rocking or exhibits another "positive" behavior. Head injured individuals often require more straightforward directions, such as: "Todd, please sit with your chair flat on the floor." This may become Todd's goal during a lesson and may need to be repeated frequently. Table 15-2 lists strategies including rules, charts, printed cues, and other direct approaches that help head injured students establish appropriate behaviors.

Traditional behavior management methods should be used in conjunction with the more direct, cognitive approaches. However, the teacher must be quite explicit when giving positive reinforcement: "Good, Todd, your chair is flat on the floor," or "Steve, remember when you had trouble joining the reading group? Today you came to the table on your own! That's great!"

Team planning (including the teacher, psychologist, other rehabilitation staff and family members) is essential if behavior management systems are to be tailored to individuals' needs and carried out consistently. Chapter 13 includes a more detailed discussion of behavior modification techniques that are effective with head injured students.

Strategies

Team members introduce strategies to help students perform more effectively in social situations as well as in academic tasks. The purposes of and general approaches to teaching strategies are described earlier in the chapter. Because the structure of social situations is less obvious than that in which students perform more formal school tasks, it may be difficult to target specific behavioral problems when students' social responses or interactions are inappropriate.

Table 15-2 presents a list of situations and behaviors that are problematic for head injured students in school and provides corresponding strategies that help them function more effectively. Individual strategies may be used in a variety of situations, and their use may be the focus of a lesson for a head injured student. As in the use of behavior management systems, strategies should be developed and carried out by the team of professionals who work with respective students.

Unstructured "Free Time"

The "rules" of social behavior are far less clear during unstructured, free periods (lunch, transitions, gym, class, holidays) than during more structured classroom activities. Lacking established routines or descriptions of expected behaviors, head injured students can become disoriented and overloaded (Boll, 1983; Rampp, 1980) and may react by crying, hiding, refusing to participate, or becoming verbally or physically abusive (Rutter, 1981). Lezak (1978) suggests that these adverse reactions can be avoided by shortening or eliminating unstructured activities (such as gym or swimming), by providing structured tasks (e.g., for free periods before, during, and after school), and by controlling environmental distractions (e.g., having students eat in the classroom rather than in the cafeteria).

Head injured students' lack of judgment becomes apparent during unstructured periods. They may randomly walk about the room, disrupting play situations or conversations, and may initiate social contacts by kicking over block buildings, dismantling puzzles, or changing the station on someone's radio. These individuals often attempt to control a play situation and may insist on portraying the dominant character (father, doctor) in any role play. During board games, they enforce their own rules, insist on being first, have difficulty waiting for their turn, or, because of confusion or overload, simply stop playing within a very short interval.

The teacher can provide guidance and model appropriate behaviors during these free periods (Kerr and Nelson, 1983). Two students may be encouraged to play a game under the direction of an adult who clearly explains the rules and demonstrates the procedures. As the head injured individual learns to take turns, follow rules, and complete the game, one or two additional peers can be included, and the adult supervision can be gradually faded out. "Stop action," described in Table 15–2, is an effective technique in these game-playing situations.

Psychosocial Intervention

Individuals who have incurred brain damage are often painfully aware of their intellectual and memory deficits (Lezak, 1978). Even if they were confident students before their accident, they may now approach school and learning with a great deal of anxiety and discomfort. Unfortunately, some individuals cannot verbalize their concerns and may exhibit avoidance behaviors that disguise their fears. These students may also have difficulty accepting criticism or suggestions about how to improve their performance. They may become extremely critical of others and thus divert attention away from what they are doing. They may even direct criticism toward the teacher with remarks such as, "You forgot to cross your 't' " or "You always help Jeff more than me!" A word of caution: Serious emotional problems are not uncommon following severe head injury (Rutter, 1981) and require referral to an appropriately trained social worker, psychologist, psychiatrist, or other qualified professional (see Chapter 14).

Classroom activities can encourage communication about and awareness of various disabilities and learning or behavioral problems. Such program activities can include watching movies or puppet shows, or reading books that deal with physical and intellectual differences and deficits. Teachers should first guide the group into a discussion of the great diversity among people, and then move into a more specific discussion about the following topics:

- Each individual's positive traits, as well as characteristics that the person might like to change or improve.
- Differences in learning styles: Students may learn more effectively from visual information or auditory information, or from a combination of the two. They may require multiple experiences to stabilize understanding of a concept.
- Everyone has a need for strategies to facilitate memory and learning (e.g., some people write down phone numbers or addresses, whereas others may repeat the information out loud to aid storage and retrieval).
- Physical and cognitive disabilities. The instructor can supply factual information and encourage empathy by exposing the group to experiences such as guiding a wheelchair, communicating through gesture, or examining a book printed in Braille.
- The consequences of impulsive acts, such as running across the street, playing with matches, or pushing someone aside to get out of an elevator. Specific questions can stimulate discussion: "What should you do if you find a pack of matches?" Pictures can be presented that illustrate individuals' solving problems inappropriately, and students can role play alternative solutions. A fireman or policeman can visit and describe how to approach problematic situations.
- The head injured students' interactions with people in the community. Friends, neighbors, and acquaintances who knew them before the accident may not be sure how to react to them now, and social contacts may decrease (Rutter, 1981). Through role play, students explore ways to encourage others to feel more comfortable with them and practice answers to questions people may ask about their injury or disability.

These discussions can help head injured students improve their self-awareness and self-concept and approach academic and life tasks with more confidence. This information can also help members of the group who have not suffered head injuries by increasing their understanding of themselves and helping them interact more comfortably with students who have incurred brain damage.

HEAD INJURED STUDENTS VERSUS STUDENTS WITH LEARNING DISABILITIES OR IN MAINSTREAM EDUCATION: A COMPARISON

To date, there are no published research reports comparing cognitive problems of "learning disabled" students to those of students who have suffered severe closed head injuries. When noting similarities between the learning styles of these two populations, the characteristics that are unique to each individual should also be kept in mind. In general, however, learning disabled and head injured students often have problems with attention, impulse control, organization of thoughts, location of objects or themselves in space, skill integration, problem solving, generalization and seeing relationships or associations, abstract concepts and complex ideas, and social judgment.

These students may benefit from *similar* teaching techniques, such as those discussed in Cruikshank, Bentzen, Ratzeburg, and Tannhauser (1961), Johnson and Myklebust (1967), and Bush and Giles (1969):

- Task analysis (analyzing and teaching skills involved in doing a task) and synthesis (integrating those skills) (Hallahan et al., 1983). For instance, reading instructions may address the following: *Visual* and *auditory* attention, discrimination, sequencing, and memory, receptive and expressive *language* concepts, and *spatial orientation or organization.*
- A multisensory approach to teaching and learning. Linking visual, auditory, language, gross motor, and fine motor–kinesthetic skills clarifies and strengthens information. *However,* head injured individuals may become distracted when this approach is used!
- Approaching learning from one processing mode (visual) more than from another (auditory) to accommodate learning styles.
- Use of strategies to compensate for cognitive deficits (Hallahan et al., 1983).
- Analyzing and synthesizing the dynamics of social situations.

Head injured students often perform *differently* from other students:

1. They can be more impulsive, more hyperactive, more distractible, more verbally intrusive because of confusion or lack of internal control.

2. Discrepancies in ability levels may be more extreme. Learning problems may exist even though some skills remain relatively unaffected by the brain injury. The level of reading comprehension, for instance, might be four years lower than that of spelling ability.

3. They often learn more rapidly than learning disabled students. If they are *relearning* material, they may need only to be reacquainted with a process or concept to integrate the information and use it effectively. Their knowledge of the spoken and written code is frequently superior to that of the learning disabled student.

4. They may have more severe problems generalizing and integrating skills or information. These problems may require more individualized teaching or reteaching of the same skills as the content of lessons changes.

5. They often do not become independent thinkers.

6. They may not be able to process even the limited amounts of information presented to learning disabled students; their comprehension deteriorates markedly as the amount and complexity of material increases.

7. More strategies need to be taught and used to compensate for impaired memory and word-retrieval problems, to aid retention of information, and to improve the quality of communication.

8. Problems with organization of thoughts, cause-effect relationships, and problem solving may be more severe.

9. They may rely on pretraumatically habituated learning strategies that are no longer effective and may resist or reject new techniques that the teacher presents.

10. They may retain the premorbid self-concept of a perfectly normal child whose automatic responses are usually appropriate and thus have difficulty realizing that their behavior patterns have changed and need to be adjusted.

11. Markedly uneven and unpredictable progress can occur because of continuing recovery (Rutter, 1981); programs must remain flexible so that possibly sharp and frequent changes can be accommodated.

For school programs to be effective, head injured students must become aware of their present levels of performance (Prigatano et al., 1984). Children as young as 6 years of age may need to realize that they are different from the way they were before the trauma. This requires a level of maturity that often exceeds developmental expectations, but school programs such as those described earlier can focus on this.

Depending on their level of recovery and their degree of confusion, older students may either sense that they are different but not understand the ramifications of that difference or, as we have mentioned, deny the need for rehabilitation. Through the use of familiar school tasks, however, the teacher can help these students to realize that they need special assistance and to become more cooperative in all parts of their program.

TEACHING VERY YOUNG CHILDREN WITH HEAD INJURIES

There are many issues that make it difficult to identify cognitive problems of very young head injured children:

- Premorbid developmental levels and intellectual potential usually have not been formally evaluated.
- Families may recall general capabilities but not details of previous performance.

- Unknown life experiences have uniquely influenced each child's information base.
- Pretraumatic abilities were inconsistent because skills were just developing.
- Learning styles and characteristic behaviors have not been established.

Although teaching is usually based on relating information to students' experiences, this approach is difficult to do with head injured young children (Chadwick, Rutter, Thompson, and Shaffer, 1981). Teachers must thus present basic experiences and learning tasks and then observe students' performance to recognize functional abilities or to target impairments. Once *present* language capabilities are known, for instance, word-finding difficulties can be identified.

Diagnostic teaching in an appropriate, *structured* preschool or primary classroom can help to evaluate students' attention and distractability, language concepts, impulsiveness, flexibility, rate of learning and performing, judgment, memory, ability to generalize, and social skills. Eventually teachers will be able to distinguish between emerging, delayed, or impaired skills and to identify learning patterns or deviations from present learning styles. With knowledge of typical developmental milestones and through the use of prescriptive teaching and task analysis, teachers can evaluate *present* functioning and develop programs in which learning skills are expanded. Teacher intervention is often necessary to keep students on-task, reduce frustration, and enhance learning.

Issues involved in formally assessing young children are discussed in Chapter 9.

PLANNING FOR DISCHARGE
TO COMMUNITY SCHOOL SETTINGS

When severely head injured students' attention, concentration, thought organization, memory, and communication skills begin to stabilize, plans can be made to place them in school programs in their home communities. There are several issues that team members must consider when making these school placements:

- These students usually need special education supports.
- Present special education categories do not accommodate the learning styles of most head injured students.
- Since test performance of head injured students must be interpreted differently from those of other students, school placements should not be made on the basis of test scores alone (see Chapter 9).

- Team members should visit the community school to identify expected behaviors that students should develop before discharge.

This topic is discussed further in Chapter 17.

CONTACTS WITH PARENTS

Parents of severely head injured students have specific concerns about the education of their children. Many of these children were in mainstream classes before the trauma, and their families assumed they would progress normally through the school system. After an accident everyone wants to believe that recovery will allow head injured students to return to their previous classrooms.

It is difficult for families to realize the child's functioning has changed, especially if he or she walks and talks appropriately, and that special education support may now be necessary. Teachers must therefore explain to them the impact that cognitive impairments have on school performance. Conferences with parents can be highly emotional, as parents may react to this information by crying, denying their child's deficits, or expressing anger at the teacher or at the program in general for not making their child better.

Teachers must understand above all that they are dealing with parents at probably the worst time of their lives. While adapting to a "different" child with a new set of needs, they are progressing through the stages of mourning for the child that they lost at the time of the accident (see Chapter 3). This emotional stress will affect their ability to comprehend what teachers are telling them. The amount of information that both teachers and parents ask for or give may vary from conference to conference. Anxious parents may repeatedly ask questions like these: "Will Johnny return to his regular class?" "What grade level will Susie be at in June?" But teachers must not make promises and must answer: "I don't know right now, because we can't predict the pace or extent of recovery" or "I *can* tell you about your child's *present* performance." Unlike other rehabilitation professionals, teachers can explain children's difficulties to parents in terms they understand: showing parents their child's classroom materials and activities often helps to clarify the student's present abilities and the need for rehabilitation services.

Teachers can help family members deal with their head injured child or sibling more effectively by relating cognitive deficits and programming techniques to the home environment (Fuld and Fisher, 1977). Attention, thought organization, and memory are used when students discuss a television show, set the table, or get clothes and materials ready for the next day. Parents should not ask a child with memory problems to do too many discrete tasks consecutively (e.g.,"Get the blue pants in your room and then empty the waste baskets"). Teachers can give them more effective ways to communicate with their child and teach them to use strategies at home that their child has learned in school.

Finally, teachers should encourage parents to make classroom observations to understand better both their child's abilities and the techniques that help the child perform more adequately. Teachers can maintain communication with the family by using the log book to record and describe daily events, significant behaviors, and treatment techniques (see Chapter 11). Knowledge of experiences that the child has at home also helps teachers and therapists establish functional and meaningful program goals and activities.

REFERENCES

Boll, T. J. (1983). Minor head injury in children— out of sight but not out of mind. *Journal of Clinical Psychology, 12*(1), 74–80.

Bond, M. R. (1975). Assessment of psychosocial outcome after severe head injury. In R. Porter and D. W. Fitzsimons (Eds.), *Outcome of severe damage to the central nervous system.* Ciba Foundation Symposium 34 (new series) (pp. 141–157). Amsterdam: Elsevier.

Bryan, T. H., and Bryan, J. H. (1978). *Understanding learning disabilities* (2nd ed.). Sherman Oaks, CA: Alfred.

Bush, W. J., and Giles, M. T. (1969). *Aids to psycholinguistic teaching.* Columbus, OH: Charles E. Merrill.

Chadwick, O., Rutter, M., Thompson, J., and Shaffer, D. (1981). Intellectual performance and reading skills after localized head injury in childhood. *Journal of Child Psychology and Psychiatry, 22,* 117–139.

Clark, F. L., Deshler, D. D., Schumaker, J. B., Alley, G. R., and Warner, M. M. (1984). Visual imagery and self-questioning: Strategies to improve comprehension of written material. *Journal of Learning Disabilities, 17,* 145–149.

Cruikshank, W. M., Bentzen, F. A., Ratzeburg, F. H., and Tannhauser, M. T. (1961). *A teaching method for brain-injured and hyperactive children. A demonstration-pilot study.* Syracuse, NY: Syracuse University Press.

Dawson, M. M., Hallahan, D. P., Reeve, R. E., and Ball, D. W. (1980). The effect of reinforcement and verbal rehearsal on selective attention in learning disabled children. *Journal of Abnormal Child Psychology, 8*(1), 133–144.

Eiben, C. F., Anderson, T. P., Lockman, L., Matthews, D. J., Dryja, R., Martin, J., Burrill, C., Gottesman, N., O'Brian, P., and Witte, L. (1984). Functional outcome of closed head injury in children and young adults. *Archives of Physical Medicine and Rehabilitation, 65,* 168–170.

Fuld, P. A., and Fisher, P. (1977). Recovery of intellectual ability after closed head-injury. *Developmental Medicine and Child Neurology, 19,* 495–502.

Gold, P. C. (1984). Cognitive mapping. *Academic Therapy, 19*(3), 227–284.

Hallahan, D. P., Hall, R. J., Ianna, S. O., Kneedler, J. W. L., Loper, A. B., and Reeve, R. E. (1983). Summary of research findings at the University of Virginia Learning Disabilities Research Institute. *Exceptional Education Quarterly, 4*(1), 95–114.

Hartlage, L. C., and Telzrow, C. R. (1983). The neuropsychological basis of educational intervention. *Journal of Learning Disabilities, 16,* 521–528.

Johnson, D. J., and Myklebust, H. R. (1967). *Learning disabilities: Educational principles and practices.* New York: Grune & Stratton.

Kazdin, A. E. (1984). *Behavior modification in applied settings.* Homewood, IL: Dorsey.

Kerr, M. M., and Nelson, C. M. (1983). *Strategies for managing behavior problems in the classroom.* Columbus, OH: Charles E. Merrill.

Lezak, M. D. (1978). Subtle sequelae of brain damage. *American Journal of Physical Medicine, 57*(1), 9–15.

Meichenbaum, D. (1977). *Cognitive-behavior modification: An integrative approach.* New York: Plenum.

Prigatano, G. P., Fordyce, D. J., Zeiner, H. K., Roueche, J. R., Pepping, M., and Wood, B. C. (1984). Neuropsychological rehabilitation after closed head injury in young adults. *Journal of Neurology, Neurosurgery, and Psychiatry, 47,* 505–513.

Rampp, D. L. (1980). *Auditory processing and learning disabilities.* Lincoln, NE: Cliff Notes.

Rose, M. C., Cundick, B. P., and Higbee, K. L. (1983). Verbal rehearsal and visual imagery. Mnemonic aids for learning disabled children. *Journal of Learning Disabilities, 16,* 352–354.

Rutter, M. (1981). Psychological sequelae of brain damage in children. *American Journal of Psychiatry, 183,* 1533–1542.

Thomsen, I. V. (1974). The patient with severe head injury and his family: A follow-up study of 50 patients. *Scandinavian Journal of Rehabilitation Medicine, 6,* 180–183.

Torgesen, J. K. (1979). What shall we do with psychological processes? *Journal of Learning Disabilities, 12,* 514–521.

Wallace, G., and Kauffman, J. M. (1973). *Teaching children with learning problems.* Columbus, OH: Charles E. Merrill.

Chapter 16

Career Development

Eva Marie R. Gobble, PhD, CRC, and James C. Pfahl, BS, CRC*

A critical responsibility of the rehabilitation team is to help head injured adolescents prepare for their future careers. Although the focus is on vocational programming, we use the term "career" broadly to include academic, vocational, avocational, familial, and civic roles (Super, 1976). Career planning, in this sense, is the process of developing the client for economic, social, and personal fulfillment (Brolin and Kokaska, 1979). (The term "client" is used in this chapter to refer to those adolescents who receive career programming in rehabilitation or school settings.) For adolescent clients, comprehensive rehabilitation should include vocational therapy with other essential cognitive and physical rehabilitation services. Vocational therapy in this context includes therapeutic activities to facilitate career development.

Head injured adolescents, like their nondisabled peers, experience the normal stress of development from dependent child to independent adult (Havinghurst, 1972). Since employment involves the individual's need for independence and a feeling of responsibility, it is a source of major anxiety. Severely head injured adolescents must additionally learn to compensate for the cognitive and psychosocial deficits that could dramatically reduce their chances for successful employment.

Effective vocational programming requires an understanding of the level of the client's career maturity. In Super's (1957) career development model, the individual progresses through five major life stages: growth (from birth to 14 years), exploration (ages 15 to 24), establishment (ages 25 to 44), maintenance (ages 45 to 64), and decline (ages 65 and up). Career

---

*Authorship listed alphabetically at authors' request.

maturity is the level at which the person has successfully resolved the major issues within a particular career stage. Although disability may have a profound effect on this process, professional guidance can enhance the level or career maturity at any given stage.

Research has shown that vocational success in young adulthood is importantly related to the career maturity of 14 through 18 year olds (Super and Overstreet, 1960), which suggests that head injured adolescents are at a critical stage of their career development. The vocational therapist must plan a program that enhances career maturity during the exploratory stage of development. The major goals to be accomplished during this stage are the following:

- Crystalization of interests
- Self-appraisal of strengths and deficits in relation to an occupational choice
- Development of work experience
- Knowledge of skills needed in occupational preferences
- Acceptance of responsibility in acquiring skills
- Development and implementation of a career plan (Jordan and Heyde, 1979)

Role exploration, occupational trials through part-time jobs, school experiences, and leisure activities are instrumental in accomplishing these goals. Sampling of actual jobs with systematic and accurate feedback helps the individual make more realistic career choices. Counseling may also be necessary to help clients integrate their needs, interests, abilities, and opportunities into a tentative career choice.

For head injured clients, occupational trials and counseling are part of a larger program of vocational therapy, which also includes direct treatment of vocationally relevant cognitive, psychosocial, and motor deficits. In this chapter, we will describe assessment and treatment components of a career development program, including vocational skills training and counseling. We will conclude with a discussion of career planning for clients with and without employment potential. The focus is on severely head injured adolescents with minimal work experience before the injury.

COMPONENTS OF A CAREER DEVELOPMENT PROGRAM

Career development programs involve assessment and treatment components that are most efficiently conducted within a comprehensive interdisciplinary rehabilitation program. The vocational therapists responsible for career development programming may have diverse professional backgrounds but must have skills in analytical instruction and counseling. Additionally, vocational therapists must have a sound knowledge of rehabilitation theory and techniques. At our agency, admission into the program is based on age (at least 15 years), level of cognitive recovery (at least middle stage of recovery, with an attention span of at least 15 minutes), and the need for vocational or avocational programming.

Assessment

The goal of vocational assessment is to identify initial strengths and deficits relevant to vocational planning, placement, and performance. Results of neuropsychological, speech-language, occupational therapy, and educational diagnostics (see Chapter 9) are integrated with vocation-specific evaluations. To focus vocational programing, comprehensive assessment should include informal and formal probes in the following cognitive and psychosocial areas:

- Initiative in setting goals
- Interpersonal skills, including communication
- Self-direction in daily living activities
- Problem-solving ability
- Learning ability for new skills and tasks
- Perceptual skills
- Memory
- Attention span, selective attention, and attentional flexibility
- Orientation to person, place, time, and task
- Organizational abilities
- Emotional lability

Physical and occupational therapists provide detailed descriptions of gross and fine motor functioning and potential. The vocational therapist then plans an evaluation that fits the client's current level of functioning. The results of the initial evaluation are not used to determine vocational placement or predict outcome. Rather they represent a baseline profile of the client's ability to integrate cognitive and motor skills with vocational tasks. The diagnostic vocational evaluation focuses on the following critical vocational behaviors.

Realistic Appraisal of Work Abilities. Career maturity reflects clients' abilities to examine realistically their skills and match those skills with an appropriate occupational choice (Super, 1957). The client's self-concept is integrally tied to self-appraisal of abilities.

Adaptability to Work Demands. In any given job the worker may be required to do any of the following:
- Maintain attention on a repetitive short cycle job
- Move flexibly from one task to another
- Meet precise standards, requirements, or duties on the job
- Follow directions from a supervisor and also independently organize a task
- Make judgments, generalizations, or decisions
- Perform under stressful conditions where working speed and sustained attention are required
- Communicate effectively with other individuals in a work setting (U.S. Department of Labor, 1972)

Self-Direction and Motivation. Employers typically expect good work attitudes and the ability and initiative to identify tasks that need to be accomplished.

Effective Interpersonal and Communication Skills. A majority of the jobs listed in the Dictionary of Occupational Titles require at least adequate communication skills (Field and Field, 1982).

Application of Academic Knowledge. Most entry-level occupations require that the worker have a minimum proficiency in the basic academic skills of language and mathematics (Field and Field, 1982).

Management of Personal and Self-Care Needs. Workers are expected to manage their personal needs and effect proper grooming.

Self-Reliance in Transportation and Mobility in the Community. Employment generally requires the ability to transport oneself independently in the community.

The assessment of these critical vocational behaviors is accomplished by a combination of informal and formal techniques. The evaluator is required to gather diagnostic information to be used later in the treatment phase. Table 16-1 presents a list of those tests and informal assessment techniques which are appropriate for gaining diagnostic and norm-referenced information for an adolescent population.

Treatment

The overall goals of vocational therapy for adolescents are somewhat different from those for adults. Rather than focusing on the establishment of occupational choices, the primary goals for adolescents are the exploration of career options, the ability to make a "tentative" but realistic career choice, and the development of critical vocational skills. Therapeutic intervention to achieve these goals includes the following:

Table 16-1. Selected Vocational Tests and Methods

Realistic Appraisal of Work Abilities	Wide Range Interest and Opinion Test (Jastak and Jastak, 1979) Career Maturity Inventory (Crites, 1978) Parts of the Social and Prevocational Information Battery (Halpern, Raffeld, Irvin, and Link, 1975) Counseling AAMD-Becker's Reading Free Vocational Interest Inventory (American Association on Mental Deficiency, Washington, DC) Prevocational Assessment Curriculum Guide (Mithaug, Mar, and Stewart, 1978) Vocational Assessment Curriculum Guide (Rusch, Schutz, Mithaug, Stewart, and Mar, 1982)
Adaptability to Work Demands and Self-Direction and Motivation	Valpar Component Work Samples (Valpar International, Tucson, AZ) VIEWS Work Samples (Vocational Research Institute, Philadelphia, PA) Singer Vocational Evaluation System (Singer Company, Rochester, NY) Microtower (ICD Rehabilitation and Research Center, New York, NY) McCarron-Dial Work Evaluation System (McCarron Dial Systems, Dallas, TX) JEVS Work Sample System (Vocational Research Institute, Philadelphia, PA) Simulated or Actual Work Placements
Effective Interpersonal and Communication Skills	Consultation with speech-language pathologists and classroom teachers Observation of client on work samples listed above
Application of Academic Knowledge	Personnel Tests for Industry: Verbal, numerical, oral directions (Langmuir, 1974; Wesman and Doppelt, 1969) Selected diagnostic academic or achievement tests Observation of selected work samples Consultation with classroom teacher
Management of Personal and Self-Care Needs	Observation of client in work simulations Consultation with primary caretaker and therapists
Self-Reliance in Transportation and Mobility in the Community	Informal assessment in the community setting Consultation with primary caretaker and therapists

- Determining specific behavioral competencies to be acquired by the client
- Reviewing the effectiveness of compensatory strategies used by the client in other therapy settings
- Selecting a prescribed treatment format which incorporates task analysis and allows for the acquisition, proficiency, and maintenance of behaviors
- Programming for generalization into the work environment

In this section of the chapter, the following aspects of treatment will be discussed: task analysis, stages of treatment, generalization, and monitoring of the client's performance.

Task Analysis

Techniques that involve the manipulation of antecedent and consequent events to increase the probability that a specified response will follow a particular stimulus (Horner and Bellamy, 1978) are helpful in improving the performance of head injured adolescents. Task analysis involves the identification of the component parts of a specified task. We have found that task analysis serves two functions. First, it helps the vocational therapist in selecting for the client the simplest possible method of completing a task. For example, a task that requires an individual to package 10 forks, spoons, and knives in a plastic bag may be analyzed in several ways. The procedure selected to perform this task should include the smallest possible number of distinct operations. It may be easiest for the client to count all of the utensils first and then place them in the plastic bag. Initially, the therapist should avoid tasks that require a variety of dissimilar operations and movements since this may be a source of confusion for the client.

Second, task analysis outlines the necessary components of instruction the client will need to receive. If treatment is designed to make use of previously acquired skills, the therapist will need to highlight how these behaviors are related to the task at hand. Additionally, in helping clients acquire new skills, the therapist must outline the steps to facilitate the learning of the behavior.

Stages of Treatment

In vocational therapy it is important that skill development be based on the following stages: acquisition, proficiency, and maintenance. During the acquisition phase, the therapist should carefully analyze the selected work tasks to identify the component skills that the client must acquire and design intervention to teach these skills. It is during this stage that the client learns new skills through repeated practice. Attention must be paid to cognitive problems that may interfere with the acquisition of the skill. Flexible experimentation with a variety of teaching strategies (e.g., shaping, forward or backward chaining, more detailed task analysis) and reinforcement systems may be necessary.

Once clients can perform the skill correctly, they enter the proficiency phase. In this phase, the therapist designs tasks to help the clients improve the speed and accuracy with which they perform the skill. During this phase we give clients the opportunity to practice their newly acquired skills in a realistic work environment.

After clients demonstrate proficiency in a skill, the therapist must plan for practice of the behavior to ensure maintenance at the designated criterion level. Maintenance activities should occur with sufficient frequency to reinforce correct task performance. The therapist should monitor whether the length of time between practice sessions has an effect on the client's performance. Some clients may need to practice skills more frequently than others to maintain the behaviors.

Generalization

Generalization is enhanced by deliberate manipulation of aspects of the treatment environment. We have found that varying the following conditions enhances the generalization of a newly acquired skill:

- The therapists who work with the client (since familiarity with only one therapist increases the chances that the newly acquired behavior will only occur in the presence of that therapist)
- The vocational task and the physical setting in which the skill is to be performed
- The stimulus used to elicit the desired skill (e.g., auditory instructions instead of written instructions)

Monitoring the Client's Performance

Throughout the stages of treatment and during generalization activities, the therapist should monitor the client's performance closely. This includes watching for signs of independence, carry-over of instruction from one situation to another, endurance, and fluctuation of performance due to variations in the work setting (e.g., increased noise level, change in work station). Problems that are noted should be addressed as soon as possible to prevent deterioration in the client's task performance. Therapists must have flexibility in their schedules to address problems as they occur. These observations of the client's performance will have an impact on the career planning process, to be discussed later.

To illustrate this therapeutic sequence, a method for teaching an accounting procedure is presented in Table 16–2. This accounting procedure would be taught first in a vocational therapy setting and later generalized to a work environment.

Counseling

The method by which the head injured adolescent acquires critical vocational skills and implements educational and vocational decisions is a primary consideration in career development, and as such, is a frequent target for counseling intervention. This intervention is necessary to help clients to integrate information about themselves and the world of work (Egner and Jackson, 1978). Often head injured adolescents are unable to integrate this information effectively due to deficits in social perceptiveness, self-regulation, attention and concentration, memory, language, and reasoning. Counseling methods that are used with this population should incorporate three components: containment of loss, self-awareness, and goal setting (Diller and Gordon, 1981; Lynch, 1984).

Containment of Loss

Recognition of loss may lead to overwhelming feelings of inadequacy or denial (Wright, 1960). These feelings often inhibit career maturity since the adolescent cannot appraise abilities accurately. Clients must be confronted with their problems and at the same time helped to focus on their remaining skills and assets. This counseling technique requires that the client can trust the therapist and express feelings without fear of disapproval or rejection. The therapist must reassure the client that it is normal to mourn one's loss and have feelings of depression. Guidance is needed to help clients restructure their thinking so that they can focus on positive aspects of their skills. Cognitive restructuring techniques (Burns, 1980) are particularly helpful in this area. Using these techniques, we help clients to explore irrational thoughts and fears and to learn how to counteract them. It generally requires that the individual have adequate ability to reason and to process language.

Table 16-2. Vocational Therapy Plan

Name of Task: Preparation of Customer's Quarterly Statement

Critical Vocational Skill Areas:

1. Realistic appraisal of work abilities
2. Adaptability to work demands
3. Self-direction and motivation
4. Application of academic knowledge

Objectives:

1. Acquisition phase: Given charge slips for three customers, the worker will (1) sort charge slips by customer name and account number, (2) order slips by the date, and (3) prepare a customer statement (five consecutive trials).
2. Proficiency phase: In a simulated work environment, the worker will sort and order the charge slips and prepare statements for 20 customers (no more than three errors on five consecutive trials).
3. Maintenance phase: In a simulated work environment, the worker, when requested, will sort, order, and prepare a statement for specified customers (one trial per customer with no more than three errors).

Materials: Set of customer charge slips, calculator, statement forms, typewriter.

Prerequisite Skills: The worker should be familiar with the following operations and procedures before beginning task:

- Use of calculator
- Use of typewriter
- Ability to sort by name and number
- Ability to order information chronologically by date

Verbal Cue to Initiate Task: "Prepare a quarterly statement for the following customers from these charge slips" (therapist points to slips).

Task Procedures (the skills that should be acquired by the student):

1. Set up work station; secure necessary equipment.
2. Sort charge slips by customer name.
3. Verify that customer name and account numbers match store account records.
4. Sort and chronologically order charge slips by date.
5. For each customer:
   - Record account information on billing statement using a typewriter.
   - Record information from charge slip in the appropriate transaction columns on the statement.
   - Add each transaction total (on calculator) to determine sum.
   - Compare calculator tape with bill statement to determine accuracy.
   - Record total amount on statement with typewriter.
6. Repeat step 5 for each customer until all charge slip packets are recorded.

Therapeutic Procedures:

1. Assess the client's entering level in outlined prerequisite skills.
2. Teach prerequisite skills as needed.
3. Task analyze each procedural step.
4. During the acquisition stage, do not progress until the client acquires each necessary skill in turn. If necessary, teach the client strategies to compensate for deficits that interfere with the acquisition of the skill. Encourage the client's independence as much as possible. If learning problems occur, use an alternative instructional technique.
5. Provide systematic feedback to clients on their performance using video tape or recording the amount of work performed on a chart or graph.

Table continued on following page.

Table 16-2 (continued).

6. Provide supportive counseling when the client experiences failure. Confrontational counseling may be indicated for the client who is overreacting to small setbacks or actively engaging in denial over work performance.
7. Encourage the client to set production and accuracy goals for each work session.
8. Help the client to make the transition from the acquisition phase to the proficiency stage with structured counseling and reinforcement.
9. Use more than one therapist with the client during the proficiency and maintenance phases.
10. When generalizing the skill to a simulated work environment, incorporate realistic distractions that a worker is normally expected to handle.

Self-Awareness

To help adolescents become aware of their abilities and limitations, systematic procedures are needed to facilitate recall and monitoring of performance. The use of videotape review and an adaptation of the interpersonal process recall technique (Heffenstein and Wechsler, 1982) have proved to be effective. This technique allows adolescents to review the quality and nature of their performance. Additionally this process helps clients set functional goals for achieving community independence. The therapist may be required to interpret the feedback that the client is reviewing on videotape. Many times, due to poor reasoning and problem-solving ability, clients may not be able to evaluate the effectiveness of their performance. Care should be taken by the therapist to present both positive and negative aspects of the client's performance. Reinforcement should be given to emphasize target behaviors.

Goal Setting

Goals are critical determinants of learning and general behavior (Rotter, 1954). Goal setting is an important variable in helping adolescents to learn new skills and to increase productivity. We cannot overemphasize that if clients feel that their treatment goals are not important or do not match their own expectations, there will be little personal investment in the rehabilitation process. In our experience a modification of a procedure developed by Gardner and Warren (1978) has been particularly helpful in counseling clients in this area. Using this counseling procedure, we guide clients to set goals for achieving critical vocational skills. To facilitate goal setting, the therapist must do the following:

- Determine the quality of the client's behavior in the vocational therapy setting. If possible the behavior should be quantified in terms that adolescents will understand.
- Give the client feedback about previous performance. Self-awareness techniques (e.g., video tape review) may be necessary to enhance the client's comprehension.
- Help the client to set a goal for the next effort. Realistic goal setting should be encouraged. As the client reaches the upper limits of ability, goals should be set at approximately the same level as prior performance. When this occurs, the therapist will need to explain why a higher goal was not set.

The incorporation of these three components into counseling will enhance the client's ability to integrate self-concept and the world of work. These approaches can be readily combined with other counseling techniques, such as rational-emotive therapy, cognitive restructuring, and reality therapy (Burns, 1980; Ellis, 1962; Glasser, 1965). See Chapter 14 for further discussion of counseling techniques for head injured adolescents.

CAREER PLANNING

Employment

As the individual makes gains in generalizing critical vocational behaviors to the work environment, the therapist is able to gauge the type of occupational settings that will be appropriate. Since adolescents are at an exploratory level of career development, plans for community reentry should focus on helping them to sample various occupational situations on a part-time basis. Subsequent involvement in a training program or full-time competitive employment should be based on the client's level of vocational maturity and cognitive ability.

To determine if a client is ready for employment or job training, we have found the prevocational and vocational inventories developed by Mithaug, Mar, and Stewart (1978) and Rusch, Schutz, Mithaug, Stewart, and Mar (1982) to be particularly helpful. These inventories help the therapist to determine whether a client is functioning at a sheltered or competitive level of employment. If the client has potential for competitive employment, the therapist should make recommendations regarding the type of occupations that would be most appropriate.

We use work adjustment samples to help determine the type of setting appropriate for an individual client. Work adjustment samples are job trials in which the client is exposed to various job demands (repetitive or varied duties, working with people, meeting precise standards, and so forth). During these samples the therapist monitors both the client's ability to apply critical vocational skills and the factors that appear to interfere with effective performance. This information is invaluable in selecting occupational options.

Another approach to selecting training or employment options is the Vocational Diagnosis and Assessment of Residual Employability Skills (VDARE) developed by Sink and Field (1981). In the VDARE approach, the therapist rates worker behaviors and then, with the aid of an inexpensive computer search, selects job options that will be realistic for that client. The vocational therapist will need to investigate these job options to determine their feasibility for the client and additionally prepare him or her for community reentry. Treatment activities should then resemble the duties that will be expected in the actual job setting.

It is critical that the vocational therapist recommend those options that best serve the interests of the adolescents. Often families and clients experience despair over shattered dreams. Although these feelings should be acknowledged, the family may need to receive supportive counseling to understand the impact of the head injury on vocational functioning. This approach helps to facilitate community reentry since family members and professionals are then working toward the same goals.

Avocational Possibilities for the Severely Handicapped

It is a challenge to rehabilitation professionals to develop career alternatives for those who lack the potential for either competitive or sheltered employment. Meaningful alternatives to work are necessary to enhance the client's feelings of self-worth. Through counseling, we encourage severely impaired patients to accept avocational activity as a realistic and meaningful goal. Again we encourage the family to support the client in pursuing these options.

Avocational programming includes the following:
- Identification of avocational interests and abilities
- Selection of plausible avocational activities
- Development of a plan to present and teach activities to the client
- Adjustment of instruction when necessary to ensure the client's mastery

The treatment techniques discussed earlier are also effective in avocational programming. The Avocational Activities Inventory (Overs, Taylor, and

Adkins, 1977) is useful in selecting appropriate avocational activities. In this inventory avocational activities have been systematically divided into nine major categories:
- Games
- Sports
- Nature activities
- Collection activities
- Craft activities
- Art and music activities
- Educational, entertainment, and cultural activities
- Volunteer activities
- Organizational activities

Together with the clients, we select activities on the basis of the client's interests and ability level.

Counseling may be needed to resolve internal conflicts and anxieties that prevent clients from identifying and selecting meaningful and realistic avocational activities (Overs, Taylor, and Adkins, 1977). Clients often need help in clarifying the purpose and place of avocational activity in their lives. Before engaging them in the counseling process, the vocational therapist must analyze their current level of cognitive and motoric functioning, estimated learning ability, interests, and values. We also investigate community resources to determine available options. Table 16-3 illustrates the type of evaluation and planning that is relevant in avocational programming.

Family support is often crucial to avocational programming. Many of the clients who are in need of avocational activities have major cognitive, physical, or social deficits that require the family or significant others to be involved in helping them participate in the activity. The therapist should determine if the family is ready to accept avocational programming and their responsibilities in this programming. Some families feel overwhelmed by this responsibility and may thwart avocational plans. Interdisciplinary team planning with social service may be necessary so that the family receives the necessary counseling to address reactions and problems if they do occur.

Until very recently, our society has considered employment to be the primary acceptable role for adults. Avocational activities have finally been recognized as career alternatives. However, community resources for the disabled are very sparse in this area. Support groups, consisting of concerned family members and professionals, are necessary to promote the development of high quality community based programs to provide meaningful avocational activities for head injured individuals who are unable to work.

Table 16-3. Case Study: Avocational Programming

Name: Cindy B.

Age: 16 years

Presenting Problems (secondary to closed head injury): Memory impairment (short-term and long-term); visual acuity and visual field deficit; spastic quadriplegia; poor fine motor control

Avocational Goal: Develop leisure time skills

Evaluation: Through consultation with the treatment team, information was gathered on Cindy's functional skills, present equipment modifications, and compensatory cognitive strategies. It was determined that Cindy could retain information after frequent presentations of the material with verbal outlining (e.g., the therapist would verbally outline how to perform a motor task while demonstrating the method). It was found that the following needed to be considered when establishing a program:

Problem	Remedial Adaptations
Memory impairment	• Presenting information repeatedly and in outline form.
Visual acuity and visual field deficit	• Positioning material at correct angle in left visual field in well-lit area.
Quadriplegia	• Adapting table surface height to accommodate wheelchair and allowing client to maintain correct body position; positioning materials so that they are within reach.
Fine motor control	• Adapting materials so that client can position them with palmar grasp or finger pushing movement.

Other Factors: Cindy was able to read and comprehend at the elementary level. Performance deteriorated with an increase in length and complexity of material to be read. Game directions needed to be broken down into one to two sentence components. Cindy appeared to process information presented in more concrete terms.

Identification of Leisure Time Activity: Through a Leisure Interest Inventory and informal interview, playing card games was selected as an avocational goal. It was also determined that Cindy had limited knowledge of the rules of card games.

Treatment Plan: Avocational activity selected: card games such as "Crazy Eights."
   Objectives:
      1. Client will demonstrate ability to play designated card game by recalling and using relevant rules and displaying the necessary manipulative skills.
      2. Client will play card game with significant other in the home environment.

Therapy Considerations and Arrangements:
   • Visually modified ("Lo-Vision") cards and a card holder were purchased at an adaptive equipment materials center.
   • Through consultation with physical and occupational therapists, correct positioning was determined for Cindy to optimize her ability to reach and handle materials.
   • The use of activity analysis in breaking down the steps to the game allowed Cindy to learn the game gradually and efficiently.
   • At the request of the therapist, Cindy's mother participated in one of the therapy sessions. The mother was given information on how to implement this avocational activity in the home environment.

Follow-up Consultation: The therapist contacted Cindy's family. It was determined that Cindy was able to play the card game with various family members and appeared to be enjoying the activity. Additionally, the mother reported that the family had expanded the rules of the "Crazy Eights" game.

SUMMARY

Career development programming is essential in helping head injured adolescents assume meaningful life roles. The focus of career development includes not only paid work but also the roles of family member, unpaid worker, citizen, and participant in avocational pursuits. Like other young adults, head injured adolescents are critically concerned with self-fulfillment. They should be given opportunities to develop into independent and self-supporting adults. The extent to which these goals can be achieved depends on the quality of available career programming. Advocacy from families and concerned professionals will be needed to help promote the establishment of more career development programs and community resources.

REFERENCES

Brolin, D. E., and Kokaska, C. J. (1979). *Career education for handicapped children and youth*. Columbus, OH: Charles E. Merrill.

Burns, D. D. (1980). *Feeling good: The new mood therapy*. New York: W. W. Morrow.

Crites, J. O. (1978). *Career maturity inventory: Theory and research handbook* (2nd ed.). Monterey, CA: McGraw-Hill.

Diller, L., and Gordon W. A. (1981). Interventions for cognitive deficits in brain injured adults. *Journal of Consulting and Clinical Psychology, 49,* 822–834.

Egner, J. R., and Jackson, D. T. (1978). Effectiveness of a counseling intervention program for teaching career decision making skills. *Journal of Counseling Psychology, 25,* 45–52.

Ellis, A. (1962). *Reason and emotion in psychotherapy*. New York: Lyle Stuart.

Field, T. F., and Field, J. E. (1982). *The classification of jobs according to worker trait factors*. Roswell, GA: North Fulton.

Gardner, D. C., and Warren, S. A. (1978). *Careers and disabilities: A career education approach*. Stanford, CA: Greylock Publishers.

Glasser, W. (1965). *Reality therapy*. New York: Harper and Row.

Halpern, A., Raffeld, P., Irvin, L. K., and Link, R. (1975). *Social and prevocational information battery*. Monterey, CA: McGraw-Hill.

Havighurst, R. J. (1972). *Developmental tasks and education*. New York: McKay.

Helffenstein, D., and Wechsler, F. (1982, February). *The use of interpersonal process recall in the remediation of interpersonal and communication skill deficits among the newly brain injured*. Paper presented at the Ohio Psychological Association Winter Workshops.

Horner, R. H., and Bellamy, G. (1978). A conceptual analysis of vocational training. In M. E. Snell (Ed.), *Systematic instruction of the moderately and severely handicapped* (pp. 441–456). Columbus, OH: Charles E. Merrill.

Jastak, J. F., and Jastak, S. (1979). *Wide range interest and opinion test*. Wilmington, DE: Jastak Associates.

Jordan, J. P., and Heyde, M. B. (1979). *Vocational maturity during the high school years*. New York: Teachers College Press.

Langmuir, C. R. (1974). *Personnel tests for industry— oral directions test*. New York: Psychological Corporation.

Lynch, R. T. (1984). Traumatic head injury: Implications for rehabilitation counseling. *Journal of Applied Rehabilitation Counseling, 14*(3), 32–55.

Mithaug, D. E., Mar, D. K., and Stewart, J. E. (1978). *Prevocational assessment and curriculum guide*. Seattle: Exceptional Education.

Overs, R. P., Taylor, S., and Adkins, C. (1977). *Avocational counseling manual: A complete guide to leisure guidance*. Washington, DC: Haewkins and Associates.

Rotter, J. B. (1954). *Social learning and clinical psychology*. Englewood Cliffs, NJ: Prentice-Hall.

Rusch, F. R., Schutz, R. P., Mithaug, D. E., Stewart, J. E., and Mar, D. K. (1982). *Vocational assessment and curriculum guide*. Seattle: Exceptional Education.

Sink, J. M., and Field, T. F. (1981). *Vocational assessment, planning and jobs*. Athens, GA: VDARE Service Bureau.

Super, D. E. (1957). *The psychology of careers*. New York: Harper and Brothers.

Super, D. E., and Overstreet, P. L. (1960). *The vocational maturity of ninth grade boys*. New York: Teachers College Press.

Super, D. E. (1976). *Career education and the meanings of work. Monographs on career education*. U.S. Department of Health, Education and Welfare, U.S. Office of Education.

U.S. Department of Labor (1972). *Handbook of analyzing jobs*. (Reprint 13). Menomonie, WI: University of Wisconsin, Stout, Stout Vocational Rehabilitation Institute.

Wesman, A. G., and Doppelt, J. E. (1969). *Personnel tests for industry — verbal and numerical tests*. New York: Psychological Corporation.

Wright, B. A. (1960). *Physical disability — a psychological approach*. New York: Harper and Row.

PART VIII
PROGRAM MANAGEMENT

As the number of head injury programs within rehabilitation facilities has grown in recent years, important questions have emerged regarding the most effective design and management of these programs. These questions are particularly pressing in areas of service delivery such as cognitive rehabilitation, where generally accepted assignments of professional responsibilities among the traditional rehabilitation disciplines do not yet exist. In Chapter 17, Cohen and Titonis describe an interdisciplinary model of head injury rehabilitation that attempts to avoid the service fragmentation that often accompanies standard multidisciplinary approaches. They recommend two levels of clinical management within large pediatric head injury rehabilitation programs: (1) general program management and coordination of services, and (2) clinical direction of specific interdisciplinary teams, such as the cognitive rehabilitation therapy team. The authors also discuss admission and discharge issues, staff conferences, and communication with families and interested third parties. They stress the acquisition of necessary community services (including school placement) and planned follow-up after discharge.

Chapter 17

Head Injury Rehabilitation: Management Issues

Sally B. Cohen, MEd, and Jan Titonis, MPH*

Head injured patients and their families challenge rehabilitation professionals with very special needs. Managers of programs for the head injured must take into account the range of deficits and rates of recovery to deliver service in an organized and timely way. These programs need to be staffed by experienced professionals in all rehabilitative disciplines and to provide a coordinated delivery system (Prigatano et al., 1984) that begins at admission and follows the patient beyond discharge from inpatient rehabilitation.

According to Berrol and Cervelli (1982), the ideal rehabilitation center system includes the following: a sufficient volume of patients, a rehabilitation staff working as a team, an integrated treatment philosophy, criteria for patient admission and discharge, an evaluation and communication system, a commitment to long-term follow-up, a commitment to cooperation and communication with community agencies, and an adequate funding and administrative system. Ben-Yishay and Diller (1983) advocate a continuum of care that extends from acute hospitalization through independent living. They describe the sequelae of head injury and note that multiple interventions are required at different stages of recovery.

In our experience, a matrix model (Wilson, 1984) works well as an overall structure in the delivery of comprehensive services (Fig. 17-1). In this model a coordinator is responsible for program management and individual case management, including admitting patients, monitoring their progress, discharge planning, and follow-up. This program coordinator need

*Authorship listed alphabetically at authors' request.

	Program Coordinator	Program Coordinator	Program Coordinator
Medical Staff			
Nutritional Services			
Occupational Therapy			
Orthotics			
Pharmacy			
Physical Therapy			
Speech-Language Therapy			
Education			
Nursing Services			
Psychological Services			
Rehabilitation Counseling			
Social Service			
Volunteer Services			

Figure 17-1. A matrix model for the management of comprehensive rehabilitation services.

not be a physician but must work closely with the medical staff. The coordinator establishes channels of communication to assure consistent programming and timely reporting of the patient's progress to family members, community agencies, and third party payers.

ADMISSION PROCEDURES

Criteria for admission to a head injury rehabilitation program are based on the facility's resources and structures as well as the patient's medical readiness for rehabilitation (see Chapter 4). Medical management issues are critical and reimbursement patterns need to be considered.

Prior to transferring the patient to a rehabilitation center, a visit by rehabilitation staff to the acute-care hospital serves the following purposes: (1) to evaluate the patient's potential for rehabilitation, (2) to gather information about the patient to share with other rehabilitation staff, (3) to provide an opportunity for rehabilitation center staff members to establish rapport with personnel from the referring hospital, and (4) to check insurance information and initiate preauthorization procedures. During this visit pertinent medical and nursing information is gathered about surgeries, medications, equipment needs (e.g., tracheostomy equipment, tube feeding equipment, wheelchair, splints), vital signs, and positioning recommendations. At The Rehabilitation Institute of Pittsburgh the program coordinator and a member of the rehabilitation nursing staff conduct this visit. Often the first contact with the family is made at this time and information is given to them regarding the rehabilitation program's policies and procedures and the rehabilitation center routine. We also discuss special needs such as temporary housing for family members from out of town, and we invite families to visit the rehabilitation center prior to admission. During their visit, the family can be given written information about head injury. Additional information regarding stages of recovery, specific cognitive problems, or specific treatment strategies is presented to family members after the patient has been admitted to the rehabilitation center.

At the time of admission it is appropriate to inform the patient's local school district and other agencies that the patient is now in a rehabilitation program. In this way the channels of communication are established at admission for transition back to the community.

INTERDISCIPLINARY TEAM

Some rehabilitation centers use a *multidisciplinary* model of service delivery in which each discipline works with the patient from its own point of view. The danger inherent in this approach is that professionals from diverse disciplines often fail to integrate their intervention. The *interdisciplinary* team model is more effective and more efficient. It is directed by the program coordinator and "views the patient as a whole, not just a placement problem, job problem, floor management problem, or a collection of intellectual deficits" (Olson and Henig, 1983, p. 3). Members of the team, working together, plan treatment programs that include only those disciplines that are current priorities for the patient. A consistent approach is critical in treating head injured patients and includes each team member using similar interactive styles, behavior management techniques, and other treatment strategies for the patient.

Many agencies have experienced difficulty in creating effective interdisciplinary treatment teams, particularly in areas such as cognitive rehabilitation, where professional qualifications, responsibilities, and boundaries have not yet been well defined. This difficulty may result in part from the fact that health professionals, more than other occupational groups, have a high need for achievement and advancement in their professions and a keen interest in their work and in the development of knowledge for its own sake. Because their work consists of solving problems they find intrinsically interesting, they tend to be inner directed rather than motivated by external rewards or punishments. Their specific goals or group identification, however, may vary. Gouldner (1957) distinguished between cosmopolitan and locally oriented employees. Cosmopolitan employees are those who have relatively little loyalty to the employing organization but a considerable commitment to specialized role skills. They are also likely to use an external reference group for orientation. Locally oriented employees are those who are very loyal to the employing organization but have relatively little commitment to specialized role skills. They are likely to use an inner reference group for orientation. Health professionals tend to be more cosmopolitan than local. Since cosmopolitan employees are oriented to their profession, they seek advancement and status in their professions more often than in their employing organization. They are easily upset by organizational requirements that interfere with their work, identifying with the goals, values, and forms of recognition of their profession. Although many health professionals do not fit this stereotype, these generalizations are widely applicable and can be helpful for those who establish and manage interdisciplinary treatment programs.

Case Illustration of Interdisciplinary Team Treatment

At the time of admission, Bob was at an early stage of cognitive recovery and was agitated, especially by touch. This interfered with participation in physical therapy, occupational therapy, speech-language therapy, and nursing procedures. Possible environmental adaptations were evaluated, and psychological and psychiatric consultations were obtained. Bob was given a single room, the lights were kept low, and staff members were instructed to speak to him calmly. The psychologist met with the treating staff to guarantee that they were approaching Bob in a consistent way. The psychologist also observed Bob to determine the times of the day when he was more amenable to direct intervention. The psychiatrist prescribed medication to control serious agitation. The established treatment approach required that the occupational therapist, physical therapist, speech-language therapist, and nursing staff devote some of their therapy time to behavior shaping. Partly as a result of this well-planned and consistently applied team approach, Bob progressed beyond this stage of confusion and agitation and became a more compliant and active participant in his rehabilitation.

The interdisciplinary model allows each discipline to learn from the others. Strategies from physical therapy and occupational therapy regarding positioning, for example, help other staff members reduce the patient's discomfort and provide the best position for feeding, reading, or table activities. Strategies from speech-language therapy help other staff members communicate with the patient most effectively, whether verbally or by means of alternative communication devices. Strategies from cognitive therapy help other staff members incorporate into their treatment sessions activities that improve the patient's processing, memory, or organizational abilities. Thus, there is program continuity for patients regardless of which professional is working with them. When effective strategies are identified by the team, the family can be involved to expand generalization of newly learned skills to more natural settings.

COGNITIVE REHABILITATION THERAPY — CLINICAL MANAGEMENT

The cognitive rehabilitation therapy (CRT) program at The Rehabilitation Institute of Pittsburgh was developed in response to the needs of head injured patients. As noted in earlier chapters, cognitive problems of these patients often include impaired alertness, attentional deficits, decreased self-control (impulsivity), disorientation, receptive and expressive language problems, memory problems, and impaired problem solving, judgment, and initiation. These patients are also often irritable and depressed. CRT provides a carefully designed series of tasks that helps patients regain maximum levels of cognitive functioning. The CRT team at the Institute is composed of speech-language pathologists, occupational therapists, special educators, psychologists, and a clinical facilitator. A special education school and prevocational-vocational services, closely tied to the CRT program, are also available to patients.

General Structure

Overall program coordination and clinical direction of specific rehabilitation programs, such as CRT, should be separate but interrelated to address the various facets of treatment that affect families, insurance companies, and community facilities as well as clinical staff members and patients. This section will focus on the structure and operation of the CRT treatment team.

The clinical treatment team of a cognitive rehabilitation therapy program must have a dynamic structure that makes possible flexible adaptations to changes in patient population, patients' recovery levels, and individual cognitive and behavioral problems that need to be treated. Although the CRT staff may be members of various departments in a rehabilitation center, their treatment focuses on cognitive rehabilitation and is monitored and evaluated by the CRT team. As was stated earlier, team planning and joint intervention enable therapists to expand their knowledge and functional skills beyond the areas in which they were trained. An occupational therapist and speech-language pathologist doing joint treatment can each bring valuable expertise to group tasks that focus on thought organization and problem solving (see Chapters 11 and 12). At The Rehabilitation Institute of Pittsburgh, the CRT team has established a format for treatment that provides group and individual therapy. Figure 17-2 outlines this program. The focus of treatment includes orientation, attention and concentration, and basic thought organization and relates thought organization and problem solving to the following areas: structured activities, prevocational tasks, community mobility, social and communicative skills, perceptual skills, and self-awareness. Treatment goals and procedures are described in detail in Chapters 10 to 12.

To focus intervention accurately, treatment team members must ask some essential questions: What general cognitive problems do patients have at different levels of recovery (see Chapter 8)? What are the specific problems of individual patients? Can the problems be ranked in order of priority? What treatment techniques will be effective or should be tried? What is the structure within which the treatment should be delivered?

Clinical Direction

It is difficult for any therapist to be aware of all aspects of a multifaceted treatment program. A clinical facilitator can help establish and maintain overall program goals, keep treatment goal oriented, and coordinate treatment approaches in different therapy settings. Since therapists are more likely to accept suggestions or questions about treatment from someone who has worked with patients, it is critical that the facilitator have a clinical background. Duties of the clinical facilitator are discussed further later in this chapter (*Maintaining an Effective Treatment Team*).

The therapist-facilitator relationship should be one of interdependence, in which both parties accept joint responsibility for programming. In less successful relationships, therapists either become overly dependent and fail to initiate direction or become overly independent and resist direction; at the same time program managers may become dictatorial and refuse to listen to or value therapists' ideas. Healthy interactive relationships within a rehabilitation treatment team occur when the program coordinator, clinical facilitator, and treating therapists communicate, cooperate, and problem solve together.

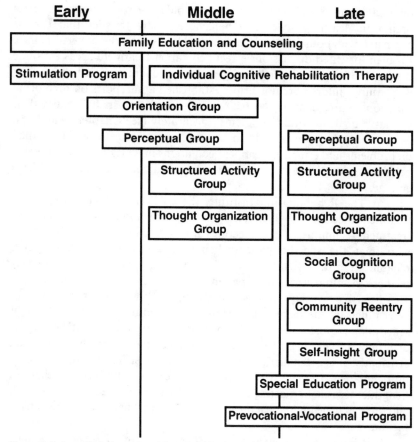

Figure 17–2. Interdisciplinary cognitive rehabilitation therapy program at The Rehabilitation Institute of Pittsburgh.

Within this framework a skillful clinical manager can do the following: help staff members identify subtle changes in patients' performance, analyze the appropriateness of program areas, rank treatment goals in order of priority, support the staff through difficult therapy procedures (e.g., treating depressed patients or discussing deficits with patients and families), make the staff accountable for treatment decisions, and bring quality assurance to the CRT program. Flexible programming requires active direction that encourages task analysis and energetic problem solving by staff members.

Approaches used to develop clinical treatment plans for very young children differ from those used for older children and adolescents. Reports on individuals 8 or 9 years of age or older provide information on premorbid learning styles and behavioral characteristics that can be compared with both general developmental levels and present performance. Problem-oriented discussions effectively target treatment areas for these people. However, because learning styles and characteristic behaviors of very young children are not firmly established and reports on premorbid functioning are scant, it is often difficult for therapists to identify their cognitive or behavioral "problems" accurately (see Chapters 9 and 15). These treatment plans should focus on present performance rather than on problems and establish treatment conditions in which therapists observe behaviors, compare performance over time, and note if cognitive problems emerge.

At The Rehabilitation Institute, the CRT clinical facilitator holds treatment meetings at which decisions are made about therapy goals and treatment techniques. These meetings are attended by CRT staff members who treat the specific patients being discussed and often by other rehabilitation staff members who also treat these patients. The frequency of these meetings varies: new patients or patients showing rapid changes are discussed weekly; others are discussed biweekly or monthly as determined by the team. Discussions last 15 minutes per patient. Tight scheduling requires therapists to focus intently on the patient's problems or program issues prior to the treatment meetings and to think and plan efficiently. It is often difficult for therapists to restrict their discussion to problem areas; frequently they are eager to discuss all aspects of therapy. Lengthier treatment meetings are held if discussions need to be extended, and these may be initiated at any time by either the therapists or the clinical facilitator.

It is important to evaluate the effectiveness of treatment meetings. When strategically planned, they *require* staff members to evaluate critically the patient's current goals and the team's intervention procedures. The effectiveness of these meetings depends upon the investment that therapists have in the team process and upon the quality of the interactive relationships among team members.

The Primary CRT Therapist

The use of a primary CRT therapist is an efficient way to accomplish documentation and reporting as well as parent training. One of the CRT therapists treating a specific patient is designated to collect information about the patient's functioning in *all* aspects of the CRT program and report it orally or in writing: to document treatment progress, share in program planning with other staff, and describe programs to families, community agencies, or funding sources. Treatment-oriented checklists describing goals, performance on specific tasks, strategies, and treatment approaches for each area of the program facilitate the gathering of information. This process guarantees that families and others receive one organized report of the total program rather than several individual accounts, which can be fragmented, redundant, or confusing.

Maintaining an Effective Treatment Team

There are many issues involved in establishing and maintaining an interdisciplinary team (e.g., the CRT team) in a department-oriented institution. The central issue is that professionals from different departments providing essentially the same service must value the unique talents and training of the other team members.

To deliver effective treatment, CRT team members must be able to do the following:

- Become accountable for *team* goals and treatment procedures, which may differ from department goals and procedures
- Accept and trust direction from outside their departments
- Be aware of how the CRT program fits into the patient's total rehabilitation plan
- Recognize how their specific therapy objectives relate to the overall CRT goals that include selecting treatment priorities and deciding that patients should move to another part of the program or that a specific component of CRT treatment should be terminated
- Have a functional approach to treatment that is meaningful to the patient
- Work efficiently within time constraints relating to individual therapy sessions and to the patient's length of stay
- Adapt to changes in treatment theories and techniques
- Maintain a caring but professional and objective approach to treatment of patients whose lives have changed as a result of the trauma
- Be able to provide treatment that may cause resistive or negative responses in patients
- Be able to deal effectively with hostile or emotional families or patients

To manage an interdisciplinary team effectively, the facilitator must proceed as follows:

- Establish credibility with therapists by making decisions that demonstrate knowledge of appropriate treatment techniques, by

supporting therapists' decisions and by actively participating in treatment planning
- Establish a mechanism for team planning and evaluation
- Clearly delineate the respective roles of therapists and facilitator and maintain expectations of compliance and cooperation for everyone
- Maintain leadership while encouraging therapists to contribute to team direction
- Require continuity in and accountability for program decisions
- Introduce new ideas or procedures to facilitate programming
- Maintain professional goals despite resistance or conflicts among the team members

It is interesting to note that when anxiety or tension is aroused within this system, the allegiance of team members may switch temporarily away from the *program* to the *departments*. Of course, this is counterproductive to team interaction. The more cohesive the team has become, the shorter the period of divisiveness will be.

STAFFINGS

Owing to the large number of head injured patients at our facility at any one time (30 to 50), patients' progress is monitored on two levels. In addition to the CRT team treatment meetings described earlier, the program coordinator chairs formal staff conferences. Three types of staffing are held: evaluation, treatment-progress, and discharge. Evaluation staffings are the first formal meetings of the total treatment team and are scheduled 7 to 10 days following the patient's admission. Therapists briefly report results of individual evaluations and rank program goals in the following broad treatment areas: mobility, motor functioning, communication, self-care, prevocational or vocational development (for patients 16 years old and older), individual psychosocial functioning, and family psychosocial functioning.

For example, a young head injured patient may present with mild left-sided weakness but adequate ambulation, significantly impaired cognitive-language skills, and low frustration tolerance. In addition, the family is in need of information and counseling regarding the patient's problems. The team may rank the goal areas as follows:
1. Communication
2. Individual and family psychosocial functioning
3. Motor functioning
4. Self-care
5. Mobility

The team reviews these rankings at subsequent staffings and, guided by the program coordinator, modifies the program as indicated by the patient's current needs and overall program goals.

Treatment-progress staffings are held monthly or as needed. The treatment team's discussion focuses on the amount and rate of progress, program needs, and plans for continued stay or for discharge. Revised priorities may emerge at a staffing, requiring changes in the patient's program. For instance, as a patient recovers, the intensity of physical therapy services may be reduced while that of cognitive rehabilitation therapy may increase. Consultation from a psychologist or psychiatrist will be recommended if the team determines that behavioral or emotional problems are interfering with the patient's ability to participate in therapy.

All rehabilitation team members participate in decisions regarding continuation of treatment. Projection for discharge is generally reached at a treatment-progress staffing. When planning discharge, the focus of the staffing is on specific patient or family training needed prior to discharge and services that will be needed following discharge. To facilitate this process, the program coordinator must be familiar not only with all aspects of the patient's program but also with community resources. The coordinator then contacts the appropriate community agencies or alerts outpatient services at our agency. At the discharge staffing, which is held close to the time of discharge, the team reviews service needs and creates a plan for follow-up.

We invite family members to attend staff conferences, although the limited time (30 minutes) is inadequate if they have many questions. The program coordinator arranges a separate meeting in those cases in which parents are unable to attend a staffing or when lengthy discussion is anticipated. Representatives from insurance and rehabilitation companies attend staffings routinely.

The reports generated from staffings become part of the medical record and are a summary of the patient's course in rehabilitation. These reports are distributed to team members and involved third parties, including referring hospitals, school districts, and insurance carriers.

PLACEMENT IN COMMUNITY SCHOOLS

As head injured students' cognitive and social skills improve, rehabilitation center staff members can begin to investigate placement in community schools. Special education supports are needed for most of these students. In mainstream classrooms there are many distractions, and the expected pace of activities, the rate at which information is presented, and the amount of material that is covered can be overwhelming to someone who must put a great deal of energy into making sense out of what people are saying, recalling yesterday's reading story, or remembering what books to take to the next class (Bryan and Bryan, 1978). These issues are discussed in detail in Chapters 8 through 12 and 15.

It is important for educators to become better informed about the cognitive disabilities and unique learning styles that can result from a head injury (see Chapter 15). School districts generally base class placements on IQ and achievement test scores; little attention is given to classroom functioning and rate of learning and working. *Test scores and classroom performance of head injured students must be interpreted differently from those of other students* (see Chapter 9). Head injured students with IQ and achievement test scores in the average range often cannot perform as "average students." They may have difficulty generalizing or remembering information and comprehending material that increases in length and complexity. These students can get lost in the content of a lesson as well as in the halls of a school; they may comprehend one page of reading but not follow a chapter of *six* pages; when stressed, they may "freeze" and be unable to respond to or remember information. Their uneven ability levels are different from the more stable performance that is expected in mainstream classes. It has been our experience that almost all severely head injured students placed in mainstream classes have needed support services eventually. Unfortunately, this is sometimes not recognized until the students have experienced failure.

Because of school laws and formal criteria for placing students in special education settings, it is difficult for community school personnel to disregard classroom labels when making placement decisions. Special education categories usually do not accommodate the learning styles of head injured students. Consequently these students may be placed in inappropriate community classrooms.

Reentry into community schools is quite difficult for head injured individuals, who now may be in different grades and even different schools from those they were in before their accidents. The effectiveness of the placements depends on how school personnel interpret and adapt to students' present disabilities (Fuld and Fisher, 1977). Students who have critical cognitive deficits but have adequate verbal skills and no physical impairments are most easily subject to mistaken impressions. Teachers and others assume that because they appear intact and their language skills are good, they can process information adequately. Inconsistent performance or impulsive, uninhibited, or fragmented responses may be interpreted as intentional or belligerent behavior. On the other hand, students with mild physical impairments and communication deficits may function at relatively higher levels cognitively. Often students in both of these categories can continue to learn comfortably in a learning disability class in which teachers use more detailed task analysis, attend to differences in learning style, give increased assistance to ensure that students complete work successfully, and teach strategies to compensate for weak cognitive and social skills. It is important, however, for the teachers to recognize similarities and differences between these students and their learning disabled (LD) peers (see Chapter 15) and to adapt educational programs to fit the head injured students' inconsistent performance and uneven progress. It is also important to have students *demonstrate* what they can do. Incorrect assumptions about students' capabilities lead to unrealistic expectations, inappropriate programs, and frustrated and anxious students *and* teachers.

PREPARING FOR DISCHARGE

Although individual considerations influence decisions to discharge patients, there are three standard criteria: no progress within a 60 day period; deteriorating medical status or medical problems that preclude active participation in rehabilitation; or sufficient recovery that treatment needs can be met on an outpatient basis. Members of the treatment team provide patients and family members with appropriate training prior to discharge. Predischarge training is discussed in several of the treatment chapters of this volume. In this section, we focus on community classroom placement.

Before head injured students are discharged, staff members from the rehabilitation center should visit potential community classrooms for the following purposes:

- To see if the physical plant is appropriately accessible for physically handicapped students
- To note curriculum content (required subjects and materials) as well as teaching techniques and expected behaviors of students (independent work required; acknowledgment of students with "problems"; amount of teacher assistance given; structured versus unstructured programs)
- To note the number of support services available (physical therapy, occupational therapy, speech-language therapy, social service) and the time permitted in "special" classes
- To note the range of students' intellectual abilities and social skills and the teachers' expectations regarding students' judgment (e.g., supervision on the playground, in gym class, in the halls, and on transportation vehicles)

The rehabilitation team can then assess the appropriateness of the placement and can train the student in skills and strategies that will help him or her to function more effectively in the new setting. A part-time trial placement in the new classroom can help staff members from the rehabilitation center and the new school evaluate the placement and provide a comfortable transition period for everyone. If this is not possible, head injured students should at least visit the new school, meet the teacher, and see the classroom; this helps to decrease anxiety of people in both settings. In addition, school personnel can observe school and therapy programs at the rehabilitation center where teachers and therapists can share specific information about programs and demonstrate treatment and teaching techniques.

Following discharge, some patients continue to require a variety of services in addition to special education. Physical therapy, occupational therapy, speech-language therapy, cognitive rehabilitation therapy, and counseling often need to continue. Some of these services are provided through school systems, others are not. Again, the need to educate community staff members is critical. Returning to the rehabilitation center for specialized outpatient services may be necessary.

FOLLOW-UP

Follow-up is an essential service. Most rehabilitation centers have some mechanism for monitoring patients' *physical* recovery after discharge. With head injured patients it is also important that *cognitive* progress continue to be assessed. An organized system of follow-up serves to prevent these patients from "falling through the cracks." Patients should return to the rehabilitation center at prescribed intervals based on their needs. Patients who have significant physical, cognitive, and psychosocial deficits require more frequent follow-up. Patients whose deficits are less severe may be seen 2 to 3 months after discharge, giving them a chance to adjust to community programming.

It is important to note the developmental level of the patient in determining follow-up schedules. Preschoolers may not succeed in preschool or kindergarten programs that are large and unstructured, and may need "special" education programs (see Chapter 15). Patients may do well in the primary grades but experience academic problems later, when more information is given and greater integration of information is required. Routine psychological and achievement testing, as noted earlier, cannot always identify these problems. Similarly, patients entering puberty may experience exaggerated problems in emotional lability and social adjustment. High school students may find that their intention to attend college full time is no longer feasible owing to cognitive problems. They will need guidance regarding part-time attendance, community college programs, or vocational training.

Those who work with head injured patients know that intervention does not and should not stop when a patient is discharged from inpatient rehabilitation. As their needs change, persons at all levels of recovery may require intervention from professionals knowledgeable about head injury. Ben-Yishay and Diller (1983) observe that "in many instances the effects of brain injury on the person's subsequent behavioral, social, and occupational adjustment only manifest long after the early hospital based medical and rehabilitation interventions have reached their maximum benefit" (p. 234).

REFERENCES

Ben-Yishay, Y., and Diller, L. (1983). *Notes toward a proposed systems approach to the rehabilitation of the traumatically brain injured* (Rehabilitation Monograph No. 66). New York: New York University Medical Center, Institute of Rehabilitation Medicine.

Berrol, S., and Cervelli, L. (1982). *Description of a model care system* (Head Injury Rehabilitation Program Final report). San Jose, CA: Santa Clara Valley Medical Center.

Bryan, T. H., and Bryan, J. H. (1978). *Understanding learning disabilities* (2nd ed.). Sherman Oaks, CA: Alfred.

Fuld, P. A., and Fisher, P. (1977). Recovery of intellectual ability after closed head-injury. *Developmental Medicine and Child Neurology, 19,* 495–502.

Gouldner, A. (1957). Cosmopolitans and locals: Toward an analysis of latent social roles, I. *Administrative Science Quarterly, 2,* 281–306.

Olson, D. A., and Henig, E. (1983). *A manual of behavior management strategies for brain injured adults.* Chicago: Rehabilitation Institute of Chicago.

Prigatano, G. P., Fordyce, D. J., Zeiner, H. K., Roueche, J. R., Pepping, M., and Wood, B. C. (1984). Neuropsychological rehabilitation after closed head injury in young adults. *Journal of Neurology, Neurosurgery, and Psychiatry, 47,* 505–513.

Wilson, J. A. (1984). How to deliver comprehensive rehabilitation using a matrix organization model. *Hospital Topics, 62*(1), 29–32.

Author Index

International League Against Epilepsy,
    136, 139
Irvin, L. K., 415, 425
Irwin, J. V., 181, 193
Isaacson, R. L., 71, 87
Ishijima, B., 66, 69

J

Jackson, D. M., 45, 67
Jackson, D. T., 418, 425
Jaffe, M. B., 188, 193
Jamison, D. L., 72, 87
Jane, J. A., *xxiii*, 36, 67, 69, 247, 274
Jasper, H., 286
Jasper, H. H., 35, 69
Jastak, J. F., 415, 425
Jastak, S., 415, 425
Jellinger, K., 15, 68
Jenker, F. L., 35, 68
Jenkins, D., 96, 115
Jenkins, P., 203, 208
Jenkins, L. W., 30, 35, 68, 69
Jennett, B., *xxii*, 73, 87, 127, 134, 135,
    139, 227, 246, 253, 269, 271, 273,
    274
Jennett, W. B., 15, 32, 68
Johns, D. F., 193
Johnson, C., 132, 139
Johnson, D. J., 404, 409
Johnson, L., 362, 379
Johnson, M. B., 261, 274
Jones, P., 248, 272
Jongeward, R. H., Jr., 224, 244
Jordan, J. P., 412, 425
Jorgenson, C., 260, 273
Jung, R., 279, 286
Junkunz, G., 376, 378

K

Kagan, N., 327, 337, 339
Kail, R. V., Jr., 220, 221, 224, 225, 244,
    245
Kallstrom, C., 266, 273
Kalsbeek, W. D., *xxii, xxiii*
Kaplan, E., 260, 273
Karmi, M. Z., 23, 68
Kassell, N., 31, 69

Kaste, M., 76, 87
Kauffman, J. M., 398, 409
Kavale, K., 237, 245
Kaye, H. H., 72, 87
Kazdin, A. E., 398, 409
Kent, C. A., 192
Keogh, B. K., 226, 245
Kerr, M. M., 389, 398, 402, 409
Kessen, W., 245, 246
Kimelberg, H. K., 26, 66, 68
Kirchner, J., 198, 209
Kirk, S., 236, 245
Kirk, W., 236, 245
Kishore, P. R. S., 24, 67
Kjellman, B., 66, 67
Klatzo, I., 24, 68
Klintworth, G. K., 32, 68
Klonoff, H., 73, 75, 76, 77, 81, 87, 270,
    273, 348, 359
Kneedler, J. W. L., 388, 404, 409
Kneedler, R. D., 226, 244, 245
Kobayashi, K., 77, 78, 86, 88
Kokaska, C. J., 411, 425
Kondo, A., 34, 68
Kontos, H. A., 36, 69
Korein, J., 185, 192
Kornhuber, H. H. 279, 286
Kottke, F. J., 167, 193
Kraner, R. E., 266, 273
Krasner, L., 348, 360
Krech, D., 277, 286
Kroner, K., 155, 163
Krumholtz, H., 355, 359
Krumholtz, J., 355, 359
Kubicki, S. T., 81, 86, 87
Kübler-Ross, E., 101, 115
Kuhl, D. E., 33, 70, 73, 74, 86, 89
Kurlycheck, R. T., 335, 340
Kuss, H. J., 376, 378

L

Lafleur, J., 45, 69
Lakin, P., 102, 115, 236, 244, 313, 339
Lange-Cosack, H., 81, 86, 87
Langfitt, T. W., 25, 26, 33, 68
Langmuir, C. R., 415, 426
La Pointe, L. L., 187, 188, 193
Larochelle, L., 45, 69
Larson, D., 24, 67

Subject Index

A

Abuse as cause of head injury, xix–xx
Academic assessment. *See* Educational assessment.
Academic deficits, 75–76
Academic placement. *See* Educational programming.
Acceleration factors in head injury, 4–18
Acne, 127
Activities of daily living, 148–149, 153, 157–158, 186–187
Admission criteria, 119–120, 430
Affective disorders. *See* Psychosocial dysfunction.
Age and epidemiology of head injury, xix–xx
Age and outcome, 71–73, 76–77, 81, 271–272
Aggressive behavior, 51, 65, 154–155, 352, 355, 365, 375–376
Agitation, 126, 154, 207, 291, 375–376
Airway, obstruction of, 122–123. *See also* Aspiration.
Akinesia, 45
Akinetic mutism, 15–18
Alcohol abuse and head injury, 374–375, 378
Amitriptyline (Elavil), 375–376
Amnesia. *See also* Memory deficits.
  anterograde, 73
  outcome and, 34
  posttraumatic 72–74, 82
  retrograde, 55
Amygdala, 51, 53
Anemia, 129
Anti-convulsant medication. *See* Seizures, posttraumatic, treatment of.
Anxiety, 52, 94–96, 99–100, 103, 105, 363–364
Aphasia, 76, 168, 179, 181, 258. *See also* Cognitive deficits.
Apraxia, 171, 178–182
Apraxia of speech, 171, 178–182, 188
Applied behavioral analysis. *See* Behavioral disturbances, treatment of.

Articulation, deficits of. *See* Motor deficits, treatment of, Motor speech treatment.
Aspiration, 122, 136, 199, 200–201, 203–205
Assessment, cognitive. *See* Cognitive assessment.
  cognitive-language. *See* Cognitive-language assessment.
  educational. *See* Educational assessment.
  medical. *See* Medical examination.
  neuropsychological, 81–85, 251–258 *See also* Cognitive assessment.
  swallowing. *See* Swallowing, deficits of, assessment of.
Ataxia, 168, 170
Athetosis, 44–45
Attention, 221
Attentional deficits 36, 81, 172, 222, 230–231, 250, 254, 270–271, 297, 311, 313, 317, 353, 387
  treatment of, 298–306, 335, 341, 390
Auditory stimulation. *See* Stimulation, sensory.
Augmentative communication, 181, 188
Automobile accidents, as cause of head injury, xix–xx
Autonomic instability, 128
Avocational programming, 422–424
Axon retraction balls, 15, 17

B

Barbiturate coma, 144
Barbiturates, 137, 144
Basal ganglia, 37, 40–45, 49, 54, 170
Behavior management. *See* Behavioral disturbances, treatment of.
Behavior modification. *See* Behavioral disturbances, treatment of.
Behavioral disturbances, 51–54, 72, 78–80, 127, 154–155, 176, 207–208, 235, 291–292, 326–328, 347–348, 350–354, 356–359, 365, 369, 371–372, 396–402